Landscapes of Disease

CEU Press Studies in the History of Medicine

Volume VIII

Series Editor: Marius Turda

Landscapes of Disease

Malaria in Modern Greece

Katerina Gardikas

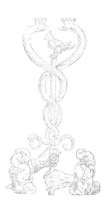

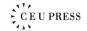

Central European University Press
Budapest—New York

Published in 2018 by
Central European University Press
Nádor utca 11, H-1051 Budapest, Hungary
Tel: +36-1-327-3138 or 327-3000 · *Fax:* +36-1-327-3183
E-mail: ceupress@press.ceu.edu
Website: www.ceupress.com

224 West 57th Street, New York NY 10019, USA
E-mail: meszarosa@press.ceu.edu

ISBN 978-6155-211-980

ISSN 2079-1119

Library of Congress Cataloging-in-Publication Data

Names: Gardikas, Katerina, author.
Title: Landscapes of disease : malaria in modern Greece / Katerina Gardikas.
Description: Budapest ; New York : Central European University Press, 2017. |
Series: CEU Press studies in the history of medicine, ISSN 2079-1119 ;
volume VIII | Includes bibliographical references and index.
Identifiers: LCCN 2017012464 (print) | LCCN 2017019737 (ebook) | ISBN
9789633861912 | ISBN 9786155211980
Subjects: LCSH: Malaria--Greece.
Classification: LCC RC163.G9 (ebook) | LCC RC163.G9 G37 2017 (print) | DDC
616.9/36209495--dc23
LC record available at https://lccn.loc.gov/2017012464

Printed by Prime Rate Kft., Hungary

CONTENTS

LIST OF TABLES

LIST OF FIGURES

LIST OF MAPS

ACKNOWLEDGEMENTS

This research was made possible by several grants: a research grant from the Rockefeller Archive Centre (2004), a grant from the Special Research Fund of the University of Athens (2005) and a grant from the J. F. Costopoulos Foundation (2005). In July 2009 I benefited from a visit to the Wellcome Trust Centre for the History of Medicine at UCL as a visiting scholar. I am particularly grateful to these institutions for their generosity. I also wish to thank the editors of the volume *Health, Hygiene and Eugenics in Southeastern Europe to 1945* and the publishers of the *Journal of Contemporary History* for permission to draw from my two articles, of which I made extensive use in chapters 2 and 3, respectively.[1]

In writing this book I have been fortunate to have benefited from the help and influence of many scholars, scientists, and other colleagues and friends who have left a mark on my work in a great variety of ways. Without their support I would not have come this far. This is the moment to acknowledge the debts I have incurred over many years and many research paths. I am particularly indebted to medical historians Dr. Marius Turda of Oxford Brookes University, Professor Georgios Antonakopoulos of the University of Thessaly and Dr. Socrates Litsios of the World Health Organization for their encouragement and support and for sharing their knowledge and experience and, particularly, for their invaluable comments and suggestions. Christian Promitzer of the Karl-Franzens-Universität of Graz also offered me his most valuable comments, for which I wish to express my sincerest thanks. I am also grateful to medical historian Professor Paul Weindling of Oxford Brookes for his generosity in offering me a wealth of valuable infor-

1   "Health Policy and Private Care: Malaria Sanitization in Early Twentieth Century Greece," in *Health, Hygiene and Eugenics in Southeastern Europe to 1945*, ed. Christian Promitzer, Sevasti Trubeta, and Marius Turda (Budapest: Central European University Press, 2011), 127–42, and "Relief Work and Malaria in Greece, 1943–1947," *Journal of Contemporary History* 43, no. 3 (2008): 493–508.

mation and references; to Dr. Tom Rosenbaum and Dr. Darwin Stapleton for their generous help in the calm and stimulating environment of the Rockefeller Archive Centre; to Bernardine Pejovic of the Archive of the League of Nations for her priceless guidance through the material; to Professor Bernardino Fantini for enlightening discussions in Geneva early enough in my research to influence its course; to Professor David Warhurst of the London School of Hygiene and Tropical Medicine for his advice and for saving me from jumping to unfounded conclusions; to Dr. Catherine Boura, former Greek consul-general in New York, for her warm friendship and support; to Professor Kostas Krimbas of the Academy of Athens for his keen interest in the progress of my work and his insightful comments; to my friends Professor Dimitris Christodoulou of the University of Thessaloniki, Dr. Kalli Simitopoulou and Professor Nikolaos Xirotiris of the University of Thrace for their criticism and encouragement and for helping me understand basic and complex scientific concepts; to my students and colleagues at the History Department of the University of Athens, who have been consistent in their support and patience with my sometimes tedious malarial stories in private chats and seminars; to Professors Christos Kattamis, Dennis Cokkinos, Dimitrios Loukopoulos of the University of Athens, the late Professor Nikolaos Matsaniotis of the Academy of Athens, Professor John Kyriopoulos of the National School of Public Health, and Professor Theodoros Dardavessis of the University of Thessaloniki, who all offered their medical expertise with great generosity; to Dr. Damian Mac Con Uladh for handling the manuscript with great care; to Mikhalis Spyridakis of the Greek Archaeological Service and Nasos Argyriou of the Institute for Mediterranean Studies for their assistance in compiling the maps; and, finally, to Dr. Helen Gardikas Katsiadakis for her pains to keep me and my manuscript coherent and for all that sisters do. My most profound debt, however, is to my late uncle Professor Stavros Papandreou, whose casual comment on the social impact of malaria set off this enquiry many years later.[2]

---

2   The software used in preparing this book comprises Nota Bene 11.5 as a research and writing tool, QGIS 2.18 for the preparation of the maps and SAS 9.4 for the statistical analysis.

INTRODUCTION

On a fine day in April 1829, a group of French scientists, members of the scientific expedition exploring the Morea, were approaching the town of Filiatra, in the southwestern Peloponnese. Much to their surprise, a band of violins and women with flowers emerged from the town to greet them. Word of their plant-collecting activity had preceded the members of the expedition, leading the locals to take the French scientists for physicians who would cure their illnesses. Panaget, the group's physician, did, in fact, visit the town's sick, while the Frenchmen were happy to share their supply of quinine and provide relief from malaria fevers. As Jean-Baptiste Bory de Saint-Vincent (1778–1846), naturalist and leader of the expedition, noted in his account of the expedition, "seeing us collect plants, everyone imagined that we were famous doctors and that we should have remedies for all ills. My stock of quinine suffered significantly from the consequences of this belief."[1]

The incident, a fortuitous encounter between the indigenous population and Western scientists, and its favorable outcome may have given the locals exaggerated expectations of contemporary Western medicine, whose healing powers they were already convinced of before the triumphal reception they prepared for the Frenchmen. Little did the villagers know how fortunate they were in not having received the full baggage of Western professional medicine which, besides the pharmaceutical treatment of fevers with quinine or infusions of the powder of the cinchona

---

1   Bory de Saint-Vincent, *Relation*, vol. 1, 360. Panaget died shortly thereafter, also of fever. On the expedition, see Osborne, "Resurrecting Hippocrates."

tree bark, also included more invasive practices against fevers such as bleeding and purging.[2]

This study explores malaria in its social and physical environment in Greece, the most malarious country in Europe, and also the one most heavily infested with *falciparum* malaria, at a time estimated to have coincided with the highpoint of the worldwide prevalence of the disease. This, according to the US malariologist Paul F. Russell, probably ranged between 1880 and 1920.[3] His colleague Lewis W. Hackett, on the other hand, set the peak of malaria prevalence at around 1850, a dating with which the Greek climatologist Elias Mariolopoulos also agreed.[4]

Before the seventeenth century, when the therapeutic use of the bark attracted attention to the disease, sources are silent about endemic fevers and fever epidemics. Furthermore, the Greek lands had, since late antiquity, for the most part, become a marginal frontier zone between competing armies, navies, religious authorities, states, and empires. They were sparsely populated and poorly urbanized. Escaping malaria in the increasingly desolate lowlands was one among several factors that induced peasants to settle within a zone, "in terms of elevation . . . above the malarial stratum but low enough for tree crops."[5] When their societies were not ravaged by war and disease, their economies were subjected to expropriations and plunder for raw materials, fighting men, and taxes. Under the Ottomans since the fifteenth century, these lands came under the command economy of a centralized empire and enjoyed longer periods of peacetime. Local organization took the form of small communities, which started to develop and occasionally prosper by the end of the seventeenth century, as they began producing for the European market and, moreover, attracted the attention of European scholars and antiquarians. On the eve of the Greek War of Independence, the few large towns in later-day Greece did not exceed 15,000 inhabitants each, while a tendency to populate the lowlands began, but was suspended because of the war. Otherwise, emigration and lawlessness regularly became the fate of the population surplus.

---

2   Roux, *Histoire*, 26–27; Hennen, *Sketches*, 190, 411–12; Faure, *Des fièvres intermittentes et continues*, vol. 1, 144; cf. McNeill, *Mosquito Empires*, 63; see also chapter 2.

3   Russell, "World-Wide Malaria Distribution," 937.

4   Hackett, "Distribution of Malaria"; Mariolopoulos, *To klima tis Ellados*, 33.

5   McNeill, *The Mountains*, 86.

Thus, before modern statehood, the land that became the hearth of Greek nation and state building was virtually a political, economic, and cultural backwater. Social relationships played out, as Eric Wolf has summarized in the concluding words of his *Europe and the People without History*, as "divergent paths of groups and classes" that "do not find their explanation in the self-interested decisions of interacting individuals. They grow out of the deployment of social labor, mobilized to engage the world of nature. The manner of that mobilization sets the terms of history, and in these terms the peoples who have asserted a privileged relation with history and the peoples to whom history has been denied encounter a common destiny."[6] This history was jumpstarted and, at the same time, sanctioned by references to antiquity in a radical narrative of national regeneration. The thriving economic and cultural centers, where the new idea of nationhood was conceived and developed, were multicultural cities elsewhere in the Ottoman Empire and Europe.

I have limited my study of malaria in modern Greece to the 140 years or so from the country's emergence into statehood in the 1830s up to the eradication of the disease in the mid-1970s. The state that emerged in 1830 out of the response of the Concert of Europe to the War of Independence comprised but a small part of these marginal lands. A state-building process had already begun even as the War of Independence was being waged, and was pursued more systematically after 1828 by Ioannis Kapodistrias, the country's first elected governor. However, it was under the Bavarian regents, who ran the new kingdom between 1833 and 1835 in the name of King Othon, still a minor when he acceded to the throne, that Greece received its most comprehensive ever state-building plan, which also comprised sanitary policies. A loan package of sixty million francs set the kingdom on its financial feet, with Britain, France and Russia jointly guaranteeing the loan—and thus the initial viability of Greece—and thereafter making sure that Greece would not destabilize European peace.

In the new kingdom, the state of health became the responsibility of the Interior Ministry, which assumed the lion's share of state-building functions. The policies of the Bavarian regents in introducing new institutions to the young state also included sanitary legislation and drew on contempo-

---

6   Wolf, *Europe and the People without History*, 391.

rary western European, primarily French, models.[7] State authorities were, moreover, responsible to carefully examine the health of sites proposed for new urban settlements.

Whatever measures and sanitary structures were put in place in the early days of the monarchy disintegrated in the years that followed, as the country failed to maintain them in the face of old and new social and environmental pressures. Greece lay exposed to endemic diseases and frequent epidemics. Consequently, the members of the medical profession became alarmed at the country's urban and military health statistics. The humanitarian crises brought about by the two world wars in the twentieth century required repeated and generous reconstruction programs, each with a significant component of foreign aid and public health expertise. Eventually, malaria was brought under control and finally eradicated by the mid-1970s thanks to the introduction of DDT and the postwar economic improvement of the country.

Endemic malaria emerged as by far the country's most common health issue and became the leading factor in the early diffusion of Western medicine in Greece. Indeed, many decades later, in the context of the refugee humanitarian crisis of 1922, a League of Nations committee visiting the country in 1923, precisely to consider ways to provide foreign expertise, noted that "the two main public health problems facing Greece" remained malaria and the public health service itself.[8]

Moreover, as malaria prevalence developed in interaction with the physical environment and the mobility of its prospective victims, the authorities designed public health measures albeit with imperfect knowledge of the physical, social, and cultural determinants of the disease. The history of malaria in Greece in this period must be told with a large degree of hindsight. We know that the story ended in eradication in the mid-1970s, although we may not know in detail how malaria in modern Greece developed as it did. On the one hand, doctors and other decision-makers explored the country—charting its geography and state of health—while, on the other, a considerable proportion of the Greek public developed a keen interest in the innovations of Western science, be it quinine, microscopy, Paris green, or DDT. Bory de Saint-Vincent's story encapsulates an early moment in this encounter.

---

7 Farr, "Medical Topographies in 19th Century Bavaria"; Ruisinger, *Das griechische Gesundheitswesen*, 53.
8 League of Nations, Health Organisation, Health Committee, *Rapport*, 8.

Malaria, once an experience shared by between one in three and one in four Greeks annually, is now considered a concern of the past, despite the recent reemergence of largely imported *vivax* cases in locations where it had been endemic in earlier days. Today, Greeks in their seventies or older come up with vivid, but no longer painful, recollections of the disease. A university professor of history remembered the embarrassment his splenomegaly caused him at school and a doctor reminisced how his father had carried him, a six-year-old boy at the time, over 30 kilometers of dirt road on foot from a remote village in Crete to hospital in Khania, thus saving him from *falciparum* malaria.[9] A medical historian among my informants told me from personal experience, that the physical suffering of malaria is so intense that one never really forgets it.[10] The eradication of malaria has, however, caused this common memory to fade and disappear from shared histories.[11]

For reasons connected with the official nature of the bulk of the written sources, the geographical coverage of this study expands in step with the accession history of new territories to the Greek state between the London Protocol of 1830 and the Treaty of Lausanne in 1923. I have made one exception, however, in the case of information collected by the French Armée d'Orient, which sheds light on malaria in late Ottoman Macedonia.[12] I have also chosen to limit the geographical scope to a "Balkan" perspective, mostly omitting the larger islands of the eastern Aegean, on account of their proximity to the Asia Minor coast, and Crete, owing to its remoteness from the Greek mainland and its exchanges with North Africa. Nonetheless, in 1907, that is, before the island's formal unification with the Greek kingdom in 1913, the Anti-Malaria League included Crete in its malaria survey and control program.[13] Moreover, precisely because of its relative remoteness from mainland Greece, in 1945 Daniel E. Wright, an American sanitary engineer from the Rockefeller Foundation (RF) working for the United Nations Relief and Rehabilitation Administration (UNRRA), drew up a ma-

---

9   I. Kh. and G. Kh., personal communications (Thessaloniki, 15 September 2006 and Athens, 23 October 2007, respectively).
10   G. A., personal communication (Athens, 22 December 2003). See also Appendix I for a firsthand account of the lived experience of malarial fevers in 1892 by a physician sufferer.
11   See chapter 4.
12   See chapter 3.
13   Theodoridis, "Paratiriseis tines."

laria-eradication experiment for Crete with funding from the Greek War Relief Association (GWRA).[14]

As for the smaller Aegean Islands, their malaria history, although quite extensive, is one of only sporadic bouts of medical attention. Besides some preliminary work by the Malariology Division of the Athens School of Hygiene on the island of Paros in the interwar years, malaria on the remote Aegean Islands attracted attention toward the end of the Second World War, when the Cairo office of UNRRA set up a schooner as a hospital ship that visited the small, doctorless islands of the Cyclades on a quite remarkable humanitarian mission.[15]

From a methodological perspective, perhaps the most serious difficulty regarding the terms of the narrative is the need to accommodate two intervening paradigm shifts reflected in the medical sources. The first such shift occurred within the time frame of my period of interest, namely the shift from miasmatic to germ theory.

Miasmatic theory, which held that fevers were caused by emanations of poisonous particles from rotting organic matter in marshes, was not in principle opposed to the prevailing Hippocratic and Galenic humoral theory. For many of these fevers, the sources used the Hippocratic term "intermittent fevers" (*dialeipontes pyretoi*) but also other descriptive terminology. Nonetheless, in the history of fevers "intermittent fevers were potentially subversive of humoral theory," as physicians located their origin outside of the human body.[16] These various fevers were understood either as manifestations of a single disease that could change from one fever type to another, or as individual disease entities, according to the notion that identified the disease with the symptom rather than with its causal agent. However, causal agents could indeed be more than one, pointing to a uniform set of internal disturbances that cures had to redress.[17]

---

14 Col. M. R. Lubbock, Deputy Chief of Mission, Bureau of Relief Services, to Buell F. Maben, Chief of Mission, "Report on Health and Welfare Divisions," June 1946, Greece #19, PAG-4/4.2.:35 [S-0524-0059], UN Archives; Report of the Director, Health Division, Health Division, UNRRA-Greece Headquarters, Historical notes, General, Greece #20, PAG-4/4.2.:35 [S-0524-0059], UN Archives. See also Vassiliou, "Politics, Public Health, and Development," 235–42 and 248.

15 See Livadas and Sfangos, *I elonosia en Elladi*, vol. 2, 223–26; Ruth Parmelee to W. S. Finlayson, 7 July 1945, Health Monthly Progress Reports February 1945–November 1946, PAG-4/3.0.12.2.3.:45 [S-0527-0709], UN Archives.

16 Lonie, "Fever Pathology," 30.

17 Geyer-Kordesch, "Fevers and Other Fundamentals," 106, 107.

Until approximately the end of the nineteenth century, references to these fevers did not necessarily nor fully correspond to accounts of malaria, the nosological entity we know today. Besides malaria, fevers often included typhoid fevers, with which they shared common symptoms such as abdominal pains. Even the Greek term for malaria, *elonosia* (swamp disease), came into usage in the 1900s and was unknown in the nineteenth century.

In the 1870s, germ theory promoted a research framework for the discovery of the specific causal agents of diseases among parasites and microbes and of their transmission mechanisms. The French military doctor Alphonse Laveran discovered one such causal agent of malaria in 1880, and Ronald Ross and Giovanni Battista Grassi independently established the role of the *Anopheles* mosquito in transmitting human malaria in 1898. Clearly, the intermittent and periodic fevers cited, for instance, in the nationwide medico-statistical survey of 1838–40, do not represent the same nosological concept as that found in the surveys conducted between 1901 and 1908, although they both broadly correspond to malaria.[18]

The second shift, inherent in any historical study of malaria today, is the product of the present-day molecular approach to disease and immunity. For lack of pertinent contemporary observations, since relevant epidemiological data are unavailable for the period before eradication, this frequently renders attempts to reconstruct some aspects of the disease history in present-day terms conjectural.

The paradigmatic shift between miasmatic and germ theories also affected the status of medical geography, an analytical and explanatory tool used extensively in malaria research. Indeed, after the discovery of the infecting agent and the transmitting vector, much of the explanation of malaria epidemiology was reduced to the mechanics of transmission with geography and the importance of place serving a secondary explanatory role.[19] The decline of medical geography coincided with the rise of bacteriology, essentially leaving only malaria and tuberculosis as diseases also susceptible to the effects of place.[20] It will be argued here that, besides affecting the continuity between the two knowledge regimes, this paradigmatic shift had serious practical implications for the Greek response to malaria; before the

---

18   On this issue, see the discussion in Dobson, *Contours of Death*, 312–17.
19   Buttimer, "Airs, Waters, Places," 215.
20   Numbers, "Medical Science," 219.

advent of DDT, the preference to use quinine to control malaria presented a modern, "scientific" alternative to mosquito control, which would have been a far more costly environmental approach.

STATE OF THE LITERATURE

The history of malaria in modern Greece is the subject of a DPhil thesis at Oxford by Maria Vassiliou.[21] The work focuses on state antimalarial policies from the late 1920s, the contributions of the League of Nations and the Rockefeller Foundation, and post–Second World War residual spraying programs, their consolidation stage and the eradication of the disease within the World Health Organization (WHO) policy framework. Recently, two articles on the history of malaria in Greece have appeared in English, one by Maria Mandyla and coauthors and the other by Costas Tsiamis and coauthors; both articles treat the creation of the Greek Anti-Malaria League and the influence of the Italian school of malariology on early-twentieth-century antimalarial programs.[22]

Additionally, two publications deserve a mention. Older but informative, a two-volume work by Gregorios A. Livadas and Ioannis C. Sfangos entitled *Malaria in Greece, 1930–1940*[23] is a contemporary account in English of the malaria situation and control work by two of the protagonists, which has been the principal source of information on Greece in the international literature. The other publication, a special issue of the Greek medical history periodical *Deltos* in 2005, offers a general review of the subject.[24]

Frank M. Snowden has authoritatively examined malaria in Italy, a country both heavily infected with the disease and an innovator in malarial research and control. In a broad chronological setting, Snowden focuses on the complex relationships among society, scientific research, the nation-state, and international developments.[25] Sandra M. Sufian, on the other hand, focused on the Zionists' malaria control programs and their nation-building and social engineering approach to the landscape and the people

---

21 Vassiliou, "Politics, Public Health, and Development."
22 Mandyla et al., "Pioneers"; Tsiamis, Piperaki, and Tsakris, "The History of the Greek Anti-Malaria League."
23 Livadas and Sfangos, *Malaria in Greece*. This is the English translation of their *I elonosia en Elladi*.
24 *I istoria tis elonosias stin Ellada*.
25 Snowden, *The Conquest of Malaria*.

of Palestine during the Mandate period.[26] More recently James L. A. Webb Jr. discussed the emergence and spread of human malaria across all continents from the dawn of humanity to the present as part of the evolutionary process,[27] while Randall M. Packard linked the understanding of the disease to social and economic context.[28] Also in a global context, J. R. McNeill has focused on the role of malaria, yellow fever, and differential immunity in defining the outcome of the wars between Western forces in the Americas and the Caribbean.[29] Finally, Christopher Hamlin, in his *More Than Hot: A Short History of Fever*, clarifies the complex conceptual and cultural history of fevers from antiquity to the present.[30]

Other recent works on modern Greek medical history have treated more general issues of public health. Dimitra Giannuli offered a critical view of the Rockefeller Foundation's achievements in Greece.[31] John Kyriopoulos's edited volume *Dimoseia ygeia kai koinoniki politiki: o Eleftherios Venizelos kai i epokhi tou* (Public health and social policy: Eleftherios Venizelos and his era) contains the proceedings of a conference held in 2007 at the National School of Public Health (ESDY) in Athens on the public health and sanitary reforms introduced by the liberal governments of Eleftherios Venizelos between 1910 and 1932.[32]

Central to this study are a number of nationwide surveys, the earliest being a general medical survey ordered by the government, conducted between 1838 and 1840, and published at the time as a supplement to *Ellinikos Takhydromos*. The Greek physician Clôn Stéphanos (1854–1915), some forty-five years later, used it in his *Grèce au point de vue naturel, ethnologique, anthropologique et médicale*.[33] More than sixty years after the first medical survey, when germ theory was already established, there followed a series of six malaria surveys carried out between 1901 and 1919. They resulted from a mobilization of the Greek medical establishment in response to fears about the general health of the nation. The mobilization had begun in the 1880s

---

26 Sufian, *Healing the Land.*
27 Webb, *Humanity's Burden.*
28 Packard, *The Making of a Tropical Disease.*
29 McNeill, *Mosquito Empires.*
30 Hamlin, *More Than Hot.*
31 Giannuli, "Repeated Disappointment."
32 Kyriopoulos, *Dimosia ygeia kai koinoniki politiki.*
33 Stéphanos, *La Grèce.* On Stéphanos's work, see Antonakopoulos, "Klon Stefanos (1854–1915)."

with medical conferences[34] and, in the early twentieth century, produced vertical campaigns specifically targeting tuberculosis and malaria. Conducted by a private body, the Anti-Malaria League, the malaria surveys sent out questionnaires to local physicians and municipal authorities throughout the country. Finally, from the 1930s to eradication in the 1970s there was a stream of malaria surveys on a local or a national scale to assess the effects of antimalarial work and to record wartime damage.

Other primary sources used in this study include official state records, published statistics, maps, personal papers, propaganda material, and a small number of personal interviews and correspondence. Research work was carried out at archives of institutions which took an active part in the fight against malaria: the Rockefeller Archive Center of the Rockefeller Foundation at Sleepy Hollow, New York; the Archives of the League of Nations at the United Nations Library in Geneva; the Archives of the United Nations Relief and Rehabilitation Administration (UNRRA) at the United Nations in New York. I have also consulted the personal papers of Ronald Ross at the Historical Archive of the Library of the School of Hygiene and Tropical Medicine in London; the personal papers of Daniel E. Wright, available online at the Special Collections in the Library of the Virginia Polytechnic Institute and State University (Virginia Tech) in Blacksburg, Virginia; the War Office documents at the National Archives in London; the Greek State Archives (GAK) in Athens and Ermoupoli; the Eleftherios Venizelos and the Alexandros Korizis collections at the Historical Archives of the Benaki Museum in Athens; the printed material collections of the Wellcome Library in London; the library of the School of Hygiene and Tropical Medicine in London; the map collection at the British Library in London; the Bibliothèque Interuniversitaire de Médecine in Paris; the Gennadius Library in Athens; the library of the National School of Public Health in Athens; the library of the Academy of Athens; the printed material at the Greek Literary and Historical Archive (ELIA) in Athens; the Hellenic Parliament Library; and the Central Library of the Aristotle University of Thessaloniki. A fair amount of material was found in the microfilmed archival collection of the Military Service Archives of the Greek Army in Athens. Furthermore, a large number of primary sources, pamphlet materials, and firsthand

---

34 Makkas and Rallis, *Praktika.*

contemporary accounts in Greek was put out by physicians involved in the fight against malaria in their effort to rouse public concern, the most comprehensive publication being the five-volume proceedings of the Anti-Malaria League titled *I elonosia en Elladi kai ta pepragmena tou Syllogou* (Malaria in Greece and the League's proceedings). Unfortunately, the archive of the Athens School of Public Hygiene (the forerunner of the ESDY) was not made available to me at the time of my research.

The study of malaria has produced a large amount of published sources dealing with the history and epidemiology of the disease worldwide, the histories of institutions, scientists, and the development of ideas as well as antimalarial drugs. Some of this literature was written by the protagonists of the antimalarial campaigns and reflects the controversies which split them into warring camps. No study of malaria in Greece is possible, however, without consulting the writings of Ioannis P. Kardamatis (1859–1942), a physician who dedicated his life's work to studying and combating malaria.[35]

Structure

My curiosity regarding malaria was triggered by its presumed responsibility for the economic backwardness of Greece.[36] This, however, is only one among a variety of approaches to the study of Greece's relationship with the disease. Another approach, already adequately covered in the recent literature, studies efforts to control malaria. This study focuses rather on the human factors that contributed to the spread of the disease. In also looking at the physical environment, it considers, furthermore, the adaptive responses of the other two sets of competing species, namely a small number of species of *Anopheles* mosquitoes and malaria *Plasmodia*—each species with its own supply of weapons and defenses—by informing the analysis with a coevolutionary approach.[37] By focusing, however, on the short term, I look into cul-

---

35   For biographical information on I. P. Kardamatis, see [Kardamatis], *Eortasmos ogdoikontaetiridos*, and Kitzmiller, *Anopheline Names*, 111–13.

36   Still at an impressionable age, in the mid-1960s, I was exposed to this idea thanks to a remark to this effect from Stavros Papandreou (1883–1969), professor at the Athens School of Agriculture. On the postwar recovery from the economic and mental effects of malaria on Greece, see McNeill, *The Metamorphosis*, 179–80. See also Nájera and Hempel, *The Burden of Malaria*. On the dynamic and nonlinear association between malaria and poverty, see Packard, *The Making of a Tropical Disease*, 179–93 and 201–15.

37   Mackinnon and Read, "Virulence in Malaria"; Mackinnon and Read, "Immunity."

tural adaptations of the population to environmental pressures—indeed, often failures to adapt—that involve relevant collective or individual choices.[38]

The central question of this study is how malaria interacted with the new social and economic realities that emerged in Greece after independence. Did nationhood and its freedoms and pressures increase or reduce the suffering of the Greeks from malaria?

This is, however, a comparative question that is confronted by a serious limitation. On account of the lack of data on fevers in the Ottoman-ruled Greek lands, it is impossible to compare the postindependence situation, for which there exists an abundance of sources, with earlier realities. I have therefore concentrated on inferences from the observable implications, that is, qualitative outcomes that help evaluate a hypothesis, of changes noted within a period of approximately 140 turbulent years of national history. For instance, on the basis of established facts of epidemiology, specific observed changes in settlement patterns, the independent variable, are consistent with implied changes in local malaria epidemiology, the dependent variable. Likewise, observed facts pointing to malaria epidemics, the independent variable, are consistent with the implications of reduced acquired immunity to malaria, the dependent variable.[39]

I argue that, to understand the complexity of the malaria situation in Greece after independence, a variety of factors needs to be considered: the fragmented landscape and unstable climate, social and economic developments, shifts in the location of malaria foci and vector breeding sites against a backdrop of a few persistent heavily endemic places, no less than wartime and humanitarian crises, and a welcome reliance on foreign aid and expertise. Furthermore, cultural factors, primarily the popularity of quinine for treatment, relief and as an affordable substitute for costly malaria control schemes, alleviated much of the suffering and reduced the number of deaths. Conversely, however, one may wonder—with no hard evidence to test such a hypothesis—whether the blanket administration of quinine might have also undermined acquired immunity, and whether

---

38 On this subject, see Greene and Danubio's edited volume *Adaptation to Malaria*. The contributions to this collection address mostly study dietary adaptations to endemic malaria—the prophylactic role of oxidants, in particular—but also deal with policy choices and marital patterns. Greene and Danubio, "Adaptation to Malaria," 391–92. For a study on malaria and human coevolution in the long term applied to sickle-cell anemia, see Durham, *Coevolution*, 103–53.

39 King, Keohane, and Verba, *Designing Social Inquiry*, 99–100 and 109–11.

it may have resulted in more virulent malaria epidemics and increased suffering and wretchedness.

The book is divided into four chapters. Chapter 1, titled "Malaria, an Ancient and Global Disease," summarizes the principal milestones in the history of malaria and malaria control, both worldwide and in Greece, traditional strategies of prevention, avoidance, and cure, including the use of quinine. Chapter 2, "The Fragmented Geography of the Disease," borrows the idea of geographical fragmentation as a defining feature of the Mediterranean environment from Peregrine Horden and Nicholas Purcell.[40] It also treats the effect of fragmentation on climate variability and the notion of the malaria season with a similar attention to variation and looks into the effects of climate and seasonal variability on the instability of the disease, the differences between endemic and epidemic malaria and on the effects of these differences on the Greek malaria experience. Chapter 3, "Malaria in Peace and War," explores the effect on malaria of regular, peacetime human activities in agriculture, colonization, industry, and urban development and on the effects of war, army mobilization, and army life, in general, and population displacement. Chapter 4, titled "Patients, Doctors, and Cures," takes a look at the patient and his relationship with treatment, physicians, and health care. The cultural transfer of medical knowledge among professionals and lay patients, the use of quinine and its social and epidemiological implications are particularly prominent in the topics discussed in this chapter.

The concluding chapter is an attempt to explore the central hypothesis of the book, that is, to examine how malaria interacted with the social and economic realities in Greece after independence. This hypothesis is broken up into a series of specific questions. Did malaria become more widespread, virulent and unstable? Did the balance between benign tertian, or *vivax*, and malignant tertian, or *falciparum* malaria, change over the years and how might the population have adapted culturally? In fact, the organization of control measures to combat malaria, particularly Greece's heavy reliance on quinine, is perceived in the context of such a cultural response, with considerable implications on the physical environment and possibly on immunity levels and public health. Not all of these questions find their definitive answer here.

---

40 Horden and Purcell, *The Corrupting Sea*.

Finally, to gain an appraisal of the changing fate of malaria landscapes as "sites of memory" in Greece, it would be useful to reflect on their physical and cultural transformations, as they responded to costly drainage and sanitization schemes. Some, like Lake Copais in Central Greece and the plains of Macedonia, became fertile agricultural land; others, like the Gialova lagoon in the southwestern Peloponnese and Lake Antinioti in Corfu, are natural reserves. Since its drainage, Lake Karla in Thessaly has been a persistent problem for ecological management and Ropa Valley in Corfu, where the British went hunting in the nineteenth century, is now an area of mixed land usage; it is mostly grazing land scattered with small businesses, accommodates a Roma settlement at one end and a golf club at the other and is encircled by vineyards and olive groves on the surrounding slopes.[41]

---

41 Gardikas, "Dystopika topia."

CHAPTER I

MALARIA: AN ANCIENT AND GLOBAL DISEASE

The Emergence of Human Malaria

When did malaria reach the Mediterranean, and Greece in particular? Did all three malaria parasites that infected the population arrive simultaneously? Did climatological change over the centuries affect malaria prevalence? Could malaria prevalence have receded and then reemerged? What are the conflicting theories and to what degree can they be reconciled or what is the source of their disagreement? For how long, in other words, has the population endured malaria and malaria-related blood disorders, i.e., sickle-cell anemia and thalassemias, and the suffering and death caused by these diseases? Answering these questions requires a brief overview of the evolution of human malaria in its site of origin: the Old World.

The first historians of malaria a century ago had access only to written sources, principally Greek and Latin, and later Chinese, Egyptian, and Ayurvedic medical and nonmedical texts. Mid-twentieth-century historical research incorporated evidence from entomology and climatology. Recently, genetic research has allowed scientists to reconstruct much of the evolutionary history of the human *Plasmodia* by combining ecological studies with evidence of evolutionary pressures from malaria. As a result of the broadening of the scope of its sources, the history of malaria, which began as a history of the classical lands, has today become a global history that takes the narrative back to hundreds of millions of years ago.[1] However, the early history of malaria is a terrain fraught with uncertainty and specula-

---

1 For a global approach, see Webb, *Humanity's Burden*.

tion.[2] This is also true with regard to the arrival of the disease on the shores of the Mediterranean, where, in fact, the narrative begins to tread on firmer ground only by the time of late antiquity.

The evolutionary history of the disease predates the encounter of malaria with humankind. The genus *Plasmodium* dates as far back as the Cambrian period, about 500 to 600 million years ago.[3] How did the four species of human *Plasmodia*[4] evolve among human groups? By virtue of their ancient history and their concomitant polymorphisms, the *Plasmodium* species have a privileged position in their adaptive arms race with humans, over whom *Plasmodia* possess a considerable evolutionary advantage. *P. falciparum*, for instance, contains one of the most polymorphic genes in existence, the gene encoding for the antigen termed merozoite surface protein 1 (MSP1), which is critical for the ability of the parasite to invade human red blood cells.[5] The extremely high degree of diversity of molecule MSP1 would have required some forty-eight million years of random mutation, but this diversity was actually achieved, not by chance, but by natural selection within the parasite's recent history of a few thousand years, thanks to the antigen's interaction with the human immune system in the process, on the part of the *Plasmodium*, to try to evade recognition and break into the human red blood cells.[6] Thus, much of the research into the history of *P. falciparum*, a history of mutual adaptation between invader and defender, has been based on the degree of polymorphism of certain antigens. As a result of research along these lines, S. M. Rich and F. J. Ayala place the origin of present-day *P. falciparum* to a cenancestor, or common ancestor, as recently as 5,000 to 50,000 years ago.[7]

The spread of malaria to new zones of, first, epidemic, and then endemic infection was determined by the migration of humans to locations of suitable altitude, temperature, and ecology and by the presence there of poten-

---

2   Cormier, *The Ten-Thousand Year Fever*, 9.
3   Ayala, Escalante, and Rich, "Evolution of Plasmodium," 55.
4   Recently a fifth species, *Plasmodium knowlesi*, naturally found in macaques in southeast Asia, has emerged as a human malaria parasite, particularly in Malaysia. Lee et al., "Hyperparasitaemic."
5   Antigens are substances, often molecules of the invading organisms, by which the host immune system detects their presence and is thereby mobilized to mount its defense. The genes responsible for coding antigens are particularly susceptible to selective pressures. Ayala, Escalante, and Rich, "Evolution of *Plasmodium*," 59.
6   Hartl, "The Origin of Malaria," 17; Rich and Ayala, "Population Structure."
7   Rich and Ayala, "Population Structure."

tially susceptible *Anopheles* mosquito vectors. Furthermore, the survival chances of a malarial species depended on its ability to maintain a continuous chain of infection by surviving long enough in its host, thereby adapting to host population density. Thus, as long as Eurasian populations of hunter-gatherers remained sparse and mobile, infections must have been unstable and limited to *vivax* and *malariae* malaria. Furthermore, as infected African migrants entered the Eurasian landmass, they encountered different species of mosquitoes than those in Africa; some of them, however, were capable of hosting and transmitting human *Plasmodia*. Another possible independent early source of human infection could have arisen from simian *vivax* malaria from apes in tropical southeast Asia that may have infected humans in the Pleistocene, before the arrival of African parasite strains of the agricultural era.[8]

Despite the fact that *vivax* malaria enjoys the widest worldwide prevalence, its evolutionary history received little attention until recently. Several of its close relatives infect chimpanzees. Current research associated the fact that human *vivax* infection is mostly absent from Sub-Saharan Africa thanks to the emergence there of the Duffy-negative mutation, which protects 90 percent of the population, with the discovery in central Africa of chimpanzees and gorillas in the wild infected with a diverse spectrum of malaria *Plasmodia* genetically similar to *P. vivax*. The research results suggest Africa as the origin of *P. vivax* along with "a much more recent timescale for human *P. vivax* infection, consistent with it having selected for the spread of the Duffy-negative mutation."[9] It is probable that "an ancestral *P. vivax* stock was able to infect humans, gorillas, and chimpanzees in Africa until the Duffy-negative mutation started to spread—around 30,000 years ago—and eliminated *P. vivax* from humans there. Under this scenario, extant human-infecting *P. vivax* represents a parasite lineage that survived after spreading out of Africa."[10]

P. vivax spread throughout the globe in the blood of migrating humans to become the most prevalent and persistent type of human malaria.

8   Webb, *Humanity's Burden*, 12 and 42–46; Carter and Mendis, "Evolutionary and Historical Aspects."
9   Sharp, "*Plasmodium Vivax* in African Apes."
10   Wellcome Trust Sanger Institute, "Out of Africa" and Weimin Liu et al., "African Origin." A recent study estimates that the mutation established itself in Sub-Saharan Africa around 42,000 years ago. McManus et al., "Population Genetic Analysis."

According to the dominant hypothesis, it spread into Asia out of Africa at the end of the Pleistocene, between 30,000 and 10,000 years ago. Its trail from West Africa to the Near East is traceable in the declining frequency of Duffy negativity.[11] In the words of James Webb, "on the basis of available evidence, human refractoriness to *vivax* malaria as a result of Duffy negativity appears to be the very earliest known chapter in human beings' genetic adaptation to vector-borne infectious disease and, indeed, the very earliest known chapter in humanity's long struggle with parasitic disease."[12] Indeed, thanks to its ability to produce latent parasite forms in the host's liver and relapse several years after the initial attack, *P. vivax* was capable of sustaining an infection among mobile and low-density populations of hunter-gatherers or seasonal migrants.[13]

Owing to its virulence, the origins of *P. falciparum* have received the greatest attention of all *Plasmodia*. Recent access to the study of primates in the wild has indeed allowed researchers to enlarge the number of observed individuals among primate species susceptible to the human parasite and to *P. reichenowi*, its closest relative. There is, moreover, a general consensus that the spread of agriculture played a critical role in African history, specifically in the evolution of modern *P. falciparum*.[14]

Despite its ancient lineage, the current population of *P. falciparum* is of fairly recent origin. Contrary to the earlier cospeciation hypothesis, which saw both species as offshoots of a common ancestor, genetic studies of apes in the African wild have demonstrated that *P. reichenowi* is in fact the ancestor of *P. falciparum*, which "evolved from the introduction of the chimpanzee *P. reichenowi* into the human lineage," i.e., by host transfer.[15]

---

11 Carter and Mendis, "Evolutionary and Historical Aspects," 573–74, 577, and 580; Rich, "The Unpredictable Past," 15548. According to an alternative hypothesis, *vivax* malaria may have spread into Asia out of Africa with *Homo erectus* one or two million years ago. Sallares, *Malaria and Rome*, 26–27. See also Mueller et al., "Key Gaps," 557–58.

12 Webb, "Malaria."

13 As the molecular evidence suggests, extensive vivax infections probably occurred tens of thousands of years earlier than large-scale *falciparum* malaria infections. Webb, Humanity's Burden, 28.

14 Carter and Mendis, "Evolutionary and Historical Aspects," 577.

15 Rich et al., "The Origin of Malignant Malaria," 14902–4; Prugnolle et al., "African Great Apes"; Ayala, Escalante, and Rich, "Evolution of *Plasmodium*," 59; Rich et al., "Malaria's Eve," 4429; Coluzzi, "The Clay Feet," 280. This is the Malaria Eve hypothesis, named after the article by Rich and his collaborators. According to their dating methodology, the age of the extant population of *P. falciparum* is 7,700 to 3,200 years. Rich and Ayala, "Progress in Malaria Research," 267–69; Carter and Mendis, "Evolutionary and Historical Aspects," 575–78.

The dating of the actual transfer remains unclear. Among the four human malarial species, present-day *P. falciparum* is the one most vulnerable to circumstances adverse to the spread of malaria, the one most likely to die out. Furthermore, the infection it produces in humans is brief in comparison to other malarial infections and, according to one argument, requires as a result a denser population to sustain continuous transmission. It could therefore hardly survive among the sparse populations of hunter-gatherers of preagricultural Africa,[16] when the original host transfer must have occurred. In the words of S. M. Rich and his coauthors, "considerable time, on the order of many tens or hundreds of thousands of years, may have elapsed from the time of the host transfer to the time when genetic changes in the parasite and/or the human lineages made possible the rapid expansion of *P. falciparum.*"[17]

So, how and when did the new species, equipped with its current virulent features, evolve from the old to become established among humans? Perhaps the one most critical development in the evolution of *P. falciparum* was the increase in population densities in Sub-Saharan Africa with the onset of agriculture and the encroachment of the tropical rainforest by humans for the purpose of food production within the past 5,000 to 10,000 years.[18] In turn, as a result of increased human densities, the mosquitoes of the *Anopheles gambiae* complex of the region that were accustomed to feeding on ungulates evolved into a mosquito species with a preference for human bloodmeals, the *A. gambiae*, even today the most efficient and dangerous transmitter of *falciparum* malaria owing to its anthropophilic behavior. In the words of Italian malariologist Mario Coluzzi, who first developed this hypothesis in 1999, "It is highly improbable that pre-Neolithic human environments provided conditions suitable to drive the mosquito's endophilic/anthropophilic habits, whereas selection for these traits is likely to be associated with developing agricultural communities with permanent and compact settlements, the rural village."[19] Coluzzi dated these speciation events and the consequent spread of *P. falciparum* to around 6,000 years ago.

16 Webb, *Humanity's Burden*, 28.
17 Rich et al., "The Origin of Malignant Malaria," 14905.
18 Carter and Mendis, "Evolutionary and Historical Aspects," 578; Rich et al., "The Origin of Malignant Malaria"; Coluzzi, "The Clay Feet," 278.
19 Coluzzi, "The Clay Feet," 278.

This hypothesis is, indeed, also consistent with recent research on the origin of *falciparum* malaria.[20]

Although the Neolithic revolution first occurred in Asia thanks to the presence there of domesticated animals, ecological conditions in tropical Africa, such as the development of anthropophilic mosquitoes, brought about selective pressures that favored the emergence of *P. falciparum* in the African Neolithic cultures.[21] It appears, therefore, that the social as well as the entomological environment contributed to considerable differences between the two continents. As a result, additional, broad differences emerged in the epidemiology of malaria in tropical Africa and Eurasia, respectively. As noted by James Webb: "Rather than the African pattern of heavy endemic *falciparum* infection, in tropical Asia patterns of malarial infections are generally more unstable and have remained so to the present day. This may be due, in part, to the fact that the anopheline vectors there had more opportunities to take their blood meals from domesticated animals. At all events, there was considerable regional variation in the stability of malarial pressure."[22]

An alternative hypothesis, subscribed to by Robert Sallares and Sir David Weatherall, dates the origin of *P. falciparum* to around 100,000 years ago.[23] According to this hypothesis, the parasite coevolved with humans, when the ancestors of humans and chimpanzees, and the ancestors of *P. falciparum* and *P. reichenowi* diverged from their respective common ancestor around five million years ago. The 100,000-year-old human parasite was equipped to survive the cooler climate of the Pleistocene among small human groups of hunter-gatherers, but "has undergone a major population expansion within the last 10,000 years." This hypothesis opposes Rich and Ayala's "Malaria Eve" hypothesis, which, as noted earlier, postulated an intervening *P. falciparum* population bottleneck several thousand years ago and was consistent with recent findings on the direct and recent descent of *P. falciparum* from *P. reichenowi*.[24]

Since the spread of both *vivax* and *falciparum* malaria and the loss of life they incurred, humans have responded with genetic adaptation. Thus, long

---

20 Ibid., 279–80; Carter and Mendis, "Evolutionary and Historical Aspects," 578–79; Rich et al., "The Origin of Malignant Malaria," 14905.

21 Sallares, Bouwman, and Anderung, "The Spread of Malaria," 313.

22 Webb, *Humanity's Burden*, 57.

23 Joy et al., "Genetic Diversity."

24 Sallares, Bouwman, and Anderung, "The Spread of Malaria," 313.

after the development of Duffy negativity in response to selective pressures from *P. vivax*, a number of single gene disorders emerged over the past few millennia through natural selection, such as the hemoglobinopathies and enzyme deficiencies that provided populations suffering from endemic *falciparum* malaria with a degree of protection from death or severe disease.

Among these sets of blood disorders, the origins of sickle-cell anemia seem to be the least elusive to advances in genetic research. It appears that the environment within the red blood cells of patients suffering from this condition is unfavorable for the survival of *P. falciparum*. This environment acts, therefore, as a protective mechanism against severe *falciparum* malaria—not from the disease per se, but from death, cerebral malaria, or severe disease.[25]

As for the geographical provenance of the sickle-cell trait, genetic analysis has shown that the gene mutations evolved independently in three different locations in Africa after the development of Duffy negativity.[26] It then spread by migration to other parts of the continent, to the Mediterranean, the Middle East, and as far east as India, where selective pressure from malaria persisted over a long period, two to three millennia.[27] The sickle-cell mutation probably spread during the first millennium BCE or in the beginning of the first millennium CE. This hypothesis is consistent with the identification of *P. falciparum* in two Egyptian mummies dating from the New Kingdom until the Late Period (1500–500 BCE).[28]

Each one of the three genetic types of the sickle-cell trait spread from its own heartland, the one reaching the Mediterranean, Greece, Italy, and Sicily being the Benin haplotype.[29] The sickle-cell trait which emerged in West Africa as *falciparum* malaria developed into a stable, endemic disease. Its evolution is associated with the development of yam cultivation, which gave rise to greater population densities close to rainforests.[30] Larger village communities contributed toward a more stable epidemiological regime for *falciparum* malaria, a development that assisted the spread of the sickle-cell

25   Weatherall, *Thalassaemia*, 183.

26   Packard, *The Making of a Tropical Disease*, 31.

27   Weatherall and Clegg, "Genetic Variability," 332 and 335. For a comparative map of malaria and the frequency distribution of the sickle-cell trait, see Piel et al., "Global Distribution."

28   Webb, *Humanity's Burden*, 37; Nerlich et al., "*Plasmodium Falciparum*."

29   Webb, *Humanity's Burden*, 37; Webb, "Malaria"; Sallares, Bouwman, and Anderung, "The Spread of Malaria," 327–28; Christakis et al., "A Comparison of Sickle Cell Syndromes in Northern Greece."

30   Webb, "Malaria."

mutation by natural selection and helped it achieve a state of balanced polymorphism. Indeed, unless *falciparum* malaria became stable and endemic, in other words as long as it only appeared in epidemic outbreaks, adaptive genetic mutations were unlikely to settle in a state of balanced polymorphism in a population.[31]

Contrary to the limited number of mutations in the case of sickle-cell anemia, thalassemias are found in an enormous variety. Sir David Weatherall, writing about β-thalassemia, said: "It appeared that anything that could possibly go wrong with the gene might be found, if enough patients with the disease were studied." The number of β-thalassemia mutations currently stands to over 200, with a different set of β-thalassemia mutations in every population, while that of α-thalassemia to approximately 100.[32] Furthermore, unlike sickle-cell anemia, thalassemia mutations evolved independently in each population within which they expanded under local selective pressures, while the degree of relative protection from malaria offered by thalassemias seems to be considerably less.[33] The time frame of their expansion to high frequencies "has been of fairly recent origin."[34] In fact, Weatherall believes that hemoglobin disorders, in general, coevolved with *falciparum* malaria "relatively recently in evolutionary terms" and that, moreover, probably "death due to malaria increased dramatically between 5,000 and 10,000 years ago, with the development of agriculture and settlements that would have greatly facilitated the transmission of the disease by mosquitoes. These observations are all compatible with the fairly recent appearance of malaria-resistant polymorphisms."[35] In other words, Weatherall's chronology of malaria-resistant polymorphisms differs significantly from that of Webb's dating of sickle-cell anemia.[36]

The geographic range of thalassemias extends to zones where malaria is or had been endemic in the past, except for Central and South America, where malaria was only introduced by the Columbian Exchange and thus

---

31 Ibid.

32 Weatherall, *Thalassaemia*, 135–36; Weatherall and Clegg, "Genetic Variability," 333. Among other possibilities, it may be found in combination with the sickling trait as sickle-cell thalassemia, and possibly even α- combined with β-thalassemia, as in the case of a patient studied by Phaidon Fessas in Greece in 1961. Weatherall, *Thalassaemia*, 139–40.

33 Weatherall et al., "Malaria and the Red Cell," 48–49; Weatherall, *Thalassaemia*, 177.

34 Weatherall et al., "Malaria and the Red Cell," 52.

35 Weatherall, *Thalassaemia*, 183–84.

36 Webb, *Humanity's Burden*, 37.

was never the site of independent appearance of thalassemias.[37] However, each malaria zone evolved its own particular polymorphism.[38]

Thus, it appears that by the first millennium BCE the dynamics of the two most common malarial diseases, *falciparum* and *vivax* infections, had essentially drawn up the disease map of the Afro-Eurasian landmass, impacting the genetic profiles of its peoples and reaching the Mediterranean shores.

MALARIA IN GREECE

Experts remain divided as to the time when malaria, *falciparum* malaria in particular, first emerged in Greece. The split is essentially between those who, following W. H. S. Jones, believe that *P. falciparum* existed there already by 400 BCE, i.e., already by classical times, and those, like Julian de Zulueta, who believe it to have appeared after that date and who differ also in their interpretation of the critical evidence contained in the Hippocratic texts.[39] Advances in research have contributed to increased levels of sophistication in the controversy.[40]

The first enquiries into the early history of malaria in the classical lands also introduced the question of chronology. They began when, on his return from a visit to Greece in 1906 at the invitation of the British Lake Copais Company, Ronald Ross (1857–1932), the British scientists responsible for discovering the role of the mosquito in transmitting malaria, assigned the young historian W. H. S. Jones to study the biological reasons that led to the decline of the Greeks. Two years after his first publication in 1907, Jones published his second, more thoroughly researched version, to correct errors in the first.[41] In true philhellenic manner, Ronald Ross headed a fundraising and propaganda campaign, which, in turn, lay behind Jones's project.[42] Jones drew on ancient Greek and Latin literary sources, but filtered his evidence through a

---

37 Ibid., 79. For a distribution map of thalassemias, see Weatherall, "Sickle-Cell Anemia."

38 Weatherall and Clegg, "Genetic Variability," 333.

39 Disagreements focused mainly on the interpretation of the term *semitertians* (*hemitritaioi*) found in the Hippocratic *Epidemics*.

40 Sallares, Bouwman, and Anderung, "The Spread of Malaria," 311–12.

41 Jones, Ross, and Ellett, *Malaria*, 1; Jones and Withington, *Malaria and Greek History*. In Italy, Angelo Celli's malaria history of Rome, *Storia della malaria nell'agro Romano* (1925) was published posthumously.

42 Ross, "Malaria in Greece," 709.

contemporary social Darwinist lens: "Most other diseases," he wrote, "however distressing to individuals, brace a people by weeding out the *unfit*; malaria plays no such useful part in the economy of nature. It seizes all, *fit* and *unfit* alike, gradually lessening the general vitality until, in some cases, it has *exterminated* the people among whom it has become endemic."[43]

Ross, for his part, believed that malaria must have arrived in Greece from Asia or Africa, taken hold within one or two centuries and transformed it into the country he visited in 1906.[44] Without drawing a distinction among parasite species and noting the importance of landscape and immunity, both Ross and Jones concluded that malaria in its tertian, quotidian and quartan manifestations had been present in Greece already in the fifth century BCE, that is, by the time of Hippocrates.[45] In Jones's words, "[t]he inference to be drawn from the Hippocratic collection is that the Greeks of 400 BC were perfectly familiar with intermittent fevers, remittent fevers, various pernicious types of malaria and malarial cachexia," although they were "not prevalent to any great extent."[46] Jones, therefore, implied that all three malarial diseases had been established in Greece by the fifth century BCE and that malaria was one among other causes of the decline of classical Greece rather than the reverse.[47]

In Greece itself, Georgios Karamitsas, professor of medicine at the University of Athens, who added a chapter on malaria to his Greek translation of Felix von Niemeyer's textbook of internal medicine, also made use of ancient Greek medical texts to draw on their epidemiological data, but did not undertake a history of malaria.[48] In fact, by drawing on ancient Greek sources Greek physicians confirmed their sense of continuity of place and race. After 1898, physicians such as Konstantinos Savvas, Ioannis Kardamatis, and Aristotelis Kouzis each wrote his own history of malaria in Greece, becoming the first Greeks to historicize the disease by setting it within the country's contemporary national master narrative: to calculate the effect of foreign domination on the nation's health.

---

43   Jones, Ross, and Ellett, *Malaria*, vi. Emphasis added. In his introduction to Jones's first book, Ross also used a value-charged racial terminology.

44   Jones, Ross, and Ellett, *Malaria*, 9–10. See also Ross, "Malaria in Greece," 706.

45   Jones and Withington, *Malaria and Greek History*, 40 and 63–64.

46   Ibid., 70 and 75.

47   Jones, Ross, and Ellett, *Malaria*, 13 and 40; Jones and Withington, *Malaria and Greek History*, 102 and 107.

48   Karamitsas, "Peri elodon i eleiogenon nosimaton."

The same year as Jones's first book though, Aristotelis Kouzis, a medical historian, could only be certain that malarial fevers existed in Greece in the fifth century BCE on the basis of the Hippocratic texts, without ruling out the possibility that it might have first appeared toward the end of the second millennium. In the fifteenth century, the Ottoman conquest deprived the country of its medical scientists and, as a result, there was no textual evidence of the disease thereafter; at the same time, desolation and physical decline brought about an increase in malaria prevalence.[49] In his malaria textbook, malariologist Ioannis Kardamatis, by contrast, presented the decline of health in post-Hippocratic Greece as the result of depopulation, which brought on the decline of agriculture and, in turn, lawlessness and insecurity among the peasantry, which peaked in the final years of Ottoman rule and the early years of independent statehood.[50] He was convinced that Greek mythology provided evidence for the presence of malaria already in the second millennium BCE, a conviction that he corroborated with details of Greek physical geography.[51] Kardamatis, furthermore, believed that the physical decline of the Greek lands in Roman times caused malaria to take over the country.[52] Thus, while ascribing different dates and political circumstances to the country's decline, both Kouzis and Kardamatis, unlike Jones and Ross, saw malaria as a consequence rather than a cause of decline.[53]

In 1948, the British geneticist J. B. S. Haldane formulated what later became known as the malaria hypothesis, which associated the high frequency distribution of thalassemia among Mediterranean populations with the likelihood of an evolutionary advantage of protection from *falciparum* malaria.[54] Haldane's malaria hypothesis marked a paradigmatic change in the search for the origins of *falciparum* malaria in the Mediterranean. Initially, osteological evidence from archeological digs suggesting the presence of hematological disorders pointed to evolutionary pressures from, and were used as a proxy for, *falciparum* malaria on prehistoric populations in the area.

---

49 Kouzis, "Tina peri eleiogenon pyreton kata tous arkhaious Ellinas iatrous," 98–99 and 108.

50 Kardamatis, *Pragmateia*, 29.

51 Kardamatis, "I elonosia en to nomo Attikis," 109 and 113; Sallares, *Malaria and Rome*, 13.

52 Kardamatis, "I elonosia en to nomo Attikis," 117, 118.

53 The causal relationship between malaria and socioeconomic decline received its classical treatment in the case of Ninfa, an abandoned town in the Pontine Marshes, in Hackett, *Malaria in Europe*, xi–xiii. According to Hackett: "We may assume that feudalism and malaria collaborated to expel the citizens of Ninfa." Hackett, *Malaria in Europe*, xii.

54 Haldane, "The Rate of Mutation of Human Genes."

In the 1960s, J. L. Angel found an extensive presence of porotic hyperostosis on human skulls from the Mesolithic period onward, i.e., from the seventh millennium BCE, in Greece and Asia Minor. He attributed these skeletal lesions to β-thalassemia and sickle-cell anemia and deduced selective pressures due to *falciparum* malaria attributing the further spread of malaria to the emergence of agriculture in the Neolithic period. This early dating for *falciparum* malaria in Greece on the basis of skeletal remains hinges exclusively on the association of porotic hyperostosis solely with β-thalassemia and sickle-cell anemia, an assumption which is highly problematic.[55] Besides, imputing a presence in Greece of sickle-cell anemia and β-thalassemia, let alone *falciparum* malaria, as early as the Mesolithic period, would contradict the dating of the spread of these disorders out of Africa by recent genetic research. Angel went as far as to propose a full chronology of *falciparum* malaria prevalence in the eastern Mediterranean on the basis of fluctuating frequencies of porotic hyperostosis among the skeletal finds of archeological excavations.[56] The dating notwithstanding, it is nonetheless true that once established on the continent, the scope of *falciparum* malaria in Europe, as well as—if to a lesser degree—the scope of the other two malarial parasites, fluctuated, as suggested by evidence in the fields of climatology and entomology.

In his seminal 1973 article "Malaria and Mediterranean History," malariologist Julian de Zulueta introduced arguments from climatological and entomological evidence to historical investigation and, later, updated its details on the basis of more recent climatological work.[57] Toward the end of the Pleistocene, i.e., the last glacial period, temperatures in southern Europe and the eastern Mediterranean would have been approximately 9°C cooler than in the twentieth century, so as to allow only a very limited presence of

---

55   Angel, "Porotic Hyperostosis"; Angel, "Ecology and Population." In her recent PhD thesis, Antonia H. Morgan-Forster offers a revision of Angel's theory. See Morgan-Forster, "Climate, Environment and Malaria." For a critical view of the etiologies of porotic hyperostosis, see Holland and O'Brien, "Parasites, Porotic Hyperostosis." In 1983 Mirko D. Grmek, in chapter 3 of his *Les maladies à l'aube de la civilisation occidentale*, subscribed to Angel's interpretation, but later revised his opinion to agree with Julian de Zulueta and Robert Sallares, that, although *falciparum* malaria may have existed in some insignificant foci in fifth-century Greece, it only became "hyperendemic" in Roman times. For other views, see Grmek, "La malaria dans la Méditérranée," 3–4. Teddi J. Setzer, in "Malaria Detection," associates porotic hyperostosis with skeletal responses to long-term anemia due to *vivax* rather than with *falciparum* malaria.

56   Angel, "Ecology and Population."

57   De Zulueta, "Malaria and Mediterranean History"; De Zulueta, "Malaria and Ecosystems."

vivax and *malariae* infections among Paleolithic hunter-gatherers. Such infections would have increased, however, as temperatures became warmer through the Neolithic times, only reaching climatic conditions as they were "throughout historical times" at around 4000 BCE.

Even so, for De Zulueta the texts of the Hippocratic corpus still referred exclusively to *vivax* and *malariae* diseases, however pathogenic their symptoms. Whatever *falciparum* malaria may have appeared in fifth-century Greece, would have been the occasional case introduced from North Africa.[58] Interestingly, De Zulueta criticized Ross's historical reconstruction and reversed his reading of the Greek landscapes of his day: "The author of this article," wrote De Zulueta, "has had the opportunity to visit as a malariologist and as a student of history many of the battlefields of antiquity in Greece and other Mediterranean lands and has often been confronted with the difficulty of how to explain the campaigns of the past with malaria conditions of the present."[59]

De Zulueta attributed the insignificance of *falciparum* malaria in classical antiquity to a different distribution of malaria vectors and specifically mentioned, among other locations, Pharsalus, the site of the battle between Caesar's and Pompey's armies in August 48 BCE, and Actium, the site of Antony's confrontation with Octavian in September 31 BCE, both highly malarious sites in modern times. In De Zulueta's analysis, the key lay in vector distribution. *A. sacharovi*, an Asian anthropophilic mosquito, which was the principal vector of *falciparum* malaria in Greece and the eastern Mediterranean, would have been restricted "to the hinterland of Asia," where temperatures toward the end of the last glacial period would have been warmer than in the Mediterranean. As temperatures rose in southern Europe during the Neolithic period, this *Anopheles* species would have moved into the Mediterranean and the Near East and established a foothold in southern Europe even later, by moving west from Asia Minor to the coasts of the Balkans, Greece, and Italy. Initially, the Asian *Anopheles* species would have been refractory to tropical strains of *P. falciparum*; this would have delayed the spread of *falciparum* malaria in Europe for centuries, possibly until "the great increase of navigation during Hellenistic and Roman times," as hu-

---

58 De Zulueta, "Malaria and Mediterranean History," 3–4 and 8–9; De Zulueta, "Malaria and Ecosystems," 9; Bruce-Chwatt and De Zulueta, *The Rise and Fall of Malaria in Europe*, 11–13.
59 De Zulueta, "Malaria and Mediterranean History," 4–7.

mans were causing ecological pressures and extensive deforestation.[60] Increased navigation activities would have caused the introduction of the new *Anopheles* species of vectors resulting in increased malaria prevalence, "so that by the end of the Roman Empire it was already a dominant health problem."[61] De Zulueta interestingly also established a possible causal link between β-thalassemia and *A. sacharovi* (and *A. labranchiae*, the anthropophilic vector prevailing in Sicily, Sardinia, and Italy) based on the fact of the geographical coincidence of the specific vectors with the particular blood disorder[62]: "It is the high prevalence and the high mortality resulting from the association of the parasite with highly effective vectors which may lead to the development of this haemoglobinopathy."[63]

Even more recently, the history of malaria in the eastern Mediterranean has benefited from advances in molecular biology, genetics, and anthropology. In his 2002 book *Malaria and Rome* and subsequent articles, Robert Sallares draws a distinction between malaria in Italy on the one hand and Greece on the other. According to his understanding of Hippocratic terminology, the term semitertians, or *hemitritaioi*, found in the *Epidemics*, refers to *falciparum* and cerebral malaria.[64] Therefore, the fifth century BCE is a *terminus ante quem* for the presence of all three *Plasmodium* species in Greece, or, in James Webb's words, "a zone of mixed infections."[65]

Thus, in setting an early date to *P. falciparum* in both Greece and Italy and the selective pressures that this disease involves, Sallares differs from De Zulueta and other scientists.[66] At the root of Sallares's early dating of the evolution of *P. falciparum* lies a hypothesis that dates the origin of the parasite to around 100,000 years ago.[67] As noted above, for Sallares, *P. falciparum* coevolved with humans when they each diverged from their respec-

---

60 De Zulueta, "Malaria and Ecosystems," 9; De Zulueta, "Malaria and Mediterranean History," 9–10.

61 De Zulueta, "Malaria and Mediterranean History," 12–13.

62 Italian researchers noted the similar distributions of malaria and thalassemia in their country. Before Haldane, B. Vezzoso already suggested that the two conditions may be causally linked, as did V. Carcassi and M. Siniscalco several years later with their detailed study of β-thalassemia in Sardinia. Weatherall, *Thalassaemia*, 178–79; Sallares, *Malaria and Rome*, 143.

63 De Zulueta, "Malaria and Ecosystems," 10.

64 Sallares, Malaria and Rome, 14 and 18; Sallares, Bouwman, and Anderung, "The Spread of Malaria," 314–19; Jones and Withington, *Malaria and Greek History*, 63–64.

65 Webb, *Humanity's Burden*, 59. For Sallares and his coauthors, *vivax* and quartan malaria reached Greece "some time between the end of the last Ice Age and 500 BC." Sallares, Bouwman, and Anderung, "The Spread of Malaria," 314.

66 Rich and Ayala, "Progress in Malaria Research," 273–74; Packard, *The Making of a Tropical Disease*, 33.

67 Joy et al., "Genetic Diversity."

tive common ancestor, *P. reichenowi* and chimpanzee, around five million years ago. The 100,000-year-old human parasite "has undergone a major population expansion within the last 10,000 years."[68]

The implications of this disagreement are wide-ranging: Sallares's theory implies that *falciparum* malaria could survive among sparse human populations "long before the invention of agriculture," whereas, according to the Malaria Eve theory, the disease requires dense human populations, and therefore a totally different historical context, namely the emergence of agriculture. For Sallares, the Neolithic period signaled not the emergence or speciation of *P. falciparum* but its establishment in Europe.[69]

Contrary to De Zulueta, Sallares points to recent climatological evidence that suggests that, from the end of the last Ice Age to around 3000 BCE, temperatures in the northern hemisphere were 2°C higher than in subsequent millennia, making the Neolithic period more suitable for *P. falciparum* to thrive in southern Europe than in the first millennium BCE, when *falciparum* malaria subsided.[70] Increased Saharan rainfall in the warm Neolithic period would have created extensive mosquito breeding sites that would have driven mosquito vectors to the southern Mediterranean shores.[71] Following Mario Coluzzi, Sallares indicates that the speciation of the African *A. gambiae* complex, the most efficient transmitters of malaria, is an ongoing process; modern strains are of recent Neolithic origin that would have boosted the spread of *falciparum* malaria, an already existing infection, into southern Europe, "its previous evolutionary history," i.e., a capacity to sustain infection among sparse populations, suggesting "that the small human population sizes of that period would not have prevented it from becoming endemic in southern Europe then."[72] Indeed, this conclusion is consistent with evidence from predynastic Egyptian mummies from about 3200 BCE, suggesting the presence of *P. falci-*

---

68 Sallares, Bouwman, and Anderung, "The Spread of Malaria," 313. This hypothesis opposes Rich and Ayala's "Malaria Eve" hypothesis, which, as noted earlier, postulated a *P. falciparum* population bottleneck several thousand years ago, a theory consistent with recent findings on the direct and recent descent of *P. falciparum* from *P. reichenowi*.

69 Sallares, *Malaria and Rome*, 23 and 26–27, particularly note 5; Sallares, Bouwman, and Anderung, "The Spread of Malaria," 312–13. See also p. 19 in this book. For their part, Rich and Ayala clearly reject the presence of *falciparum* malaria in the Hippocratic texts. Rich and Ayala, "Progress in Malaria Research," 273–74.

70 Sallares, *Malaria and Rome*, 102.

71 Ibid., 28–29.

72 Ibid., 29–30.

parum "on the periphery of the Mediterranean world already in the fourth millennium BC."[73]

Assuming, therefore, that demographic and climatic conditions in Neolithic southern Europe were suitable for *falciparum* malaria, were there also susceptible and efficient anthropophilic malaria vectors around to transmit the infection? Sallares resolves the issue raised in 1973 by De Zulueta regarding mosquito refractoriness to tropical *falciparum* malaria as follows: the disease arrived in Greece from the Levant before the time of the Greek colonization of Italy in the eighth century BCE, where the Greeks, in turn, introduced the infection.[74] *P. falciparum* had, therefore, ample time to overcome the refractoriness of its principal vectors, namely *A. sacharovi* in the Levant and *A. labranchiae* in North Africa, before crossing over to Greece and Italy, respectively. At any rate, the introduction of its principal vector, *A. sacharovi*, must have preceded that of *P. falciparum*.[75]

More evidence about the transfer of *P. falciparum* to southern Europe has emerged from studies of hereditary blood diseases that reflect selective pressures from exposure to *falciparum* malaria, specifically sickle-cell anemia, α- and β-thalassemias, and G6PD deficiency. The Greek colonists carried with them to southern Italy and Sicily the mutations currently found in both countries: in the case of the sickle-cell trait, it is of the Benin haplotype that evolved in Africa; the β-thalassemia IVS-I-110 (G→A) mutation is estimated to have developed in Anatolia under selective pressure between 6500 and 2000 BCE, is common in Greece and is also found in areas of Greek colonization in Italy.[76] It has been suggested, therefore, that it may have originated in Greece or Anatolia and moved westward to Italy with colonization after the eighth century BCE.[77] As for the variant mutation of the G6PD deficiency, it probably evolved only once in the Mediterranean and then spread from the point of origin.[78] Thus, for Sallares and his coau-

---

73 Ibid., 31. The evidence consists of the presence of an antigen (histidine-rich protein II) expressed by trophozoites of P. falciparum. See, however, p. 21, n. 28 in this book.

74 According to Sallares, *Malaria and Rome*, 35, Italy additionally received falciparum malaria from North Africa.

75 Sallares, *Malaria and Rome*, 33–34; Sallares, "Role of Environmental Changes," 22; Sallares, Bouwman, and Anderung, "The Spread of Malaria," 318–19.

76 Tadmouri et al., "History and Origin of [Beta]-Thalassemia."

77 Sallares, Bouwman, and Anderung, "The Spread of Malaria," 326.

78 Sallares, *Malaria and Rome*, 39 and 144; Sallares, Bouwman, and Anderung, "The Spread of Malaria," 324–28.

thors, the eighth century BCE, the beginning of Greek westward colonization, is a *terminus ante quem* for the presence of *P. falciparum*, malaria resistant mutations and *A. sacharovi*, the susceptible vector. In other words, first
A. sacharovi spread from the Near East to Greece, bringing *falciparum* malaria and resistance mutations to *falciparum* malaria with it to Greece, before the spread of *A. labranchiae* arrived to Italy from northern Africa. The
sickle-cell Benin haplotype then arrived in the eastern and western Mediterranean with migrants or slaves from central Africa.[79]

Antonia Morgan-Forster, who revisited Angel's findings and theory on the
basis of updated climatological data, suggested that, while the Mesolithic climate and environment of mainland Greece and a certain level of resource exploitation could conceivably have led to malariogenic conditions for all three
human *Plasmodium* species, the absence of suitable *Anopheles* species "would
suggest a sufficient exposure to vector habitats to support a low to moderate
disease burden" at least of the more tolerant *vivax* and *malariae* species.[80] The
Neolithic physical and social environment, however, with warmer and humid conditions and the spread of agriculture and urban centers would have
allowed endemic malaria to take hold, a new situation consistent with the increase in the frequency of porotic hyperostosis in the osteological evidence.
The Bronze Age, by contrast, was cooler, with an "erratic climate of the Middle to Late Bronze Age," and, therefore, potentially less malariogenic. Still,
socioeconomic conditions and man-made opportunities for *Anopheles* to
breed and travel would have generated an increase of malaria. Indeed, ancient DNA evidence from Egypt, contemporary with the Greek Bronze Age,
indicates the existence of *falciparum* malaria in an area with frequent trade
relations with the Greek lands. Morgan-Forster's interpretation finds most of
the above consistent with Angel's theory and findings.[81]

Once established in southern Europe, the distribution of *P. falciparum*
would have been affected by a great variety of environmental and social factors, one of the most important being variations in temperature, contracting
as the temperature grew colder after the Holocene climate optimum of the

---

79 Sallares, Bouwman, and Anderung, "The Spread of Malaria," 327–28. However, Christakis et al., "A
    Comparison of Sickle Cell Syndromes in Northern Greece," 390, and Loukopoulos, "Hemoglobin," 175,
    referring to northern Greece, suggest that the arrival of the Benin haplotype of sickle-cell anemia oc-
    curred in Byzantine times.
80 Morgan-Forster, "Climate, Environment and Malaria," 279, 282.
81 Ibid. See also p. 21, n. 28 in this book.

Neolithic period, rising again, at least in Italy, during the Roman Empire[82] and falling during the Little Ice Age of the early modern period. As Sallares notes: "the effects of even small temperature changes would be most significant in geographical areas on the periphery of the distribution of *P. falciparum*, such as southern Europe, rather than in the tropics."[83]

The distribution of malaria also spread under the influence of silting, sediment deposition, as in the case of the ancient Ephesus, flooding, as in the case of the burial of Olympia in late antiquity, and alluvial depositions and anthropogenic soil erosion brought about by intensive agriculture, as in the case of the Aetolian state in Hellenistic times. As Sallares has noted: "The significance of this heterogeneity of landscape history for the history of malaria is that it is necessary to envisage a series of local histories for malaria."[84] In the same vein, criticizing Bruce-Chwatt and De Zulueta, who treated both Greece and Italy as a unified area, Sallares and his coauthors remarked: "Since many types of mosquito are incapable of transmitting malaria to humans, mosquito breeding sites do not occur everywhere, and many mosquitoes do not fly further than a few hundred yards from their breeding sites, malaria can only be really understood by microanalyses, conducted at a very local level, of geography, hydrology, climate, competition between different species of mosquito for breeding sites, and human activities."[85]

POSTANTIQUITY, THE MEDIEVAL, AND THE EARLY MODERN WORLD

Until it peaked in the mid-nineteenth century, the worldwide spread of malaria was not a linear process. Climatic fluctuations as well as ecological and social factors contributed to its distribution. In fact, until that date there exists very little evidence by which to trace the spread of the disease. Furthermore, in the early twentieth century there emerged an additional factor that affected the extent and distribution of the disease, namely systematic malaria control interventions guided by modern science.

---

82   Recent research has revealed the presence of *P. falciparum* mitochondrial DNA in adults from Imperial age cemeteries in southern Italy. Marciniak et al., *"Plasmodium Falciparum."*
83   Sallares, *Malaria and Rome*, 102.
84   Sallares, "Role of Environmental Changes," 24–25.
85   Sallares, Bouwman, and Anderung, "The Spread of Malaria," 312. This point will be raised in chapters 2 and 3.

In his highly influential *Plagues and Peoples*, W. H. McNeill presented a broad scheme in which intensifying trade and communication in the beginning of the Christian era broke down earlier distance barriers. An unintended corollary was the homogenization of infectious diseases across the southern parts of Eurasia and the Mediterranean into a newly formed disease pool.[86] Indeed, De Zulueta and Webb's interpretations of the history of *falciparum* malaria are consistent with this pattern of developments.

The global trade networks of that era carried African slaves, with a considerable burden of *falciparum* malaria, to countries across Asia as far as China and into the Mediterranean. Equally important, in terms of disease distribution, were the military and political consequences of the Islamic expansion throughout the Mediterranean and much of south Asia after the seventh century CE. It created a new world of mobility and migration that "brought about an increased mixing of infections, although the levels of malarial infections across the entirety of the Islamic world remained unstable, and societies from Morocco to Indonesia remained subject to epidemic outbreaks."[87]

One of the most important shifts in the spread of malaria was likewise the work of humans. Unable to cross the barrier of *falciparum* malaria and exploit tropical Africa, the white man enslaved fellow humans and transferred them from their homeland to the Americas. In doing so he also transported malaria in the bloodstream of black Africans to the New World. In this new environment, the *Plasmodia* found native susceptible *Anopheles* species and spread successfully.[88] Contrary, therefore, to the case of Europe, where tropical African strains of *P. falciparum* had initially met refractory mosquitoes, the New World apparently presented no such biological constraints to the transatlantic transfer of malaria, which must have occurred in the Caribbean and tropical South America "early in the Columbian Exchange."[89]

North America, on the other hand, received the infection only gradually, as European settlers and African slaves increased their presence there. Only when development drove settlers into the wilderness, to build dams

---

86 McNeill, *Plagues and Peoples*, 124–29.

87 Webb, *Humanity's Burden*, 64–65; see also McCann, *Historical Ecology of Malaria in Ethiopia*, loc. 849.

88 Russell, *Man's Mastery of Malaria*, 173.

89 Webb, *Humanity's Burden*, 79; McNeill, *Mosquito Empires*, 95.

and block natural drainage, thus creating conditions favorable to the local *Anopheles, A. quadrimaculatus*, did malaria spread and become a serious problem in the area that became the United States, particularly in the south. This, however, did not happen before the eighteenth century.[90]

MALARIA CONTROL AND MODERNITY

Beginning in nineteenth-century northern Europe, malaria began to recede from the temperate zone. In England, this gradual process had already begun by the end of the seventeenth century. With plague epidemics also on the ebb in the eighteenth century, medical attention, to quote Christopher Hamlin, "transferred to epidemic fevers."[91] From that time on, sources become more informative as the prescription of cinchona bark for fevers brought the epidemic outbreaks of malaria into the historical and medical foreground. Similarly, in the nineteenth century, the use of quinine and other cinchona alkaloids, the first disease-specific cure in Western medicine, sheds even clearer light on the identification of past malaria infections.[92]

Much of the decline that occurred before the scientific advances generated by nineteenth-century germ theory is attributed to reasons beyond human intervention.[93] Malaria control, however, increasingly became a social and state concern, with individuals drawing on ancient as well as innovative methods. Persistent failures, however, occasionally led to skepticism over the merits of scientific discoveries, undermined overoptimistic, reductionist models of epidemiological analysis and have, more constructively, suggested linkages between the disease and its social determinants.

Drainage is the oldest of all control measures, already engaged in by the ancient Greeks, Romans, Abbasids, Ottomans and still constituting sound practice.[94] Of variable effectiveness, such interventions involved enormous outputs of manpower and technical and financial commitments. However, whenever they succeeded in saving lives, drainage works essentially corrob-

---

90 Russell, *Man's Mastery of Malaria*, 173; Humphreys, *Malaria*, 21–29; McNeill, *Mosquito Empires*, 199ff.
91 Hamlin, *More Than Hot*, 91.
92 Webb, *Humanity's Burden*, 12.
93 The decline of malaria in Europe was the subject of Bruce-Chwatt and De Zulueta, *The Rise and Fall of Malaria in Europe*.
94 Webb, *Humanity's Burden*, 15–16 and 61–62.

orated miasmatic theory by substantiating the causal relationship between wetlands, marshes, and emanations of rotting particles on the one hand and malaria on the other.

Progress in the field of treatment occurred in the seventeenth century with the discovery that the bark of the cinchona tree, which grew in the Peruvian Andes, had properties that were more powerful than traditional oxidant febrifuge treatments, such as wormwood, willow, wine, foodstuffs, and spices.[95] Use of the Peruvian drug in Europe increased, particularly among the men of the warring European armies and navies dying of fevers in the tropics. Its usage expanded even further after 1820, when two French chemists, Joseph-Bienaimé Caventou and Pierre-Joseph Pelletier, isolated quinine and cinchonine, the two principal active ingredients of cinchona powder or the "bark," and made it possible to standardize its quality and administration and generate a debate on the correct dosage.[96]

The selective nature of causal reasoning intrinsic to the miasmatic theory of disease was overturned by germ theory and its search for specific causes. Working within this new scientific paradigm, in October 1880, Alphonse Laveran (1845–1922) identified the parasite that caused malaria in a patient in the French Army hospital in Constantine in Algeria.[97] The discovery was completed, when in 1898 Ronald Ross and Giovanni Battista Grassi (1854–1925) independently proved the Anopheles mosquito to be the vector that mediated the transmission of malaria from human to human, and when Italian scientists Camillo Gogli (1843–1926), Angelo Celli (1857–1914), Ettore Marchiafava (1847–1935), and Amico Bignami (1862–1929) proved the existence of three distinct species of human Plasmodia; J. W. W. Stephens added a fourth such parasite in 1922.[98]

After 1898, malaria control in Europe and the colonial tropics entered a new, optimistic era. Often driven by the scientific nationalism of competing empires,[99] scientists and public health practitioners generated innovative strategies that involved both environmental and public health measures.

---

95   Dobson, "Bitter-Sweet Solutions for Malaria," 78–79.
96   Litsios, The Tomorrow of Malaria, 15; Smith, "Quinine and Fever," 354–67.
97   Laveran had witnessed what later emerged to have been gametocytes of falciparum malaria and named the parasite Oscillaria malariae.
98   Snowden, The Conquest of Malaria, 37; Litsios, The Tomorrow of Malaria, 18–20. On the differences between the approach of Rossi and that of Grassi, see Fantini, "The Concept of Specificity," 44–46.
99   Snowden, The Conquest of Malaria, 37.

Draining, sanding, oiling, and Paris green all aimed at destroying *Anopheles* at the larvae stage, and an early mosquito-eradication program was devised that sought "species sanitation."[100] By contrast, a different school of thought, inspired by the German bacteriologist Robert Koch (1843–1910), recommended sterilizing the human reservoir of *Plasmodia* through the use of quinine sanitization. Indeed, an increased international demand for quinine, largely generated by colonial and military needs, led to the establishment of cinchona plantations outside South America, specifically in the hills of the Himalayas and in Java. As a result, quinine became more widely affordable as its price began to fall in the 1880s.[101]

Drainage projects acquired a fresh importance among mosquito-control strategies in Europe and the United States, as the fight against malaria had become vital for the competing imperial powers and affected their international standing. Following a relentless antimosquito campaign carried out by William C. Gorgas (1854–1920) with the financial backing of the US Congress, the construction of the Panama Canal, which had failed earlier because of malaria and yellow fever, was completed in 1914. Sharing the same approach to malaria control, Ronald Ross recommended its application at Mian Mir, a British military cantonment near Lahore in the Punjab. By 1904, the British experiment had failed, amid much controversy. As a result, a number of British malariologists, most notably S. P. James, became convinced that malaria control had to focus, rather, on the administration of quinine and general social and sanitary improvement.[102] These early disputes largely shaped the approach to malaria control for the greater part of the twentieth century.

Italian malariology achieved a prominent status in the international field. Not only was Italy a heavily malarious country, it was also one with a long medical tradition and incipient imperialist ambitions. It developed its own national school of malariology after 1880 with the support of powerful interested parties, banks, and philanthropists.[103] There were, nonetheless, serious dissensions within the Italian school, which were largely socio-

---

100 Bradley, "Watson, Swellengrebel and Species Sanitation," 144–46; Fantini, "The Concept of Specificity," 46.

101 For a fascinating account of the history of quinine, see Honigsbaum, *The Fever Trail*. On the subject of medicine and empire, see Worboys, "Manson, Ross and Colonial Medical Policy"; Watts, *Epidemics and History*.

102 Bynum, "An Experiment That Failed"; Litsios, *The Tomorrow of Malaria*, 42–44.

103 Snowden, *The Conquest of Malaria*, 4 and 41.

political in origin. The two camps centered around the figures of Angelo Celli on the one hand and Giovanni Battista Grassi on the other. Essentially, Grassi envisaged the strategy of the radical cure or human reclamation (*bonifica umana*) by sterilizing patients' blood with quinine in the months of no transmission, much like the system advocated by Koch. By contrast, Celli favored protecting the entire rural population with free quinine and thus breaking the transmission cycle. In applying Celli's system, the Italian state ensured the free supply of quinine to the rural poor in the malarious districts.[104] More importantly, however, Celli, himself a republican MP, inspired a vigorous social movement among the medical and educational professions that also integrated the school system into the national antimalarial scheme. According to Frank Snowden, Celli's

> antimalarial campaign was the most ambitious public health initiative in Italian history, and the medical profession embraced it wholeheartedly. To reach the population most at risk from malaria, doctors launched what the Socialist paper *Avanti!* described as the most extraordinary movement in the history of the profession—an immense and generous program of "going to the people." Inspired by the vision of the Rome School, doctors and medical students went into the countryside to encounter the poor at their workplaces, homes, and shelters. Their purpose was to educate the people in the fundamentals of the mosquito theory and to administer quinine.[105]

The impact of the discoveries of the etiology of malaria on Greece was immediate. The medical elite and philanthropists mobilized to tackle the country's most prevalent disease and, in 1905, came together to form the Anti-Malaria League. Much of the activities and the policies they advocated, particularly reliance on quinine, were modeled on Italian practices[106] and driven by malariologist Ioannis Kardamatis and his "almost fanatical evangelism on the subject of malaria."[107]

Before the end of the First World War, malaria control in Europe had relied on local, regional, corporate and, above all, national initiatives. The

---

104 Snowden, *The Conquest of Malaria*, 50–52. The Greek state adopted the Italian system until the 1930s. See Tsiamis, Piperaki, and Tsakris, "The History of the Greek Anti-Malaria League."

105 Snowden, *The Conquest of Malaria*, 62. On the role of schools and teachers, see ibid.,77–78.

106 Tsiamis, Piperaki, and Tsakris, "The History of the Greek Anti-Malaria League."

107 Kitzmiller, *Anopheline Names*, 111–13.

ideas, however, around social welfare were changing under the influence of a new way of addressing social problems that was inspired by similar ideas in the United States.[108] These were the same ideas that had led to the creation of the League of Nations, which was established not only to prevent war but also to address social injustices, for the sake of preserving peace and forestalling social unrest. Malaria epidemic outbreaks in Europe in the aftermath of the war contributed to the internationalization of the approach toward the disease. Malaria control thus entered a new, internationalized, phase through the work of the Malaria Commission of the League of Nations Health Committee, and through the more global interventions of the International Health Division (IHD) of the RF. Malaria control has remained an international concern ever since, with the World Health Organization (WHO) inheriting the functions of the League of Nations Health Committee after the end of the Second World War.[109]

Meanwhile, the division into proponents of a social versus an entomological approach to malaria epidemiology was inherited by specialists in the interwar years and came to be known, respectively—and with a degree of oversimplification—as the "European" and the "American" approach. The former view prevailed among the members of the League of Nations Malaria Commission and bore the legacy of the early-twentieth-century failures mentioned above, influenced, moreover, by the hardships and the reemergence of malaria in interwar Europe and the need for attention to strategies of prevention. The latter was largely the view of the malariologists of the RF's IHD, whose worldwide network—ill-matched for the enormous task before it—had begun to investigate malaria for the first time as a global issue. Typically, its members transferred from Brazil to Greece, as in the case of M. A. Barber, and from Greece to China, as in the case of M. C. Balfour (1896–1976). They were, in Warwick Anderson's words, "pragmatic cosmopolitans."[110]

The early 1930s were, moreover, marked by the solution of one of the unexplained problems of malaria distribution that plagued malaria research, namely the observed "anophelism without malaria" in the Netherlands and

108 Weindling, "From Moral Exhortation," 116.
109 Nájera, "Malaria Control," 14–18 and 59.
110 Anderson, *Colonial Pathologies*, 229; Nájera, "Malaria Control," 21–24; Evans, "European Malaria Policy in the 1920s and 1930s"; Farley, *To Cast Out Disease*, 278–80.

other parts of Europe. In 1931, the IHD's Lewis W. Hackett (1884–1962), the Italian malariologist Alberto Missiroli (1883–1951), and their German colleague Erich Martini (1880–1960) revealed that one of the *Anopheles* species responsible for the transmission of malaria, *A. maculipennis*, turned out, in fact, to be a complex of several distinct species, only two of which were responsible for transmitting the parasites.[111]

The presence of the IHD malaria experts in Greece lasted from 1930 to 1938 and came about in the context of the sanitary reforms of Eleftherios Venizelos's liberal government of 1928–32. The purpose of the mission was experimental and educational, its scientific approach was both local and universal, and its effects were long term rather than immediate. The IHD team produced much research work on local malaria ecology and epidemiology and trained a new generation of Greek experts, who were able to carry out serious antimalarial work in the immediate postwar years.[112] In the short term, however, by 1940 only the most accessible parts of Greece had benefited from the control measures owing to the high labor cost of Paris greening. In Thessaly, the country's most malarious region, antimalaria work began as late as 1936.[113] In fact, shortly before the war, Lewis W. Hackett had planned a League of Nations tour of southern Europe for the purpose of studying the expense parameters of malaria control.[114]

The interwar Italian experience brought together the Italian school and the RF's IHD, under the leadership of malariologists Alberto Missiroli and Hackett, in implementing a malaria-control experiment that was at the same time entomological, engineering, hygienic, and social in its approach. The *bonifica integrale*, as it became known, was backed by Mussolini's totalitarian regime and its utopian view of agriculture, and it consisted in carrying out an ambitious land reclamation project in the Roman Campagna.[115]

Meanwhile, with the irregular outbreak of malaria epidemics, demand for quinine was becoming erratic and destabilized the quinine market. As a result, in order to protect their common interests, plantation owners and

---

111 Fantini, "Anophelism without Malaria," 99–101.

112 Although not a history of their activities per se, much of the team's work is reflected in Grigorios Livadas's two-volume *Malaria in Greece*, 1930–1940.

113 See chapters 2 and 3.

114 CH/Malaria/260 p. 3, doc 33983, dossier 911, box R 6168, 8C (Health–Malaria), C (1933–1940), League of Nations Archive. The tour never materialized.

115 Stapleton, "Internationalism and Nationalism"; Snowden, *The Conquest of Malaria*, 149–77.

manufacturers on the island of Java forged an agreement in 1913, which was represented by the Kina Bureau in Amsterdam. The function of the Kina Bureau was to protect the price of quinine by regulating supply. It controlled virtually the entire world supply of quinine in the interwar years.[116] In reaction to this development, the German and British chemical industries embarked on research to develop alternatives in the form of synthetic antimalarials.[117]

While several of the issues encountered during the interwar years remained open, the Second World War destroyed all physical progress in malaria control in Europe. During the wartime years, however, DDT, a new, potent insecticide, initially used against lice in typhus control, and eventually in fighting *Anopheles*, emerged. Its cost-effective application, known as residual spraying, revolutionized vector control and tended to subsume all other antimalarial strategies in the aftermath of the war.

Greece, where wartime and occupation hardships had destroyed any progress attained in the 1930s, was one of the first places where the new antimosquito DDT campaign was applied. The DDT campaign took place in the context of the UNRRA contribution to postwar reconstruction. In his official history of the administration, George Woodbridge noted with regard to the remarkable impact of the campaign: "It can justly be said that [malaria] has been reduced from a major economic problem in Greece to one of minor significance. This accomplishment alone would justify the UNRRA work in Greece."[118] No more than ten years after the departure of UNRRA from Greece, George Macdonald referred to local malaria and celebrated the "fertility of knowledge and practice" arising "from the prevalence of malaria and the quality of the people who studied it" and suggested that, thanks to the success of DDT campaigns in Italy, Greece, Crete, Sardinia, and Cyprus, "it would be difficult now without highly specialized and up-to-date local knowledge to say where within the area malaria can be found complying with the many descriptions which have been made of it in the past."[119]

---

116 Webb, *Humanity's Burden*, 149; Van der Hoogte and Pieters, "Quinine, Malaria, and the Cinchona Bureau." Before the Dutch Kina Bureau, the global quinine market had been dominated by a cartel formed in 1894 by three German pharmaceutical firms. See Van der Hoogte and Pieters, "Quinine, Malaria, and the Cinchona Bureau," 5.

117 Greenwood, "Conflicts of Interest." Synthetic antimalarials, in turn, provided a solution to the needs of the Allied Forces after the fall of Java to the Japanese in 1942.

118 Woodbridge, *UNRRA*, vol. 2, 134. See also Gardikas, "Relief Work and Malaria in Greece."

119 Macdonald, *The Epidemiology and Control of Malaria*, 74.

With spectacular initial effects in the temperate zone, DDT held the promise of global malaria eradication, not merely control. Many indeed feared the demise of malariology as a scientific field. The World Health Organization adopted a global malaria-eradication program in 1955, but excluded Sub-Saharan Africa from the initial stage of its application.

The global malaria-eradication program, however, ran into trouble on several fronts. It had been conceived in the simplistic cultural context of scientific modernism under the conviction that, in its universal validity, scientific progress could be pursued in disregard of local diversity and social and political particularities. The complex ecologies of malaria and local epidemiology that malariologists had studied with such precision in the interwar years lost their relevance in the new spirit.[120] Moreover, *Anopheles* resistance to DDT began to spread and catch up with the spraying schedules, while poor countries—the ones suffering most from malaria—lacked basic health infrastructures and were unable to fund the consolidation and surveillance stages stipulated in the program. Thus, although a large number of countries in the temperate zone, including Greece and Italy, benefited from the eradication campaign, the WHO was compelled to abandon eradication as its official policy in 1969 and replace it with an unspecified malaria control strategy, for which, however, it failed to provide guidelines. Thereafter, in the 1970s and 1980s, malaria returned in lethal epidemic backlashes, particularly in areas where resistance of *P. falciparum* to antimalarial drugs had emerged in the meantime.[121]

For all the controversies dividing malaria specialists before the outbreak of the Second World War, they had nonetheless achieved a consensus on implementing public health and social policies of rural development and naturalistic malaria control at a conference in Bandung in 1937. In the Cold War atmosphere of postwar politics, however, the Western powers controlling the United Nations and the WHO failed to act on the interwar Bandung consensus and tackle sensitive, malaria-related social issues. Reliance on DDT vector control seemed at the time to provide a politically safe alternative.[122]

---

120 Webb, *Humanity's Burden*, 169; Packard, "'No Other Logical Choice'"; Nájera, "Epidemiology"; Nájera, "Malaria Control," 42–44.
121 Nájera, "Malaria Control," 63; Litsios, *The Tomorrow of Malaria*, 128–31.
122 Litsios, *The Tomorrow of Malaria*, 137–41 and 146; Litsios, "Malaria Control," 272–73.

After more than two decades of international irresolution on the subject, in October 1992, a WHO ministerial conference in Amsterdam adopted the Global Malaria Control Strategy, which proved a turning point in incorporating both physical and cultural management. By acknowledging the adverse effect of the social and economic realities of the modern world and the centrality of local ecology and experience, it initiated new international strategies that have come to include epidemiological and ecological malaria research, appraisal of social determinants, local involvement, educational and economic realities, and the status of women.

In the aftermath of the Amsterdam conference, the revival of malaria research under the new molecular paradigm has further undermined the old divisions. Sobered by oscillations between progress and regression, today, in the words of J. A. Nájera: "The recognition of the complex relations between malaria and development is inducing antimalaria programs to search for a strong working collaboration with programs aimed at poverty alleviation and socioeconomic development, at a more fundamental level than the mere protection of project objectives."[123]

In conclusion, while malaria is still an extremely grave global problem the following figure shows that the rate of malaria mortality has decreased throughout the twentieth century, with the exception of Sub-Saharan Africa.[124]

Currently, the results of the Malaria Atlas Project (MAP), provide an invaluable tool to visualize the complexity of the global distribution of malaria risk and transmission. The project has revealed that, between 2000 and 2015, control interventions have reduced the amount of *falciparum* malaria in Africa by 40 percent.[125]

Yet, despite encouraging developments, such as the number of countries in the process of eliminating malaria, several wider threats give cause for alarm. The possible effects of global warming on vector proliferation, the likelihood that the worldwide economic recession might impact on control strategies and funding are serious dangers. Truly dangerous situations appear, however, with the emergence of *P. falciparum* resistance to artemisinin

---

123 Nájera, "Malaria Control," 82.

124 The figure is based on data on geographical regions adapted from Carter and Mendis, "Evolutionary and Historical Aspects," Table 3.

125 The project's website is located at www.map.ox.ac.uk; see also Bhatt, "The Effect of Malaria Control" and Hay et al., "The Global Distribution."

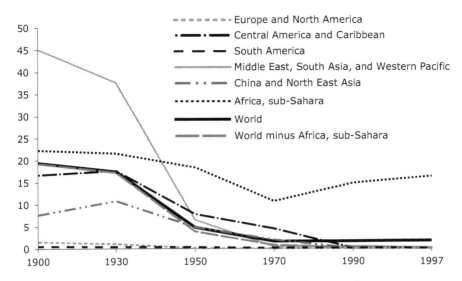

Figure 1.1. Annual malaria mortality per 10,000 in the twentieth century

Source: Carter and Mendis, "Evolutionary and Historical Aspects," 579.

combination therapy (ACT) in Cambodia, the Lao People's Democratic Republic, Myanmar, Thailand, and Vietnam[126] that spreads in southeast Asia and, perhaps worst of all, in Africa, signs of cross-species infections that point to malaria reservoirs in primates in the wild.

Nonetheless, despite serious sources of concern, significant progress is visible on a global scale indicating that the contemporary antimalarial strategies are having a measurable effect. According to the WHO's *World Malaria Report 2015*, malaria deaths fell by 48 percent among all age groups, and by 58 percent among children under five, with Nigeria and the Democratic Republic of Congo accounting for more than 35 percent of these deaths in 2015. Between 2000 and 2015, malaria incidence fell by 37 percent globally.[127]

126 To prevent the buildup of parasite resistance to artemisinin derivatives, the latest antimalarial drugs, antimalarial treatment currently consists of administering drugs in combination in a treatment policy known as artemisinin combination therapy (ACT). On resistance to ACT treatment, see Fortner, "Drug Resistant Malaria." See also World Health Organization, *World Malaria Report*, xiv.
127 World Health Organization, *World Malaria Report*, x and xiii.

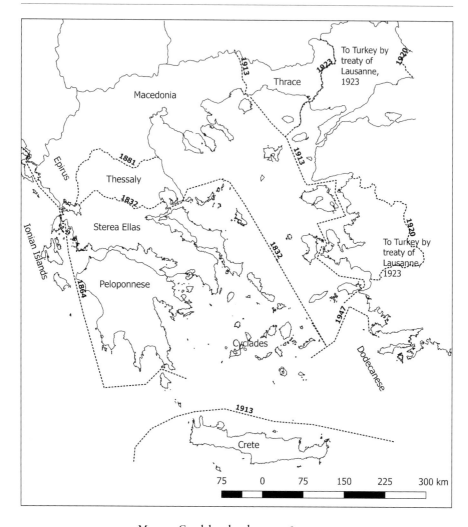

Map 1.1. Greek border changes, 1830–1947

CHAPTER II

THE FRAGMENTED GEOGRAPHY
OF THE DISEASE

Western physicians received the idea of the medical importance of place from the Hippocratic corpus. Leonhard Ludwig Finke (1747–1837) essentially created the field of medical geography in the 1790s by adding an anthropological dimension to the traditional approach.[1] At the same time, British colonial expansion in the eighteenth century, with its health implications both for the military and for civilians, generated a British interest in the geography of disease, particularly of fevers, not only among professionals but also among the lay public.[2] British, French, and Spanish military strategists had also become aware of the sanitary effects of foreign "climates" on their invasion and defense plans, most notably with respect to the greater Caribbean and Central America, as shown by J. R. McNeill in his book *Mosquito Empires: Ecology and War in the Greater Caribbean, 1620–1914.*[3]

This environmentalist approach, which also had a strong climatological component, accommodated the diseases of an expanding geographical experience, particularly of fevers such as yellow fever and intermittents, into an already familiar explanatory framework.[4] This framework was later to lose its importance, however, in the context of the nineteenth-century Humboldtian view of medical geography, which, rather than explore the great variety of human disease experience, sought to uncover the universal natural laws governing disease on a global scale.

---

1   For an appraisal of Finke as a medical geographer and anthropologist and an introduction to his methodology, see Finke, "On the Different Kinds of Geographies."
2   Bynum, "Cullen," 140–41; Dobson, *Contours of Death*, 10.
3   McNeill, *Mosquito Empires*, 188–89.
4   Bynum, "Cullen," 142–43.

The early students of disease in the Greek lands adopted an explor-
atory approach that was closer to Finke's method than to "Humboldtian
medicine."[5] Subsequently, with the rise of the germ-theory paradigm in the
late nineteenth century, when the importance of place in the theory of disease lost its relevance, geography continued to play a part in the etiology of
only two diseases: malaria and tuberculosis.[6]

This chapter considers the fragmented geography of malaria in Greece,
borrowing the idea of fragmentation as a defining feature of Mediterranean
history from Peregrine Horden and Nicholas Purcell. According to these
authors, the history of the Mediterranean is marked by the division of its
environment into *microecologies*.[7] The following passage about Greece from
Bory de Saint-Vincent's *Relation* emphasizes the country's fragmentation
very eloquently:

> It is understandable that in a mountainous, very fractured, country, where
> great ruptures have produced isolated basins that do not communicate with
> one another, a great amount of diversity, based on different interests, hab-
> its and even needs, must have gained root among the inhabitants of these
> basins; here, more than elsewhere, barriers set by nature, even between areas
> circumscribed by geology, have rendered men, often at very small distances,
> complete strangers to one another: thus emerged these primitive ancient
> states of the Peloponnese, so famous in history, each with its own separate
> patriotism, whose typical spirit will always reappear, no matter what kind of
> civilization one may try to introduce to this bizarrely rugged peninsula, so
> long as well-traced communications along the high mountain passes, good
> paved roads across the precipices or the marshes, and solid bridges above the
> rivers or the torrents, do not erase the physical barriers.[8]

Other authors also noted the same feature of the Greek lands. The French
diplomat Henri Belle on his tours of Central Greece in the early 1870s observed in connection to the topography of Mount Oeta: "The existence of
these closed valleys is one of the strangest and most frequent topographi-

---

5   Buttimer, "Airs, Waters, Places." The distinction between Finke and the Humboldtian school of medical
    geography is analyzed in Rupke, "Humboldtian Medicine."
6   Numbers, "Medical Science," 219.
7   Horden and Purcell, *The Corrupting Sea*, 79. See also Sallares, Bouwman, and Anderung, "The Spread of
    Malaria," 311–12.
8   Bory de Saint-Vincent, *Relation*, vol. 1, 29–30.

cal features in Greece."[9] Some seventy years later, Grigorios Livadas (1894–1977), one of the leading Greek malariologists, began his two-volume account of malaria control in the interwar years by drawing attention to the "complex structure of the Greek lands."[10] For the same reason, Marshall C. Balfour, the leading malariologist of the IHD of the RF in Greece, also considered it necessary to produce a variety of regional studies, in order to encompass an adequate range of profiles and mosquito ecologies in his experimental approach to malaria epidemiology in Greece, which he found "a very complicated subject."[11] Interestingly, Melville Douglas Mackenzie, a member of the League of Nations commission that visited Greece in 1929, compared the topography, climatology, and population distribution to that of Sardinia, the island that would later witness the fiercest postwar *Anopheles*-eradication campaign in Europe.[12] More recently, Greek historian George Dertilis has drawn attention to the effects of the fragmentation of the Greek lands and the great length of the indented coastline on isolating populations and, thus, both exposing them to and, at times, protecting them from the hazards of disease, scarcity, and famine.[13]

In this context, I shall investigate the geographic, climatic, and social environments of stable and unstable malaria in Greece and situate malaria in its various landscapes. Landscapes are understood not merely in a physical sense but also as "a human–environmental interactive sphere, transforming over time"; landscapes are shaped both conceptually and ecologically by the cultural interaction among humans and by evolutionary transformations that also involve other species,[14] and constitute places "upon which past events have been inscribed, sometimes subtly, on the land."[15] In the words of Carole Crumley:

9   Belle, *Trois années en Grèce*, 137.

10 Livadas and Sfangos, *I elonosia en Elladi*, vol. 1, 5.

11 Entry 3092, 9 November 1930, Strode diary 1930, Rockefeller Foundation Archives (RFA), Rockefeller Archives Center (RAC) and M. C. Balfour to M. Ciucă, Geneva, 13 October 1933, 5820, 903, R6164, 8C, League of Nations Archives.

12 League of Nations, Health Organisation, Health Committee, *Explanatory Memorandum*, 58. On Sardinia, see De Zulueta, "Forty Years of Malaria Eradication in Sardinia"; Brown, "Malaria, *Miseria*, and Underpopulation"; Tognotti, "The Spread of Malaria." On the 1929 visit of the League of Nations commission to Greece, see Liakos, *Ergasia kai politiki*, 326–28; Theodorou and Karakatsani, "Health Policies in Interwar Greece."

13 Dertilis, *Istoria tou ellinikou kratous*, vol. 1, 233–34.

14 Cormier, *The Ten-Thousand Year Fever*, 12.

15 W. Ballé, "The Research Program in Historical Ecology," *Annual Review of Anthropology* 35 (2006): 77, quoted in Cormier, *The Ten-Thousand Year Fever*, 12.

Broadly defined as the spatial manifestation of the relations between humans and their environment, . . . "landscape" offers several advantages. It is a common unit of analysis in several diverse fields (geography, archeology, ecology, geomorphology, architecture, art, regional planning) and thus helps integrate diverse evidence; and it allows changes to be traced through time. The study of changes in the temporal and spatial configurations of landscapes (a traditional pursuit of archeology), in conjunction with work in cognition, offers a practical means of integrating the natural and social sciences and the humanities.[16]

State Building: The First Medical Institutions

Understanding the broader social context within which health and disease in Greece were observed and framed must take into account the social and institutional circumstances that shaped the nascent Greek state. Whatever indigenous state building the Greek revolutionary authorities and the regime of governor Ioannis Kapodistrias had attempted, much of it was undone after his assassination in September 1831 and the turbulence that ensued. King Othon arrived in the country on 25 January 1833, with a three-man Bavarian regency that ruled in his name until he came of age on 1 June 1835. The real business of state building effectively began with the arrival of these foreign men. Georg Ludwig von Maurer (1790–1872), one of the regents, later recaptured his first encounter with Nafplion, the capital until December 1834, as follows:

> In the first days after our arrival, we could see many houses still smoldering in the distance. One dared not hazard far from the town. The town had no paving. There were many ruins in the town itself. The streets were so narrow that carriages could not pass through. The Square of the Planes was full of rubble from the ruined houses. . . . The aqueduct that carried water from Aria leaked at many points and most of the excellent water spread out to produce small swamps. The moat around the walls was a stinking swamp, and yet it was inhabited by several Greek families and pigs. The fortifications and the arsenal lay in the greatest disrepair.[17]

---

16 Crumley, "Foreword," xiii.
17 Maurer, *Das griechische Volk*, vol. 2, 21–22.

International concerns about the viability of the young Greek kingdom not-withstanding, economic development, education, and health were among the immediate concerns of the new governing elite, who, besides the Bavarian regents and their entourage, were mostly foreign-educated Greeks. They saw themselves as the new kingdom's reformers, administrators, lawyers, teachers, and physicians.

By the eighteenth century west Europeans began to perceive fevers as a social, not merely a personal, concern and expected state institutions of prevention.[18] Thus, as in much else, the Bavarian regents modeled the Greek health institutions on the French blueprint. Indeed, Bavaria itself had introduced its centralized medical administration between 1799 and 1808 in the context of the bureaucratic reforms of Count Maximilian von Montgelas, while still under Napoleonic influence.[19]

In the case of Greece, the top-down reform program introduced the state's proverbial "medical gaze" indirectly from France, to an agrarian society that could never have generated it itself. Examples of such institutions included the sanitary responsibilities of the municipal police, created through a series of decrees from 1833 to 1836.[20] In fact, despite references to a medical police in the legislation, this service developed incompletely as one among several functions of the municipal police with no specifically assigned officers, except for the case of the municipality of Athens, which appointed one medical officer, the *astyiatros*.[21]

With plague and cholera epidemics threatening from across the eastern sea and northern land boundaries, and endemic diseases breaking out in epidemics, legislating for health institutions and sanitary measures where none existed and acquainting themselves with the country became an immediate priority for the new government. A public health decree issued on 31 December 1836 made it the responsibility of the medical police to protect citizens from contagious diseases, specifically listing typhus, plague, cholera, smallpox, leprosy, trachoma, venereal disease, scabies, pulmonary tu-

---

18 Hamlin, *More Than Hot*, 89–92.

19 Farr, "Medical Topographies in 19th Century Bavaria," 237; Ruisinger, *Das griechische Gesundheitswesen*, 53.

20 Diligiannis and Zinopoulos, *Elliniki nomothesia*, vol. 3, 54 and 193; Ruisinger, *Das griechische Gesundheitswesen*, 131–37. Ruisinger argues that these top-down reforms proved unequal to the needs of the country.

21 The first city medical officer of Athens was A. I. Klados; see Klados, *Efetiris (Almanach) tou Vasileiou tis Ellados*, 184. The almanac lists no other city medical officer.

berculosis, pertussis, and rabies.[22] Although in place since the years of the revolution, quarantine measures were sporadic.[23] The new regime only organized its quarantine system in 1845.[24]

In contrast to the threat of contagion, endemic diseases received a different approach. They were considered diseases of place, for which no state at the time had a ready response. With the scientific dispute between contagionists and anticontagionists unresolved, endemic diseases required centralized scientific attention. Indeed, malaria, the disease of bad airs and poisonous emanations from swamps, was the environmental disease par excellence.

Thus, apart from public health institutions such as the medical police and quarantine, the regents also set up a state scientific medical apparatus. The first state physicians were appointed to each prefecture following a decree of 30 October 1833 and, like their Bavarian counterparts, the *Gerichtsärzte*, they were charged with extensive powers of control, reporting obligations and forensic duties. Among other tasks, the prefecture physician was responsible for keeping track of and reporting "the symptoms and course of usual as well as unusual diseases," advising on appropriate sanitary measures and taking note of events and conditions related to medicine, physical history, and climatology "for the purpose of compiling a complete medical topography for the prefecture as soon as possible."[25]

All this was clearly in tune with the dominant medical-geographical public health framework of the times and the ideas of Johann Peter Frank (1745–1821), the German hygienist, and very much with the practices in force in the Kingdom of Bavaria itself.[26] The Greek Royal Medical Council was modeled on the French pattern and came into being by a decree of

---

22 Diligiannis and Zinopoulos, *Elliniki nomothesia*, vol. 3, 272–313.

23 Legislative Committee to Executive Committee, Nafplion, 11 October 1825, *Arkeia Ellinikis Paliggenesias*, vol. 8, 340, doc. 980; Dimakopoulos, "I epi tou Agonos yper tis Dimosias Ygeias Kyvernitiki Politiki"; Ruisinger, *Das griechische Gesundheitswesen*, 42.

24 Law XXII, 25 November 1845, *FEK* [Government Gazette] 31, 7 December 1845 and decree of 25 November 1845, *FEK* 37, 31 December 1845. See also Leconte, *Etude économique*, 312–13.

25 Diligiannis and Zinopoulos, *Elliniki nomothesia*, vol. 3, 219–22. In 1845, the responsibilities of the prefecture physicians were revised by a decree of 5 December (*FEK* 35, 29 December 1845). On the Bavarian service, see Farr, "Medical Topographies in 19th Century Bavaria," 239. For further details on the provincial organization of the Greek medical service, see Ruisinger, *Das griechische Gesundheitswesen*, 64–75. A full century later, between 1924 and 1930, the Greek Service of Hygiene and, subsequently, the Antimalarial Service founded in 1930 both undertook a similar data collection project on the geographic scope and intensity of malaria. Kopanaris, *I dimosia ygeia en Elladi*, 203–5.

26 Farr, "Medical Topographies in 19th Century Bavaria," 237.

13 May 1834; among its several functions, it was responsible for offering the state its medical expertise and for licensing all medical professionals.[27] This scientific apparatus infused into the emerging indigenous medical research an organicist, rather than a taxonomic, Humboldtian, approach, which subsequently informed Greek medical-geographical literature and medical education and led to the examination of the natural and man-made environmental context of disease.[28]

The medical profession was to be self-regulated under state supervision. As for medical education, in May 1835 the Bavarian regents inaugurated a medical school, the first of the four constituent faculties that were to form the University of Athens two years later.[29] The same small medical elite that had constituted the Royal Medical Council also founded the Athens Medical Society, under royal patronage, on 5 June 1835,[30] and two years later staffed the medical faculty of the university, which was inaugurated in May 1837. Ioannis Vouros (1806–1885), for instance, trained in Vienna, Halle, and Berlin with a brief stay in Paris,[31] served as secretary to the board of the Medical Council, as chairman of the Athens Medical Society, and was appointed professor of internal medicine at the University of Athens in 1837. Yet, even after these initial measures, the country possessed an extremely small number of trained health professionals. The state almanac for 1837 listed 85 trained physicians by name and town of practice and 130 licensed traditional doctors.[32] The nationwide survey of the years 1838–40 recorded by name 69 professional physicians, 122, i.e., almost twice as many, traditional doctors and surgeons, 41 pharmacists, approximately 700 midwives, 321 phlebotomists, and 61 inoculators.[33] Thereafter, however, the university

27 Diligiannis and Zinopoulos, *Elliniki nomothesia*, vol. 3, 193–97. For more on the council, see Antonakopoulos, "The Royal Medical Council of Greece." The French Medical Council was established on 14 August 1822.

28 An organicist approach to disease, according to Anne Buttimer, is one that took into account both "the body's adaptation to bio-physical milieux, but also of a person's involvement in social community and eventually identification with place." Buttimer, "Airs, Waters, Places," 213.

29 This early medical school offered courses in surgery, pharmacology, and obstetrics free of charge to unqualified practitioners. Pentogalos, *Skholeia iatrikis paideias*, 45ff; Lappas, *Panepistimio kai foitites*, 71.

30 The founders of the Athens Medical Society would study the country's diseases and remedies in similar way to contemporary medical societies in Europe and the United States. See Mitman and Numbers, "From Miasma to Asthma," 393. For more on the founding of the Athens Medical Society, see Ruisinger, *Das griechische Gesundheitswesen*, 81.

31 Kouzis, *Istoria tis Iatrikis Skholis*, 23; Ruisinger, *Das griechische Gesundheitswesen*, 313–14.

32 Klados, *Efetiris (Almanach) tou Vasileiou tis Ellados*, 150–52.

33 Several regions, however, mostly remote areas of central and western Greece, were not covered by the

overcompensated by producing an average of 85 medical degrees annually, until 1891.[34]

It is widely accepted that, after the deposal of King Othon in October 1862, the new regime let public health institutions fall apart because of a lack of funding.[35] Reacting to this development, on 3 December 1873, the members of the Patras Medical Society demanded the revival of the institution of prefecture and district physicians; it denounced their abolition as a crime against public health, which left the entire legislation "on epidemics, quarantine, inoculation, medical topography, etc." with no responsible authority to implement it and called on the government to create public health councils in each prefecture. Apart from blaming the post-1862 liberal regime, the Patras physicians also criticized the medical élite for not protecting the interests of the public.[36] A former secretary of the Royal Medical Council, I. Vamvas deplored the state of public health before a conference of Greek doctors held in Athens in 1882. According to Vamvas, the Royal Medical Council had lost its advisory powers to the state and the entire system had become obsolete, at a time when the country's more recent neighbors were advancing in public health.[37] State spending on public health declined after 1864 and, as a result, private initiatives tried to fill the void.[38]

As with much of the state-building tasks facing King Othon's regime, there was a great deal of urgency in the establishment of these early medical institutions. In their first summer in office, the government received news of fever outbreaks from towns, fortresses, and the countryside in what appears to have been a nationwide malaria epidemic. The lowlands and productive land in the plains had turned into swamps that were taking their toll on the health of the villagers as a result of abandoned drainage works after more

---

survey, namely the provinces of Parnassis, Lokris, Messolonghi, Valtos, Nafpaktia, Vonitsa and Xiromero, Gortynia, Megalopolis, and the islands of Tinos and Andros; furthermore, Clon Stéphanos, in his *La Grèce*, listed the Fthiotis issue among his sources, but I was unable to find a copy of it.

34 Lappas, *Panepistimio kai foitites*, 402–3.

35 Kouzis, "Ai meta tin idrysin tou Vasileiou tis Ellados," 88–89.

36 *Asklipios* 12, issue B' (1874): 120–25. Also, Karamitsas, "Oliga tina peri ton en Athinais dialeiponton pyreton," 143.

37 Vamvas, "Peri dimosias ygeias," 313. Public health being low in its priorities, the government spent money in the field only when epidemics struck. League of Nations, Health Organisation, Health Committee, *Patras*, 19. Indeed, even in the interwar period, it took a dengue epidemic in 1927 and 1928 in Athens for the municipality to appoint a nonpermanent health officer, P. Papamarkou. League of Nations, Health Organisation, Health Committee, *Hospital and Health Survey*, 11.

38 Liakos, *Ergasia kai politiki*, 316–17.

than a decade of neglect, warfare, and exposure to the effects of inclement natural forces. Writing of the rivers and streams and the state of the Morea landscape in May 1828, Bory de Saint-Vincent drew a vivid image of such contrasting extreme forces of nature:

> All the rivers of the Morea, the largest as well as the smallest, are subject to the same ill-effects as the shores of Elis, in other words, they are surrounded by lagoons and marshes, to which they owe . . . their unhealthiness; it is only in the winter and when the heavy rainfall flows like a canal, that they bring their tribute directly to the common reservoir, breaking their barriers and over-whelming the obstacles created by the action of the waves: at all other times, the soil and the rubble they carry accumulate on beds of sand and pebbles and end up by blocking their outlet, stopping and breaking up upon contact of their flow with the counterflow. The Alpheios, the Pamisus, and the Eurotas are the only rivers not to become completely blocked; however, barriers arise so that even the smallest boats can no longer enter them after the end of June.[39]

These desolate landscapes were dangerous for nonimmune, susceptible for-eigners. The indigenous population, however, also encountered physical hardship upon their return to normal everyday life at work in the fields and towns, or in search for a new place to settle. In Corinth, for instance, where the garrison of the Akrokorinthos fortress and the town had already been suffering over several consecutive summers. In response to the outbreak of intermittent fevers, the government in nearby Nafplion sought the opinion of the former garrison commander, Panagiotis Notaras. A Corinthian nota-ble, Notaras knew his hometown to have been a lot healthier in the past and attributed its present crisis to its "many ruins." Some amount of fevers had also existed under the *Tourkokratia*, caused mainly by the abundance of wa-ter; unfortunately, however, the waterworks now lay in a state of ruin and "were blocked at an hour's distance from the town," which was currently surrounded by marshes. Although the situation in Akrokorinthos itself was now even worse than in the town with fevers peaking in August and Sep-tember, under its Ottoman garrison the fortress had been a regular settle-ment with houses, gardens, and trees, which the locals believed had kept the area healthy in the past. To deal with illness, the fortress now possessed

---

39   Bory de Saint-Vincent, *Relation*, vol. 2, 25.

a hospital.[40] The town of Khalkida, in Euboea, also experienced a serious epidemic of intermittent fevers in the summer of 1833.[41]

The following year, toward the end of the summer, a lethal epidemic struck the provinces of Thebes and Livadeia, which peaked in October.[42] Nor were the islands spared. Thus, upon his appointment as state physician to the prefecture of the Cyclades in 1834, Vouros toured the islands and collected information from his local colleagues. That year's epidemics of intermittent fevers had been particularly extensive. On the island of Syros the town elders of the Roman Catholic community of Ano Syros knew from experience that, in their normally dry island, a rainy winter would be followed by saturated fields and pastures in the summer, which would cause "serious epidemics." Although notified, the newly appointed civilian authorities did nothing; as a result, "no one was spared there." The city of Ermoupoli was hit hard; there, incidents of intermittent fevers outnumbered all other diseases by five cases to one. By contrast, on the same island, in the community of Galisa, whose elders had been more successful in alerting the authorities, drainage ditches helped to avert an epidemic. On all of the remaining islands of the Cyclades, even those as small as Ios, communities near saturated fields suffered from that year's epidemic of "intermittent," "typhoid," and "pernicious" fevers. The latter were so severe that they often killed after "two or three fits," an observation consistent with cerebral *falciparum* malaria.[43]

In several instances on the mainland, plains had become inundated since the departure of their Muslim landowners. The plain of Taka around Tripolitsa (Tripoli) had been last drained by Kiamil Bey.[44] The province of Ileia had been regularly drained by its Muslim rulers with canals, which were still visible in the 1830s. In Ottoman times, canals were opened and kept clear by

40 P. Notaras to War Ministry, Corinth, 3 August 1833, "Reply regarding the climate of Akrokorinthos and the town," doc. 150, subfile Medicinalwesen, f. 203, Interior Ministry, Othon's administration, Greek National Archives (henceforth GAK). Colonel Paraskevà to War Secretariat, Nafplion, 1/13 August 1833, "Rapport concernant le climat de Corinthe," doc. 152, subfile Medicinalwesen, f. 203, Interior Ministry, Othon's administration, GAK. Similar drainage works from the Ottoman times were reported in Elis (Ileia), Copais, Stymfalia, Lake Taka, and Athens. *Tourkokratia* (Turkish domination) was the term used in the Greek source to denote the period of Ottoman rule.

41 Pallis, "Periergos therapeia noserou idrotos," 130.

42 More on this epidemic on p. 87 in this book.

43 Vouros, "Nosologiki katastasis." A century later, the islanders of Ios still suffered heavily from malaria but some control had been achieved recently. Kontos, "I nisos Ios," 452.

44 A. Polyzoidis, Interior Minister to King Othon, Athens, 26 October/7 November 1837, doc. 034, f. 232, Interior Ministry, Othon's administration, GAK.

corvée labor, but now the blocked canals caused flooding, loss of agricultural revenue and disease.[45] Similar signs of neglect were evident in the swamps around Athens, whose urban waterworks had been last cleaned in 1814.[46] In the summer of 1835, a few months after it became the seat of government, Athens, which had hitherto known only sporadic and mild incidents of malarial fevers, was visited by a serious epidemic of intermittent fevers.[47] For instance, Panagis Skouzes, a member of a leading Athenian family, remembered coming down with fever in his youth, in the 1790s, while leaving Athens for a visit to Khalkida.[48] A possible explanation for the 1835 epidemic may be sought in the intensive building activity that accompanied the transfer of the capital from Nafplion. The situation may also have been compounded by the annual flooding of the *elaionas*, the olive groves surrounding the town. [49]

Each year, neglect led to a cumulative worsening of the situation that resulted in the peasants increasingly losing cultivated land. In Livadeia, out of the twenty ancient drainage canals, whose traces were still visible in the early 1830s, only one remained in working condition. Of the older canals in the area of Feneos, in Korinthia, one was blocked for twenty years and the second for ten years. With no outlet, the water level kept rising until twelve surrounding villages had been submerged, while the remaining villages faced a serious threat. The German philhellene and philologist Friedrich Thiersch (1784–1860) commented that "despite all the calamities the country suffered under the Turks, the conduits of the Greek lakes had never been neglected" and cited the cases of lakes Copais, Feneos, and Stymfalia. The old men of Stymfalia remembered that in the summer of 1776, Ottoman officials had 500 men at work on an ancient drainage tunnel. Thirty-five feet below, they came across the ancient entrance gate to the remaining part of the tunnel. At this point the roof collapsed, killing two workers; the project was abandoned, leaving a vivid mark on local memory.[50]

---

45 Dalezios to King Othon, Athens, 22 March 1843, "On the drainage of the plain of Elis," doc. 041, f. 232, Interior Ministry, Othon's administration, GAK. There is evidence that the peasants were invited to work on the drainage project in exchange for promissory notes for state lands; Draft decree "On the drainage of the malarious plains of the municipalities of Elis and Myrtoundia," Athens, 18/30 July 1843, doc. 042, f. 232, Interior Ministry, Othon's administration, GAK.

46 E. Riedel (translation), Athens, 25 June 1845, doc. 067, f. 231, Interior Ministry, Othon's administration, GAK.

47 Mavrogiannis, "Protai grammai mias topografias," 542–43.

48 Skouzes, *Apomnimonevmata*, 99.

49 See About, *La Grèce contemporaine*, 196–97, on the building activities that accompanied the successive transfers of the seat of government.

50 Thiersch, *De l'état actuel de la Grèce*, vol. 2, 19–20.

Official reports from the prefecture of Ileia called for the complete drainage and reclamation of cultivable but totally inundated land of its eighty-two villages and attracted royal attention; King Othon visited the area in May 1840, gained personal experience of its "pitiful condition" and ordered a drainage study. The peasants were willing to offer labor to drain land in the immediate vicinity of their villages, but were reluctant to offer work for land further away. The full draining of the area would not only benefit agriculture but also the grazing of animals, which were being plagued by leeches and bled to death. Moreover, the local governor expected that reclaimed land would attract land-hungry peasants from the mountain communities of the districts of Gortynia and Kalavryta, who were now purchasing overpriced land in the mountains. The interior minister maintained that the project would be "colossal, the largest such project ever undertaken by the Greek government" despite its limited means. Thanks, however, to preexisting drainage canals of the *Tourkokratia*, the whole project would be feasible, argued the minister, with additional secondary canals to be executed by the villagers.[51]

The Greek authorities had a poor appreciation of the country's sanitary conditions. Earlier medical geographies painted a bleak picture of these lands. Writing in the early 1790s, principally on the basis of ancient and contemporary medical and nonmedical sources, Leonhard Ludwig Finke, the father of medical geography, wrote of the Peloponnese: "the land is empty of people and in many locations undeveloped: there are, moreover, no few marshy and inaccessible places, such as, for instance, Navarino."[52] Finke also warned travelers visiting Greece about the nosological implications of the local winds and heat and about the existence of intermittent fevers, which were particularly deadly in the autumn, exactly as reported in Hippocrates.[53]

The early 1830s saw a number of publications that touched on the new country's perilous medical state. John Hennen (1779–1828), a British Army physician, in his posthumously published *Sketches of the Medical Topography of the Mediterranean Comprising an Account of Gibraltar, the Ionian Islands, and Malta*, gave a medical-geographical account of the Ionian Islands and their hazardous landscapes, while in Friedrich Thiersch's work there is some

---

51 [D. Khristidis], Interior Minster, to King Othon, Athens, 6 November 1841, doc. 53, f. 232, Interior Ministry, Othon's administration, GAK. The term *Tourkokratia* was used in the Greek source.

52 Finke, *Versuch*, vol. 3, 96.

53 Ibid., vol. 1, 115–17 and 131–32.

interesting medical topographical information, particularly on the central Peloponnese and Boeotia.[54] However, not only was systematic information unavailable but, overall, traditional doctors in Greece did not seem to pay much attention to the dangers of malignant fevers. Writing in 1827, shortly after Lord Byron's death in Messolonghi in April 1824, John Macculloch had very strong words for the poet's Greek doctor: "That a physician should not have perceived the disorder to be remittent fever . . . in a land and season of malaria . . . is nearly incredible."[55]

In fact, the Athens Medical Society, whose members had left the city during the 1835 summer fever epidemic, notified the Interior Ministry upon their return, in January 1836, that it was publishing a medical journal, aptly named *Asklipios*, to study "the nature of the prevailing diseases in Greece, climatic conditions, therapeutic methods, etc." and to communicate its observations to Greek and European colleagues.[56] For the sanitary reformers, Greece was a medical terra incognita. Writing about the country's medical topography, the physician Konstantinos Mavrogiannis (1816–1861) noted that "Greece is a book whose first page we have not read yet, a book of elevated lessons and unexplored truths. It is not a blank piece of paper on which all we need do is transcribe whatever we have seen in printed books. We must read from it the live characters that are engraved in nature."[57]

In the minds of early-nineteenth-century Greek and Bavarian reformers, independent statehood signaled for Greece a clean break with the Ottoman disease regime. "Little has been achieved in Greece of what man has devised to free himself from the direct power of nature and to harness this power for his own needs. . . . But now a new era is beginning," declared Mavrogiannis confidently, with disease control in mind. Greece was an ideal country to study the origins and means to control endemic diseases thanks to its very

---

54 Hennen, *Sketches*; Thiersch, *De l'état actuel de la Grèce*, vol. 2, 16–27.

55 Quoted in Bruce-Chwatt and De Zulueta, *The Rise and Fall of Malaria in Europe*, 35. However, a few Greek translations of medical books with chapters on fevers made their appearance after 1745; see chapter 4.

56 Vernardos Roeser, Chairman, N. Kostis, Secretary of the Athens Medical Society, to Interior Ministry, Athens, 15 January 1836, doc. 004, f. 204, Interior Ministry, Othon's administration, GAK; [Introduction], *Asklipios* 1 (1 August 1836): iv. For a list of its first members, see Klados, *Efetiris (Almanach) tou Vasileiou tis Ellados*, 161–62.

57 Mavrogiannis, "Protai grammai iatrikis topografias," 295. The article appeared in two parts, the second published in *Eranistis*. At the end of the second part, the author promised a third part, in which he intended to discuss the situation in the Peloponnese. However, I was unable to trace this third installment, which is not mentioned in Clôn Stéphanos's bibliography either; perhaps it was never published.

backwardness.[58] Indeed, in the very capital, the early days of Othon's reign, summers brought on lethal diarrhea epidemics, greatly affecting children, which were partly attributed to "latent" intermittent fever attacks. Although the Athens Medical Society offered a prize for a study of the epidemics, no such study appeared.[59]

Endemic diseases, particularly intermittent fevers, the Hippocratic and Galenic term for the periodic fevers of malaria, represented a public health puzzle for the Greek medical authorities, who were guided by miasmatic theory. According to their way of thinking, though, relevant public health measures were the responsibility of municipal, not central, authorities. The latter were responsible for quarantine regulations and other legislation targeting epidemic diseases of high mortality; threats from abroad, specifically plague, cholera, and yellow fever; and local, purportedly contagious or "otherwise dangerous," diseases such as anthrax, smallpox, leprosy, typhus, cancer, and syphilis.[60]

THE FIRST NATIONWIDE SURVEY

What was the actual state of health of the population, what were the main diseases, their geographic distribution, causes and means of treatment? Above all, in the prevailing mode of medical-geographical thinking of the day, how was health related to place and fragmented geography, that is, with features of the landscape, climate, production, and social habit? To investigate these questions on a national scale, the government embarked on an ambitious survey, conducted by the state physicians between 1838 and 1840.[61] State officials compiled a set of "medico-statistical tables" that aggregated data from the community level up to that of the top-level administrative division (*dioikisis*).[62] The tables were published in the supplements of

---

58 Mavrogiannis, "Protai grammai iatrikis topografias," 293–94.

59 Nonetheless, the epidemics disappeared owing, it was thought, to Queen Amalia's tree-planting project and to the rise of doctors' systematic attention to intermittent fevers. See Goudas, "Erevnai peri iatrikis khorografias kai klimatos Athinon," 15–16.

60 Diligiannis and Zinopoulos, *Elliniki nomothesia*, vol. 3, 323–25.

61 Mavrogiannis, "Protai grammai iatrikis topografias," 293. Recording medical topographical data was one of the duties of the prefecture physician prescribed by the decree of 30 October 1833. See p. 50 in this book. Interestingly, according to Ian Farr, the Kingdom of Bavaria failed to carry through a similar comprehensive medical survey, until the 1848 Revolution largely rewrote the kingdom's social agenda. Farr, "Medical Topographies in 19th Century Bavaria," 239.

62 Between 1836 and 1845 the *dioikisis*, or administration, had briefly replaced the *nomos*, or prefecture, as the country's highest administrative level.

the government's semiofficial journal, *Ellinikos Takhydromos* (Greek Courier), between 1839 and 1841. It was a wide-ranging, horizontal investigation that conformed to contemporary medical-geographical thinking.

IDENTIFYING FOCI OF ENDEMICITY

The wealth of detail in the survey offered Mavrogiannis the opportunity to conduct an initial analysis of endemic diseases, with special reference to intermittent or periodic fevers (*dialeipontes* or *periodikoi pyretoi*), which were clearly by far the most prevalent disease.[63] Mavrogiannis, however, criticized the survey for not quantifying its analysis of prevailing diseases, for lack of detail, for covering a period of local observation that was too brief for any useful scientific analysis, and for presenting information on prevailing diseases out of its epidemiological context. He added, though, that the safest way to measure the intensity and severity of intermittent fevers in a community was to count the individuals with occlusions of the spleen and liver (*emphraxeis tou splinos* and *emphraxeis tou ipatos*), presumably referring to enlarged spleens, the hallmark of endemic malaria.[64] According to Mavrogiannis, the survey also failed to examine correlations between endemic diseases, for instance between intermittent fevers and tuberculosis or pneumonia.[65] Sensitive to the country's fragmented geography, Mavrogiannis further elaborated the tabular structure of the survey and described the significant degree of variability in the incidence of fevers in the Peloponnese:

> Of course, not all of the Peloponnese is covered in marshes nor do intermittent fevers prevail everywhere to the same degree; it possesses many mountains and many salubrious locations in these mountains. . . . When we examine the medical topography of the Peloponnese, we shall see that its central part, the regions of ancient Arcadia, and among its shores Trifylia, Pylia, Lakonia, and Lakedaimonia, is healthy, with the exception of their marshy villages. However, because the causes of endemic diseases exist in the whole of the remaining littoral and in many parts of the interior, they form large

---

63 Mavrogiannis, "Protai grammai iatrikis topografias," 300–304. Furthermore, he noted that, wherever intermittent fevers were not prevalent, people suffered from respiratory inflammations and pulmonary tuberculosis. See Mavrogiannis, "Protai grammai mias topografias," 535.

64 Mavrogiannis, "Protai grammai iatrikis topografias," 317.

65 Ibid., 319.

foci whose effect reverberate, albeit to a lesser degree, throughout the entire Peloponnese and gives the prevailing diseases their particular character. In some years, in fact, as if escaping from their foci, these disease-generating causes also spread to the mountainous areas and these are then also afflicted as severely as the plains.[66]

Whether Mavrogiannis, who was not one of the surveyors or a member of the Royal Medical Council, had firsthand experience of the Greek countryside, or not, he confirmed what he also found by studying the survey, namely that not only adjacent municipalities but also adjacent communities within the same municipality could differ as to their endemic diseases, depending on their respective "topographical terms." For example, in the municipality of Dorio in the province of Trifylia in the southwestern Peloponnese, the villagers of Soulima (Ano Dorio), which was located on a mountaintop and exposed to northerly winds, were healthy and physically robust, whereas those of Agrilia, located on the mountain slope, were exposed to southerly winds, suffered from intermittent fevers, splenomegaly, and were pale and weak.[67]

To highlight the fragmentation of the malarial topography, he titled the second part of his article "Scattered topography (*Topographiki diastixis*) of the unhealthy parts of the Peloponnese."[68] He also pointed out the distinction between endemic fevers and irregular epidemic outbreaks and "between normal and extraordinary epidemic years" as important outcomes of the survey and drew attention to the fact that, even when the survey designated a location as healthy, this did not indicate that it was always or completely free of fevers.[69]

On the basis of his examination of the medico-statistical tables, Mavrogiannis established that the unbroken chain of swamps and lagoons on the littoral of the Peloponnese from Corinth to Trifylia was extremely unhealthy; the inhabitants suffered from severe endemic intermittent fevers,

---

66 Ibid., 320–21. This observation is no different from a remark by IHD malariologists, M. A. Barber and J. B. Rice, a century later, in 1934, when they offered the following recommendation regarding the planning of malaria research in Greece: "Since considerable variation occurs in different villages, a group of villages is better than a single village as a control." See Barber and Rice, "Malaria Studies in Greece: The Seasonal Variation," 20, in Bar-4, folder 19, box 3, 749 I, RF 1.1, RAC.

67 Mavrogiannis, "Protai grammai iatrikis topografias," 323.

68 Mavrogiannis, "Protai grammai mias topografias."

69 Ibid., 542–43.

"mostly complicated malignant periodic fevers with . . . chronic effects."[70] Equally affected were the plains in the interior of the Messinian and Laconian gulfs. In the latter, the municipality of Karyoupolis was practically uninhabited, its population having dropped dramatically over the previous twenty years. Its principal town had 154 residents but 17 others had died within a year.[71] Similarly unhealthy marshlands also populated the eastern side of the Peloponnese.

Topographical features such as lagoons occasionally served as fisheries, thus benefiting the inhabitants by supplementing their food supply but, at the same time, put their health at risk of malarial fevers, as in the case of the municipality of Araxos, near Patras. Besides its two large swamps, Araxos also had a fishery in Lake Papas; all three contributed toward a highly dangerous environment. "The municipality is so unhealthy," noted Mavrogiannis, "that it remains deserted [erimos], with no villages or permanent residents. Only the inhabitants of the municipality of Panakhaia descend in October, remain there throughout the winter in temporary huts, departing toward the end of April, thus avoiding the miasmatic influence from the swamps in the summer."[72]

Mavrogiannis singled out marshes and lakes as the immediate contributing factors to intermittent fevers, even at considerable altitudes. The few exceptions to this general rule, intermittent fevers with no nearby marshes, led him to draw a distinction between endemic and epidemic fevers. He also differentiated between severe, malignant (kakoitheis), complicated (epipeplegmenoi) intermittent (dialeipontes) fevers close to marshlands, on the one hand, and simple, benign (evitheis) fevers such as those experienced in the dry areas of the Peloponnese, on the other.[73]

THE NINETEENTH-CENTURY REGIME

What happened over time, however, to these numerous and extensive *foci* of endemic malaria? Much of what was published in Western medical geographies was not based on firsthand travel experience but on the earlier literature;

---

70 Ibid., 537.
71 Ibid., 547.
72 Ibid., 538. See more on fisheries and their effect on malaria in chapter 3.
73 Mavrogiannis, "Protai grammai mias topografias," 553.

it was for the great part not updated and reflected the situation in the 1830s. Thus, in his 1881 edition of *Handbuch der historisch-geographischen Pathologie*, August Hirsch singled out several Greek areas for endemic malaria, on the basis, however, of information from sources varying in time.[74] Conditions, however, were far from static, as already suggested in Mavrogiannis's account.

Throughout the nineteenth century the country's epidemiological profile was being shaped in response to the social and environmental pressures which accompanied statehood. Three factors of social change are worth emphasizing for their impact on the disease environment and, especially, on the epidemiology of malaria in Greece.

Perhaps the most important change was the colonization of the plains by the mountain populations, who broke with the premodern preventive practice of avoidance, in order to participate in the promising market of export crops, primarily in currants. This settlement trend had already begun in the years before the revolution, was disrupted by war, only to expand throughout the nineteenth century; its growth accelerated after the mid-1860s until it crashed in the 1890s. In the last decades of expansion, the movement to the plains was reversed, as populations proceeded to colonize and cultivate more marginal mountain zones. These developments defined the Greek national economy and gradually restructured settlement patterns beyond recognition in response to international market demands. Nonetheless, as demonstrated in the case of Elos, treated below, many highly malarious regions had a history of many centuries in the same location.[75] At the same time, indigenous market forces and communications requirements connected the large number of old communities, which still constituted the bulk of the country's settlements, more intensely than in the past, bringing about increased mobility and transfer of human infections.

One state-building project with serious implications for public health was the army reforms introduced in the 1880s.[76] Once reformed and enlarged, the army enlisted all males, exposed them to the same homoge-

---

74 Such places were Livadeia, Thebes, Locrida, Lake Topolias or Copais, Attica, Zituni (Lamia), Nafpaktos, Vonitsa, Khalkida in Euboea, Corinth, Aigio, Tripolitza (Tripoli), Mistras, Navarino, Methoni and much of coastal Peloponnese, Crete, as well as several Ionian Islands, particularly Cephalonia, Lefkada, and Corfu. Hirsch, *Handbook*, vol. 1, 212–13.

75 Kalafatis, *Agrotiki pisti kai oikonomikos metaskhimatismo*, vol. 1, 130–33. See also the section on colonization in chapter 3.

76 Veremis, "O taktikos stratos stin Ellada," 170; Kostis, *Ta kakomathimena paidia tis istorias*, 451–59.

nized disease environment and, finally, released them to carry home whatever they had contracted during their service, be it malaria, tuberculosis, or syphilis. Indeed, more than anything else, it was the health of the army and its social implications that finally prompted Greek physicians to collectively take action at the turn of the century.[77]

In addition to the colonization of the plains and conscription, a further source of population movement contributed toward the deteriorating malaria situation: refugees fleeing persecution and ethnic cleansing, particularly in the early years of the twentieth century, the First World War, and the exchange of populations between Greece and Turkey in 1923. This phenomenon has been documented in other Balkan countries as well, as waves of refugees, forced into consolidated national boundaries, crisscrossed the region. Although undocumented, it is indeed reasonable to suspect that population displacement during the Greek War of Independence must have exacerbated the malaria situation in the 1820s.[78]

Amid all these changes, it is understandable that intermittent and other types of fevers never lost their central place in Greek medical discourse. Ten years after the first survey, the Greek medical establishment still focused on intermittent fevers. In November 1858, the Athens Medical Society held a competition to encourage a study on the causes that transformed intermittent into malignant fevers, as its members presumed, on the variations of malignant fevers in Greece and on their best treatment.[79] Anastasios Goudas, the Athenian physician, attributed past summer epidemics of intermittent fevers in Athens to a variety of reasons; winds carried malarious emanations over the marshes of the Kifissos River and over a lake at Marathon to the northeast of the city; particularly in July and August, winds carried miasmatic substances from partially dried marshes. Hugely underestimating the complexity of the problem, Goudas expected, however, that Skarlatos Soutsos, who owned an estate there, would succeed in fully draining the Marathon lake and in thus relieving Athens from malaria. A further source of malarious emanations, according to Goudas, lay under the city itself, in the blocked drainage pipes of ancient Athens.[80]

---

77 See chapter 3.
78 More in chapter 3.
79 *Asklipios*, Period II, 3 (November–December 1858): 274–75.
80 Goudas, "Erevnai peri iatrikis khorografias kai klimatos Athinon," 31–32.

Several decades of medical experience and investigation revealed that malaria was ubiquitous in Greece and beyond contemporary state boundaries. As a physician told his colleagues at the Athens medical conference of 1882, "the disease is endemic in Greece, from Aimos [the Balkan Mountains] to Rhodes and Cyprus, and appears in epidemic outbreaks in marshy villages, as in Levadeia, in arid towns, such as Athens, in mountainous ones, such as Arakhova on Parnassos, and generally in all corners of the Greek lands."[81] However, by that time, the state had lost the capability to systematically record sanitary conditions, especially after the post-1862 liberal regime had failed to appoint public physicians.[82]

According to the incidental evidence from contemporary medical literature, the country experienced nationwide epidemics in 1849, 1859, and, again, in 1860 and countless local epidemic outbreaks of varying severity.[83] Following a very dry summer, an epidemic of intermittent fevers attacked more than half the population of Sparta in September 1860; in October, the epidemic spread to the rest of the district of Lakedaimon. Despite some mortality, most patients recovered. Both the season and the reported symptoms are consistent with the presence of *falciparum* malaria. In the district of Xirokhori in Euboea, practically the entire population suffered from fevers in August; eight patients were reported to have died, while the islands of Andros, Naxos, and Thira (Santorini) each experienced a violent epidemic in October. Serious epidemics in Marathon and other rural municipalities in Attica prompted the government to take exceptional measures, send out a doctor and a pharmacist to treat the sick, presumably with quinine.[84] Interestingly, all locations from which epidemics were reported in 1860 are located in the drier eastern part of the country. The fact that western Greece did not attract the attention of the Athens Medical Society need not imply that the region remained unaffected. It may, however, suggest that malaria in western Greece was highly endemic and considerably more stable.

In his early 1880s work on the physical state of the Greek population, Clôn Stéphanos (1854–1915), still working within the miasmatic paradigm, provided no data on recently acquired Thessaly. He had studied the "med-

81 See Loukas Bellos's comments on Gavaris, "Peri epidimias ikterodous aimatourikou pyretou en Sparti," 164.
82 Karamitsas, "Oliga tina peri ton en Athinais dialeiponton pyreton," 143–44.
83 Kardamatis, "I elonosia en Elladi kata to 1905," 184–91.
84 "Peri tis dimosiou ygeias tou kratous apo 1 Iouniou mekhri 31 Dekemvriou 1860."

ico-statistical" tables of the 1838–40 survey, subsequent secondary sources, and also collected information from provincial doctors firsthand. Like Mavrogiannis in the 1840s, he furthermore found an interest in the dynamic balance between epidemic and endemic malaria but also introduced social and economic parameters to his approach, such as poor nutrition, a line of causation consistent with the persisting Galenic etiology of fevers, and lack of access to treatment, particularly in his account of "cachexie palustre," a manifestation of stable, endemic malaria among adults, consistent with increased levels of immunity to severe malaria. Stéphanos wrote:

> Despite the fact that the circle of influence of malaria is quite extensive, the foci within which it appears with intensity are *quite narrow*. . . . Nonetheless, owing to the *unequal distribution* of the various conditions that enhance or compound the effects of the infection, these effects do not appear everywhere to be proportionate to the importance of these foci. Thus, malarial cachexia appears, at its most intense, in several villages neighboring the Helos swamp in Laconia, in the area of Lake Moustos in Kynouria as well as certain villages of Argolis, where patients are completely deprived of any suitable treatment, where they only eat pitiful vegetables and where the consumption of wine and meat is almost unknown.[85]

He then went on to explain that cachexia had largely receded in frequency and intensity over the previous ten or twenty years, that is, in the 1860s and 1870s, as, on the one hand, the extent of marshlands had considerably diminished thanks to increased cultivation, while, on the other, sanitary conditions had greatly improved, implying a general rise in living standards, a view only partially shared by his contemporary, Georgios Karamitsas, professor of medicine at the University of Athens.[86] Karamitsas merely observed some improvement without, however, offering an explanation. In the past, he argued, many marshlands and large alluvial tracts of land remained uncultivated for a long time but were, nonetheless, subject to all kinds of excavating activities; no less dangerous were "swamps with mixed sea and freshwater, lakes that dry out in the summer becoming marshes suitable for the generation of the marshland miasma" and "bad air." Yet "lately, it seems that in most places in

---

85 Stéphanos, *La Grèce*, 501; emphasis added.
86 Karamitsas, "Oliga tina peri ton en Athinais dialeiponton pyreton," 143.

Greece there is a reduction, not so much in the frequency, as, indeed, in the quality of marshland diseases, because their heavy and pernicious forms have become more rare."[87] Furthermore, as Stéphanos noted, outdated and ineffective treatments of malaria had been replaced by the enthusiastic adoption of quinine usage. "The Greek peasant now rates quinine as equal to bread," Stéphanos wrote.[88] This may indeed explain Stéphanos's observation that, although malaria prevalence had not diminished, pernicious fevers had become more rare thanks to the spread of quinine medication.

The Impact of Fragmentation

To what extent, therefore, was the fragmented distribution of intermittent fevers merely an accident of the country's recovery from the War of Independence, as suggested by Clôn Stéphanos, and, therefore, limited merely to the early years; or was it an inherent feature of Greece's malaria epidemiology that persisted until the Second World War? Concomitantly, to what degree did spatial fragmentation contribute to instabilities in malaria incidence and a presence of malaria in both endemic and epidemic forms?

Related to the question of the spatial distribution of malaria endemicity and malaria epidemics were the diverging approaches taken by European and American malariologists to the question of its ultimate causes. In the interwar years, these issues gave rise to two schools of thought. The environmental or "American" approach, with Lewis Hackett as its most prominent figure, focused on the causes of mosquito abundance to understand the epidemiology of the disease. The "European" approach, represented by the majority of the Malaria Commission of the League of Nations, saw socioeconomic roots in malaria epidemiology.[89] Challenging the wisdom of both schools in searching for patterns by aggregating spatial data, the British malariologist S. P. James, a member of the Malaria Commission and one of the main proponents of the socioeconomic approach, however, dissociated social and economic realities from endemicity and, in fact, called for an extremely localized, even itemized, treatment. For James,

---

87 Karamitsas, "Peri elodon i eleiogenon nosimaton," vol. 2, 739.
88 Stéphanos, *La Grèce*, 502.
89 For a genealogy of the ideas behind each approach, see Zylberman, "A Transatlantic Dispute." Zylberman also explains how diverse opinions within the European camp actually were. Ibid., 280.

[i]n general epidemics are due to social and economic factors, which escape the control of a preventive public health organization. In this respect, all that can be usefully accomplished at present consists in an effort to predict the appearance of these epidemics and to take measures that will reduce their effect to a minimum, making sure that the specific measures to treat the disease exist everywhere. On the other hand, endemic diseases constitute a permanent difficulty, which must be fought by means specific to each locality where it appears and *even by means particular to each dwelling*. This point is perhaps the most important among those on which we should draw attention.[90]

In dealing with the issue of fragmentation posed by aggregation, on the one end of the spectrum, and itemization, on the other, this study is an attempt to adopt a medical-geographical approach with an emphasis on landscape, thus including society, culture, and local particularities in its compass. To examine the importance of fragmentation for malaria with regard to the Greek lands, I have selected a small number of malarious locations on the basis of criteria applied to a series of four successive, nationwide surveys. These surveys were conducted by a malaria committee appointed by the first national conference of the Athens Medical Society in May 1901 and then by the Anti-Malaria League between 1905 and 1907. This data-collection activity arose from the alarm felt among the Greek medical profession at a perceived deterioration in public health when, at the same time, germ theory promised a solution. The defeat of the Greek Army by the Ottomans in 1897 added to the general concern over what was seen as the nation's physical decline.

In 1901, the Athens Medical Society's national conference, attended by some 460 participants, established a malaria committee that would study the disease and its causes, compile a nosological map, and make policy recommendations, thus adopting a vertical approach to disease control.[91] No more than seventy-six physicians responded to the first survey, which covered issues relating to the nature and distribution of malaria, and to environmen-

---

90 S. P. James, "Le paludisme en Europe. Impressions générales recueillies au cours d'un voyage d'études en Yougoslavie, en Bulgarie, en Grèce, en Roumanie et en Russie," p. 17, Geneva, 18 September 1924, Organisation d'Hygiène, H.C. 230 (vol. 245), League of Nations; underlined in original. Cf. Evans, "European Malaria Policy in the 1920s and 1930s." On the concept of "eminently local epidemiology", see Zylberman, "A Transatlantic Dispute," 285–86.
91 Vladimiros and Franghidis, "To 'Panellinion Iatrikon Synedrion'"; Papastefanaki, "Dimosia Ygeia," 160.

tal and climatic conditions that favored its spread. The Anti-Malaria League, created in 1905, carried out three further surveys, in 1905, 1906, and 1907.[92] In all, some 777 physicians replied to at least one of the four surveys, or approximately one-third of all Greek doctors practicing in most of the country's 443 municipalities. The survey material thus affords generous information on features of malaria in their area of medical practice. It was later consulted by Norman White, who visited Greece with the Medical Commission of the Health Committee of the League of Nations, which was sent to study malaria in Greece in 1924. According to White, the malaria situation had not changed in the intervening twenty years. However, as will be shown in chapter 3, these intervening years were mostly a period of war, population displacement, and socioeconomic stress, unsuitable for malaria control.[93]

In general, Greece reminded foreign malaria experts of the tropics or southeast Asia. Ronald Ross compared malaria endemicity in Copais to that in India and Africa. P. Armand-Delille, serving in Macedonia in the French Armée d'Orient, noted that epidemiological conditions there were "fully comparable to a tropical country."[94] In 1972, M. C. Balfour, summarized his nine-year-long experience of malaria in Greece in the 1930s as one of a "higher endemo-epidemicity than I observed in the Orient."[95] Overall estimates of the country's average malaria morbidity varied only slightly over the half century before the Second World War.

During the First World War, Ioannis Kardamatis, secretary-general of the Anti-Malaria League, surveyed state engineers and medical and municipal sources of information in a sixth nationwide malaria survey, compiled the data in tabular form, and published it in 1924.[96] It included a nationwide, itemized presentation of all lakes as well as large and small swamps, along with averages of malaria prevalence of the populations at risk. Moreover, for comparative purposes, he aggregated this detailed record up to the level of the country's division into "Old" and "New" territories, meaning lands acquired after 1913. He concluded that in the new territories, the total expanse

---

92 Savvas and Kardamatis, "Apantiseis dimarkhon." To complete the nationwide coverage of the survey, in 1908 the League obtained additional numerical information on malaria prevalence from the municipal authorities with the help of the Interior Ministry. Savvas, *Peri tis en Elladi kai Kriti sykhnotitos*, 3–4.

93 Norman White, Rapport sur la situation sanitaire en Grèce, spécialement en ce qui concerne le paludisme, 22 August 1924, p. 12, CH/s.c.malaria/13, Health Organisation, League of Nations.

94 Armand-Delille, Paisseau, and Lemaire, "Le paludisme," 870.

95 M. C. Balfour, "Observations on Greece in 1972," p. 2, folder 8, box 2, D. E. Wright papers.

96 Kardamatis, *Statistikoi pinakes*.

of the 938 swamps larger than 1,000 square meters was 3,043.6 square kilometers, whereas the 831 swamps of Old Greece covered an area of merely 960.8 square kilometers, or one-third of those in New Greece. In terms, however, of malaria morbidity, his figures pointed to the reverse, namely that Old Greece was considerably more malarious than New Greece.[97]

Thus, including Eastern Thrace, held by Greece briefly at the time of Kardamatis's data collecting, the country was covered by a total of 4,004.4 square kilometers of lakes and swampland.[98] I have recalculated Kardamatis's aggregate morbidity averages, which differ slightly from my own calculations: 31 percent annual malaria morbidity for Old and 24 percent for New Greece and a general average for the entire country of 28 percent. Granted though that his data collection in the new territories was, by Kardamatis's own account, problematic, this conclusion must be open to question. Nonetheless, it helped him highlight the importance of small water collections in providing *Anopheles* with breeding sites and their significance as the principal source of malaria.

A more recent, post–Second World War, aggregation was compiled in 1945 or 1946 in map form by UNRRA's sanitary engineering section in Greece under Daniel E. Wright (1903–1973). With Eastern Thrace having returned to Turkey since Kardamatis's original research in 1919 and much of the land reclamation projects in Macedonia still incomplete, in Wright's calculations, out of a total of 1,013 square kilometers of Greek swampland, 509 square kilometers corresponded to New Greece and 504 square kilometers to Old Greece.[99]

The Greek Antimalarial Service (Anthelonosiaki Ypiresia), created in 1930 as part of Venizelos's public health scheme, estimated broadly that, in the early 1930s, the country's parasite index varied between 10 and 25 percent depending on the year and season. Spleen indices were extremely high, ranging between 50 and 100 percent in rural areas and 10 and 30 percent in cities.[100]

---

97 Ibid., 175–77.
98 Ibid.
99 Map "Greece, UNRRA Sanitation Section 'The Swamps of Greece in km2,'" Greece #22, Malaria and Sanitation, PAG-4/4.2.:35 [S-0524-0059], UN Archives. The map divides Greece into eleven regions which correspond to broader hydrological drainage basins. The main purpose of Wright's estimates was to serve as a guide to his nationwide DDT air-spraying program. Therefore, the definition of what constituted a swamp may differ between the two estimates; what is indicative, however, is the balance between Old and New Greece. More on latitude and its effect on climate and malaria prevalence on p. 123 in this book.
100 Kopanaris, *I dimosia ygeia en Elladi*, 207–8; Vassiliou, "Politics, Public Health, and Development," 114.

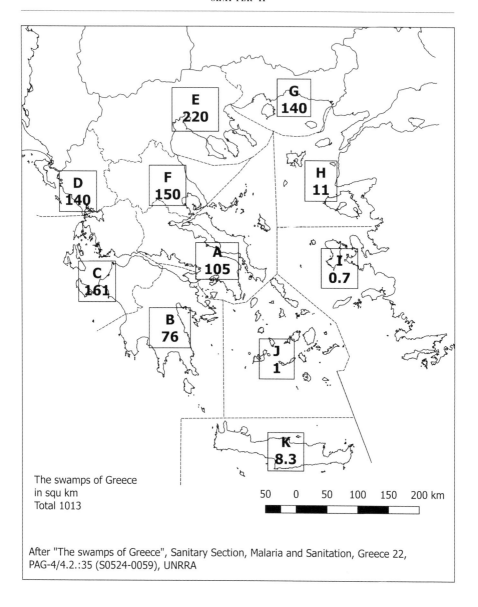

The swamps of Greece
in squ km
Total 1013

50   0   50   100   150   200 km

After "The swamps of Greece", Sanitary Section, Malaria and Sanitation, Greece 22,
PAG-4/4.2.:35 (S0524-0059), UNRRA

Map 2.1. Lakes and marshes, 1944

Finally, in 1933, generally a mild malaria year, the Malariology Division of the Athens School of Hygiene under M. C. Balfour conducted another nationwide, quantified investigation of spleen measurements and blood smear examinations of schoolchildren over a sample of 69 locations, namely thirty-eight villages and thirty-one towns from "each major plain, valley, plateau and other topographical regions of the country," comprising a total of 195,390 inhabitants.[101] The 1933 survey also compared the major geographical divisions in terms of malaria prevalence and drew the conclusion that,

[a]lthough wide variations exist between individual communities, there is a general *uniformity of averages* among the major divisions of the country. The general average spleen index for 8,184 examinations was 35.6 percent, while the average blood index for 7,662 examinations was 17.4 percent. It may be observed that Macedonia and Thrace, Old Greece, Peloponnesus and Crete agree fairly well with the general average. If the samples can be accepted as satisfactory, Epirus shows appreciably higher and the Ionian and Aegean Islands definitely lower spleen and blood rates than the average.[102]

Balfour drew, moreover, a distinction with respect to altitudes between, on the one hand, the fifty-seven towns and villages in his sample within 250 meters of sea level and, on the other, the twelve communities above that limit. Those below 250 meters represented averages of spleen and blood indices of 38 and 18 percent, respectively, while those above 250 meters fared considerably better with averages of 25 and 13 percent in spleen and blood measurements.[103]

Averaging by definition generates uniformity; it does not prove it. This study, nonetheless, focuses on variability and instability. It is, however, interesting to note that despite the crude estimates of the first Greek malariologists, namely Konstantinos Savvas and Ioannis Kardamatis, these es-

---

101 Balfour, "Malaria Studies in Greece," 314. Balfour's analysis focused mainly on the seasonal and annual fluctuation of malaria in Greece; therefore, for more on the subject, see p. 130 in this book.

102 Ibid., 314–15; emphasis added. Parasite indices were consistently lower—on average approximately half—than spleen indices; Balfour explained that in Greece "the spleen findings usually present an average picture of conditions which existed during the previous three or four years. . . . The blood index of a group is more susceptible to change, and it more nearly reflects the conditions which existed during the months immediately preceding the examination." In other words, parasite indices are more sensitive to epidemic outbreaks and to malaria control work. Ibid., 310.

103 Ibid., 322.

timates were upheld by later research, indeed by the Malariology Division of the Athens School of Hygiene. In fact, it was commonly accepted during the Second World War that before the war annual malaria prevalence ranged between one and two million cases.[104] With their validity broadly confirmed, it is worth correlating these early estimates with measurements of rates of hemoglobinopathies collected in the 1970s.

Already in the 1930s, long before J. B. S. Haldane suggested an evolutionary connection, a number of Greek doctors associated β-thalassemia, or Cooley's anemia, with malaria. In 1936, pediatrician Konstantinos Khoremis (1898–1966) speculated that malaria might cause thalassemia and offered quinine as a cure.[105] A year later, Ioannis Kaminopetros (1898–1963), director of the Pasteur Institute in Athens, rejected Khoremis's approach and posited the idea that β-thalassemia was an incurable hereditary condition. He also observed osteological lesions among his thalassemic patients.[106] To prolong their lives he tried treatment with malaria therapy, that is by inducing malaria in his patients, and noted that none of their young red blood cells contained plasmodia. This led Kaminopetros to suggest that plasmodia failed to penetrate the young red blood cells owing to some yet unknown effect of malaria. Although this was as far as Kaminopetros could argue, he was indeed onto something promising.[107]

In the early 1950s, building on the preliminary work of the interwar years, postwar medical research in Greece, particularly among hematologists and pediatricians, took an interest in epidemiological studies in hematology, especially β-thalassemia and sickle-cell anemia, and looked into the malaria hypothesis recently advanced by J. B. S. Haldane. Moreover, in 1977, a Greek Army medical team under the late Nikolaos Skhizas screened 15,550 army recruits for these hemoglobinopathies and produced a study of their distribution across the country.[108]

---

104 For example, Health Report on Greece, prepared by A.M.L. (Greece) with the cooperation of Combined Economic Warfare Agencies, 1 June 1944, Reports Medical and Health, July 1943–February 1946, 658, PAG-4/3.0.12.3.1.0.:9 [S-0527-0730], UN Archives.
105 Khoremis and Spiliopoulos, "Peri tis aitiologias kai therapeias," 83 cited in Kaminopetros, *I erythrovlastiki anaimia*, 71. I wish to thank Professors Kostas Krimbas and Dimitrios Loukopoulos for bringing Kaminopetros's work to my attention.
106 See Kaminopetros, *I erythrovlastiki anaimia*, 16 and 31–33.
107 Ibid., 71–72.
108 Skhizas et al., "Sykhnotis."

The unit of analysis adopted for this study is not an administrative entity, like the municipality, province, or prefecture, but the area of practice covered, broadly defined, by the physicians responding to the surveys, in other words the coverage of their own narrative. Concentrating on these early-twentieth-century nationwide surveys is, I believe, additionally helpful because they are the richest as well as most systematic records of malaria prevalence in Greece and, equally importantly, were conducted, not from the perspective of the state but, rather, of the local physicians, most of whom had a long-standing personal and family relationship with their area of practice. One should note, however, that there were no formal guidelines to these structured questionnaires with regard to terminology, for instance, and respondents were free to submit their personal experience and evaluations.

To create a basis for the narrative, I identified cases from among those areas whose doctors answered at least three out of the four questionnaires. From this set of areas, I then selected six cases with different topographies to study the manifestations of malaria in each over time. My criteria in selecting these six cases were the variation in severity and intensity of malaria as well as in geographical distribution over the country, in terms of latitude, longitude, and altitude. I then further extended the core narrative with additional material, such as the medico-statistical tables of 1838–40, Kardamatis's wartime malaria statistical tables, and other narrative and archival sources to reconstruct an epidemiological profile of each area. Owing, however, to the dates of the four core surveys that prescribed the selection, this analysis does not include Macedonia and Crete, which became part of the Greek state after the Treaty of Bucharest (1913), nor Thrace and Epirus, which became Greek under the Treaty of Sèvres (1920). Furthermore, in a caveat to his own work, Kardamatis noted that the wartime data collection occurred under "exceptionally difficult" circumstances; at the same time, he lacked the staff to communicate with the non-Greek-speaking communities in the newly acquired territories of northern Greece.[109]

I attempted to see whether the six frequency classes of malaria prevalence in a map compiled in 1908 on the basis of the League's surveys may be statistically associated with the frequencies of β-thalassemia and sickle-cell carriers observed in 1977. The nonparametric analysis of variance (Kruskal-Wallis) test produced significant results for β-thalassemia, signifying that

---

109 Kardamatis, *Statistikoi pinakes*, 8.

the probability that the association of the β-thalassemia frequencies with the six ranked classes of malaria prevalence of 1907 may be random is less than one in 10,000; in other words, that it is safe to infer that the association between frequencies of β-thalassemia and of malaria prevalence is nonrandom.[110] This finding suggests that centuries of selective pressures from *falciparum* malaria on the populations of the Greek lands are reflected to a significant degree in the regional variability of malaria frequencies in modern times.

The six cases selected for the analysis that follows represent a variety of landscapes. The first case, Elos, in the southeastern Peloponnese, represents an inhabited marshland with a history of malaria from antiquity to after the Second World War; Lake Topolia or Copais in Central Greece was a proverbial malarious site that underwent a costly venture of drainage and land reclamation; Petalidi, in the southwestern Peloponnese, is a hilly, relatively prosperous agricultural district; Sopoto (now Aroania), south of Kalavryta in northern Peloponnese, exemplifies a mountainous area with valleys and an abundance of rivers and streams; Gerli, present-day Armenio, to the east of Farsala in the heart of the Thessalian plain, lay on the fringe of the shallow Lake Karla; finally Fanari, also in Thessaly, was the main town at the edge of the rolling plain of Karditsa, at the foot of the Agrafa range.

By means of the narratives contained in the responses to the surveys, I reconstructed six epidemiological profiles to test the hypothesis that across the country malaria was unvarying over the time frame of this study. The hypothesis was not confirmed; on the contrary, with stable, endemic malaria on the retreat, the picture that emerges is consistent with mostly unstable, epidemic malaria, one that is associated with a low level of acquired immunity. The low case mortality rates though, as some physicians observed, was entirely due to the extensive use of quinine.

As a last, seventh, case, I have added an account from postwar Euboea, which illustrated a ground-level, itemized approach to the local causes of malaria.

---

110 Savvas, *Peri tis en Elladi kai Kriti sykhnotitos*. For a technical explanation, see Appendix III.

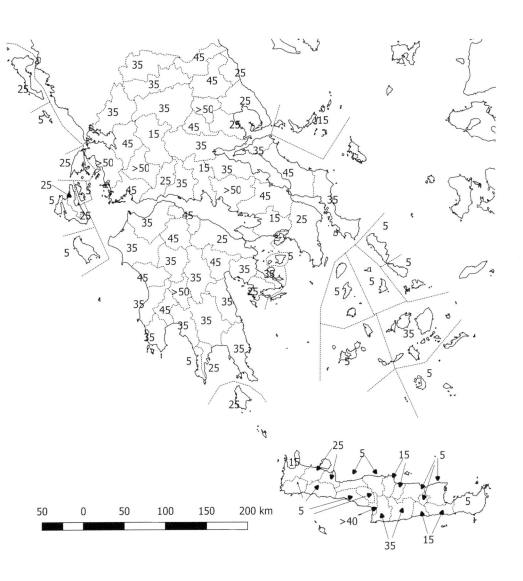

Map 2.2. Malaria prevalence, 1908

Source: *Savvas, Peri tis en Elladi kai Kriti sykhnotitos.*

Elos

Marching through the district of Elos on 1 July 1828, the physical science section of the French Scientific Expedition in the Morea set out to discover the estuary of the River Evrotas (Eurotas), directly south of the site of ancient Sparta. What on Earth were they thinking! "I had never seen such thick clouds of these atrocious insects," wrote Bory de Saint-Vincent of these "execrable diptera," which attacked the group every evening and deprived them of their sleep. The team attributed their fevers to insomnia, that is, only indirectly to mosquito bites, abandoned their exploration and withdrew to Monemvasia, effectively driven out of the area by swarms of mosquitoes.[111] Another section of the expedition encountered the same fate by the swamps of Lake Kaïafa, from where they retreated hastily to Olympia.[112]

Around the same time, Thomas Alcock, a British visitor to Sparta, saw the hand of history at work in the same disease-ridden, neglected landscape. "[Sparta] is now much affected with malaria," he observed,

> and the whole plain is considered unhealthy. . . . Previously to the revolution the Greeks had no encouragement to labor for a harvest which others might reap; and since that period Sparta has been the seat of warfare, and has therefore remained neglected. The river Eurotas, which, kept in a regular channel, was once a beauty and a blessing, now runs waste in a variety of branches, flowing over the whole plain, and causing malaria from its evaporation, whilst olives, oleanders, orange and mulberry trees, grow so thickly, that the circulation of the air is impeded, and the decomposition of the leaves produces the ill effect that now exists.[113]

With the years of turbulence behind them, as recorded in the 1839 survey, the men and women in the low-lying area of Elos produced cereals, maize, melons and watermelons, cotton, tobacco, and dairy products; they also had

---

111 Bory de Saint-Vincent, *Relation*, vol. 2, 343. The mosquitoes encountered throughout the marshlands of the Peloponnese in the summer and mid-autumn were a new species to Gaspard Auguste Brullé (1809–1873), the expedition entomologist; he named it *Culex kounoupi Br.* after the local name for mosquito, produced a drawing and described it as "just as much a nuisance as it is pretty; after mid-May to the end of the hot season, she spreads in the air in large swarms, particularly in the vicinity of water." See Brullé, *Section des sciences physiques*, 289 (no. 623), pl. XLVI, fig. 1. For a recent comprehensive hydrological appraisal, see Fatouros, *Limnon periigisis*, 285–86. An environmental study of the area is available online: Filotis, "Ekvoles."

112 See Bory de Saint-Vincent, *Relation*, vol. 2, 17–18.

113 Alcock, *Travels in Russia, Persia, Turkey and Greece*, 183–84.

silk worms and collected leeches and reeds.[114] The swamp at Skala blocked the outlet of the River Vasilopotamos to the sea, where there was a fishery. In Skala itself (roughly 18 meters above sea level)[115] there were remnants of an old dry dock, or *skala*, about half an hour's walk from the sea shore. Skala was "extremely unhealthy." The same was also true of Leïmonas (c. 16 m) and Seïdali (present-day Agioi Taxiarkhes, c. 16 m), by the River Evrotas. Together with Stefania (c. 33 m) and Trinissa by the sea, the remaining two villages recorded in the municipality of Trinassos, the population amounted to no more than 883 inhabitants or 237 families. Equally poorly populated was the neighboring municipality of Elos with 763 inhabitants, or 200 families. The main village of Elos, or Dourali (c. 16 m), was on flat ground, fertile but marshy and extremely unhealthy, and surrounded by the villages of Ala-ïmbei (Panigiristra, c. 18 m), Myrtia (c. 23 m), Tsasi (Peristeri, c. 75 m), Filisi (c. 23 m) and, on a slight elevation and slightly less unhealthy, Gramiza (c. 224 m). All these villages suffered from endemic intermittent, choleric and occasionally malignant fevers, rheumatisms, rotting teeth, helminthic diseases, rashes, and chloroses,[116] attributed to the extensive marshes, humid homes, poor nutrition and, most importantly for N. A. Foteinos, the recording state physician, personal filth and excessive consumption of salted fish. At the time of the survey, despite the general poverty, Skala had a resident licensed physician, Ioannis Rigopoulos, who also served the people of Elos, and sold medicines to his patients, as was the usual practice.[117] In the surrounding municipalities on higher grounds, fevers were less frequent, unless heavy rains caused flooding that destroyed the produce and brought on diseases "because of the emanations released from the floodwater, mostly intermittent and chlorotic [*khlorodeis*] fevers, which occasionally turn out malignant." Vlakhiotis (c. 57 m) and Vriniko (Asteri, c. 30 m), both lay "on a rocky but unhealthy slope, surrounded by a torrent, called Mariorema, which along with other torrents produces the lake in the swamp"; these two

---

114 Foteinos, "Iatrostatistikoi pinakes ton dimon tis dioikiseos Lakedaimonos." In Ottoman times, at the end of March 1805, Leake had observed that the villages produced cotton and maize, two crops with high water requirements. Leake, *Travels in the Morea*, vol. 1, 196.

115 Elevations were obtained from www.geonames.org.

116 Helen King treats this medical cultural construct in *The Disease of Virgins*. The term was used in reference to the paleness of girls at puberty; here it must be related to the anemic complexion of malaria sufferers.

117 Interestingly, however, although they had no other resident health professional, each community had its own unlicensed midwife.

communities were considered exceptions to the general healthiness of the municipality of Akrion, which had a total population of 1,239 inhabitants or 285 families. Palaia Panagia, Vezani (Ano Glykovrisi, c. 197 m), Niata (c. 324 m), and Gouves (c. 331 m), the other communities of Akrion, lay at higher altitudes. Yet, even these communities "on rare occasions" suffered from "periodic fevers." Palaia Panagia and Vezani were also served by a licensed physician, Andreas Maniatakis, who probably resided in Molaoi. Interestingly, the survey does not mention any seasonal variation of the fevers for the two malarious municipalities, where intermittents were recorded as "endemic." By contrast, in the municipalities of Melitini, Krokeai, and Kydonia, which were located at higher altitudes, intermittent fevers were reported to appear in the spring and autumn.[118]

All these places of suffering appear in the 1700 census ordered by Francesco Grimani, the Venetian *provveditore generale* of the Morea. In other words, the Elos settlements have a long history.[119] Not only had malaria not driven the inhabitants away, as it had the members of the French Scientific Expedition, but they had endured disease over many centuries. One could well suspect that it had, indeed, protected them from invading armies and extortionary officials, much in the way that Africa had become the "white man's grave."

By the time Stéphanos was preparing his publication, which drew on published material and local medical sources of information in the late 1870s and early 1880s, Elos was one of the few remaining locations of intense endemic malaria in the country, along with the Sperkheios estuary, Argolida and Lake Moustos in Kynouria, and Lake Copais in Boeotia.[120] At the same time, the district had a large number of adults with malarial cachexia and was one of those few foci that could infect with malaria "otherwise healthy" villages on the slopes of Taygetos.

Deadly malaria epidemics occurred in Lacedaemon in 1850, 1870, and again in 1880, where doctors had learned to rely on the prompt administration of quinine for treatment.[121] At around the same time, unlike the Evrotas

---

118 Foteinos, "Iatrostatistikoi pinakes ton dimon tis dioikiseos Lakedaimonos." See also Mavrogiannis, "Protai grammai mias topografias," 547–48.

119 Panagiotopoulos, *Plithysmos*, 286 and 309–10.

120 Stéphanos, *La Grèce*, 493–95 and 499–502. His local informant was a Dr. Galatis.

121 Valassopoulos, "Nosologiki geografia," 75.

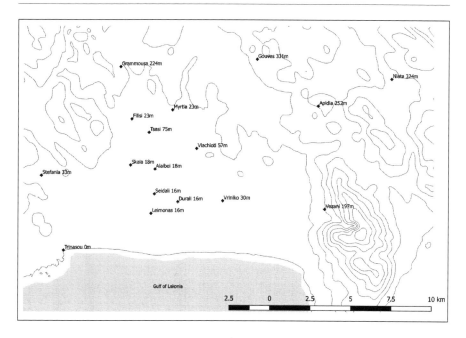

Map 2.3. Elos, 1901–7
The contour lines represent a difference of 100 meters in elevation.

estuary district, the Sparta region saw a general improvement in agriculture, particularly viniculture, and in health. The severity of malaria endemicity centered in the low-lying country, where reigned "marshland cachexia, the great enlargement of the bowels and especially the spleen that was observed among many inhabitants, particularly those in the malarious foci who resembled pregnant women."[122]

Malaria fevers lasted all the year round, with less frequency, though, between December and April, and peaked in September and October. In the early 1880s many instances were considered chronic cases.[123] The Evrotas estuary was particularly dangerous for traders, workers, and other visitors. "Such people visiting these malarious villages for the first time, even in the winter, have been attacked by malaria fevers, when the inhabitants would not have suffered in the least."[124] Clearly, unlike the visitors, locals were protected by an immunity acquired over years of exposure.

122 Gavaris, "Peri epidimias ikterodous aimatourikou pyretou en Sparti," 159–60.
123 Grigorakis, "Peri eleiogenon pyreton en Gytheio," 166–67.
124 Ibid., 168.

By the early twentieth century, with a prevalence in the Elos district and along the Evrotas generally exceeding 90 percent, malaria attracted the attention of doctors in the capital. Between June and July 1901, two physicians from Athens conducted an investigation in the area, collecting information from the local doctor and the inhabitants.[125] By the time of their visit, the two physicians had espoused the new malaria paradigm, but they considered the possibility that mosquitoes were not the only transmission factor of *Plasmodia*; they also appear informed about the controversy between Italian malariologists Ettore Marchiafava and Amico Bignami, on the one hand, and Camillo Gogli, on the other, over the existence of more than one *Plasmodia* species.[126]

According to their report, flooding changed the landscape from one year to the next and also from season to season. Mosquito abundance was directly related to flooding. The thirteen villages of the area had been relatively malaria-free for three consecutive years, but following the heavy rains in the spring of 1901, the two extensive marshes of the Vassilopotamos and Phorvas rivers flooded most of the plain. The alkaline soil of the marshland was impenetrable owing to a thick forest of tamarisk.[127]

The villagers were visited by "light" malaria in early June and severe malaria as early as July. In normal years, the swamp dried out in late May, leaving only the Evrotas and Vassilopotamos rivers and the fishery filled with water, but the plain remained quite lush and rich in vegetation. In the winter, the marshes extended from the swamps of the Evrotas estuary as far as the sea and the Theodoropotamos, a tributary of the Vassilopotamos. However, in August 1901, the flooding was such that in the nearby small plain of Gytheio the shore of Lake Plimari reached the edges of the extensive vineyards. As a result, all the inhabitants of the neighboring villages and all farm laborers fell ill with malaria, even at 200 meters above the surface of the lake. Even the locals were surprised at the abundance of mosquitoes.[128]

The two physicians focused on Dourali and its surrounding villages, which had a total population of 3,000 inhabitants. With regard to their general condition, the two doctors noted that the inhabitants were "not very

125 Triantaphyllakos and Oeconomou, *Le paludisme*, 30.

126 Ibid., 28–29.

127 Ibid., 3–4 and 14.

128 Ibid., 11–16.

comfortable, in terms of resources, although they enjoy the produce of the plain, the fields and the vast olive groves of the surrounding hills." Worse off were those whose crops were destroyed by flooding. Although fewer people died than in the past, malaria was still their most serious cause of misery, leaving them faint and unable to work.

In the three years prior to the visit of the two Athenian doctors, most adults and even children were reported to have spent the summer free of infections; in that year, though, in Dourali, apart from the priest and a local idiot, all inhabitants had fallen ill with malaria.[129] A spleen examination performed in October 1896 on the local schoolchildren from eight villages[130] demonstrated that spleen enlargement decreased with distance, or the flight range of mosquitoes, from the floodwaters of the Vassilopotamos and Phorvas rivers, a fact confirmed by the locals themselves,[131] who had also observed that the annual appearance of the mosquitoes occurred at times defined by proximity to these floodwaters: the first adult mosquitoes emerged in late May and the first malaria cases appeared at the same rates, beginning in early June. "That means that as the inhabitants of Vriniko were being infected, at Dourali one had not yet started using mosquito nets and the inhabitants of Vlakhiotis had not even witnessed mosquitoes," they wrote. At the same time, infected harvesters, already in the plain since late April, were leaving for their homes in the malaria-free villages of Mount Parnon.[132]

Like most of the country, in the epidemic year of 1905 Elos experienced a great deal of suffering from malaria. A. Karamikhas, the doctor and mayor, could not report how many of his constituents had died of malaria, but did confirm that it had been the worst year in his thirty years of practice.[133]

After a brief respite during the following dry year,[134] and an excessively rainy winter in 1907 in some of the villages in the Elos municipality, the entire population had come down with malaria, all 306 inhabitants of Vriniko, for example. "From birth they never ceased to suffer malaria attacks, so that anyone observing them will see clear signs of incessant attacks of malaria. .

---

129 Ibid., 5–6.
130 Namely, Stefania, Dourali, Leïmona, Skala, Vlakhiotis, Tsasi, Filisi, and Myrtia. Ibid., 7.
131 Ibid., 6–8.
132 Ibid., 11.
133 In Vezani, Vriniko, Dourali, and Tsasi, almost the entire population had fallen ill. "1905. Ai peri tis kata topous elonosias pliroforiai ton iatron," 402.
134 Savvas, Kardamatis, and Dasios, "1906," 561–62.

. . Generally enlarged spleens, many below the navel." They made constant use of quinine. In the nearby village of Vezani, all but a tenth of its 380 inhabitants had caught malaria. This healthy percentage lived on a slightly elevated location, at 250 meters, on a hill called Kourkoulas.[135] Mosquitoes had become so abundant that all villagers slept indoors and under bed nets.[136] Likewise in Alaïbei, Filisi, and Tsasi, almost all, i.e., 90 percent had malaria, but Vlakhiotis's better performance of 45–50 percent was attributed to the work of its resident physician, Ilias Tsakonas. This improvement was a mere transitory relief, however. Many decades later, a visit from the British Royal Army Medical Corps in March 1945, immediately after the German occupation, singled out Vlakhiotis as "particularly" malarious.[137]

In 1906, villages slightly removed from the swamp, or some 8 kilometers away, such as Apidia with its 625 inhabitants and Gouves with its 239 inhabitants, also suffered heavily (85–90 and 70–75 percent, respectively). In the more prosperous village of Niata, c. 324 meters above sea level, about 55–60 percent of its 1,204 inhabitants had malaria; as was the case in Gouves, they were in the habit of purging themselves with castor oil to treat their fevers.[138] Myrtia extended over the slope of a hill with a splendid view over the olive groves and vineyards of the plain and the gulf, but after heavily rainy winters the marsh came within 2–3 kilometers of the village.

During 1906, which had been a dry year with a moderate malaria prevalence of 25–30 percent, cases lasted throughout the winter; this and the large amount of rain affected the level of infections the following year. The local doctor reversed the question: "You should rather ask 'How many escaped malaria?' because no one in our village or the surrounding villages was spared."[139] According to a Myrtia-based doctor, G. A. Verdos, the villages closest to the swamp—Dourali, Vriniko, and Vezani—where some of the inhabitants lived in straw huts, were the worst affected.[140]

In the extensive marsh of Elos, an area of some 15 square kilometers adjoining the sea was used as a fishery, a *vivari*, where the water reached a meter

---

135 Savvas and Kardamatis, "Apantiseis dimarkhon," 499.
136 Ibid., 502.
137 A. J. Pitkeathly, 185 Fd. Amb. RAMC, to H.Q. Tigerforce, Medical Report on Arcadia, Messina and Sparta, 14 March 1945, Rural Reports General, PAG-4/3.0.12.2.3.:11 [S-0527-0675], UN Archives.
138 Savvas and Kardamatis, "Apantiseis dimarkhon," 500.
139 Ibid., 500–501.
140 Ibid., 489.

in depth in the winter, when it also collected the runoff from the Mariorema and the neighboring swamps. Under such circumstances, presumably, its salinity fell and must have become even more attractive to *Anopheles* and more dangerous to humans. As it was considered a lake, it was state property and had never been considered for drainage.[141]

In the four communities of the municipality of Trinassos, on the western side of the Evrotas estuary, local physician Ilias Tsarpalis reported that, owing to an excessively rainy winter, more than 70 percent of the villagers had fallen ill with malaria, or more than the normal 50 percent; Stefania and Skala, however, had suffered even worse. Fresh infections had set in by mid-March, but malaria had continued the year round. Case mortality was 5 percent.

The area was most dangerous for nonimmune visitors. The two doctors who visited Elos in the summer of 1901 reported the infection of two topographers and an inspector of public revenue for Lakedaemon three days after spending "three nights by the Vassilopotamos estuary with no precaution against the innumerable *Anopheles*"; of ten soldiers who fell ill within one to three days of their arrival in Elos; of several cereal merchants, whom "the hospitality of the inhabitants kept more or less protected from the mosquitoes," but who all fell ill after their departure and of their own servant, who stopped taking her quinine and contracted fevers five days after leaving Elos. One of the two doctors, "who tried to escape the mosquitoes more than everyone else, after a few rare bites, fell ill 20 days after our departure with very intense fever attacks."[142]

The data collected by Kardamatis during the First World War, between 1915 and 1919, refers to the largest marshes of Trinissa that were estimated to cover an area of 25 square kilometers, the municipality suffering an average annual malaria prevalence of 70 percent; several more marshes arising from the Vasilopotamos and Evrotas rivers in the municipality of Elos, covering an area of 5 square kilometers; a swamp called Vrova and the fishery, or *vivari*, extending over 0.5 square kilometer and contributing to an annual malaria prevalence of 55 percent.[143] Nothing appears to have changed dramatically since the previous surveys, although the averaging conceals the annual fluctuations.

---

141 Ibid., 502.
142 Triantaphyllakos and Oeconomou, *Le paludisme*, 15.
143 Kardamatis, *Statistikoi pinakes*, 138 and 162.

Malaria took its toll on the Asia Minor refugees who settled in the wider area, specifically in the province of Lakedaimon.[144] On the basis of a survey of malaria prevalence for the years 1923 and 1924 conducted by the Anti-Malaria League in October 1924, assuming that its figures represent a satisfactory approximation, the broader province-level data reveal a vast difference between natives and refugees.[145] Furthermore, by 1923, malaria prevalence among the natives was smaller than the rest of the Peloponnese (32.3 percent)[146] and considerably less than the wartime average, when the entire prefecture of Lakonia had a 27.76 percent malaria prevalence and when the province, with 33.21 percent, was close to the 1907 percentage of 35 percent.[147]

Over a period of six years, between 1933 and 1938, from October to December, the Malariology Division of the Athens School of Hygiene conducted its nationwide annual spleen and parasite indexing, which included the 846 inhabitants of Skala in the surveys. The results revealed an alarmingly high level of malaria prevalence.[148] The area continued to have consistently high levels of endemic malaria.

Under the German occupation, some malaria control with Paris green, the arsenic-based larvicide that had been introduced in malaria control in the interwar years, continued each year in Sparta. New stations were created in Gytheio and Molaoi in 1942 and 1943.[149]

The UNRRA sanitary engineering section for the Peloponnese gave the area priority in summer 1945, quite early in its antimalaria campaign. The section established a DDT spraying team in Skala, where the sanitary engineer, Captain O'Brien, joined by his more experienced Greek colleague Nassos Comninos, "surveyed the region's *Anopheles* larval beds and planned the

---

144 The province included the marshland villages of Leimonas and Seidali, Skala, and Stefania.

145 Kardamatis, "Ekthesis ton pepragmenon pros peristolin tis elonosias kata to etos 1924," 410. The census figures for 1928 reveal a minute refugee presence in the province of Lakedaimon, a mere 1.1 percent and in the prefecture of Lakonia 0.9 percent. Only Skala had as many as 17 and Elos 18 and Panigyristra 23. See République Hellénique, Ministère de l'Économie Nationale, Statistique Générale de la Grèce, *Résultats statistiques*, 193–94, 201, and 206.

146 Livadas and Sfangos, *I elonosia en Elladi*, vol. 1, 58.

147 Kardamatis, *Statistikoi pinakes*.

148 Balfour, "Malaria Studies in Greece," 318; Livadas and Sfangos, *I elonosia en Elladi*, vol. 1, 162. Also, Zeiss, *Seuchen-Atlas*, Maps VII/4 and VII/4a. For an explanation of the difference of the two indices, see note p. 71, n. 102 in this book.

149 Malaria Control in Eastern Peloponnese, Programs Vol. IV Engineering Malaria Port, PAG-4/3.0.12.2.3.:9 [S-0527-0673], UN Archives.

Year	Cases examined	Splenic index	Parasite index
1933	99	80%	38%
1934	95	89%	58%
1935	94	89%	64%
1936	100	77%	34%
1937	84	63%	25%
1938	98	83%	54%

Table 2.1. Spleen and parasite indices, Skala, 1933–38
Source: Livadas and Sfangos, *I elonosia en Elladi*, vol. 1, 162.

campaign to destroy them," initially with Paris Green. By September, "DDT arrived and preparations were made for the all-out campaign with this powerful new chemical, which acted against both larva and adult mosquitoes." By the summer of 1946, these two men had "arranged protection for two-thirds of the villages of *the most highly malarious areas of the Peloponnesos* and thus saved thousands of persons from further suffering with this terrible disease."[150] In Trinissa, for instance, the local doctors reported that DDT spraying had reduced "the cases of acute malaria by comparison to previous years by 95 percent without exaggeration."[151] The swamps of Elos, Skala, and the Evrotas River area, a total of more than 4.2 square kilometers, benefited largely from DDT aerial spraying carried out in 1946. For better access, Elos was also provided with an airplane landing strip.[152]

The purpose of the campaign had not been to eradicate the *Anopheles*. As a WHO report noted in 1956, though malaria had disappeared from Elos as a result of insecticide spraying, throughout the entire prefecture of Lako-

---

150 Major G. Haber, "Final Report of Sub-Region 'B,'" pp. 19–20, Health Division Historical Report, Greece #35, Region "ABJ," PAG-4/4.2.:36 [S-0524-0060], UN Archives, emphasis added; W. Boyd, "Region 'ABJ,' Health Division, Historical Report," 30 November 1946, p. 44, Health Division Historical Report, Greece #35, Region "ABJ," PAG-4/4.2.:36 [S-0524-0060], UN Archives; A. Comninos to G. B. Haber, Kalamata, 2 February 1946, 657 Sanitary Reports, August 1945–September 1946, PAG-4/3.0.12.3.1.0.:8 [S-0527-0729], UN Archives.

151 [Illegible signature], to UNRRA Director General of Sanitation, Sparta, 24 August 1946, Correspondence concerning Engineering and Sanitation, PAG-4/3.0.12.2.3.:10 [S-0527-0674], UN Archives. A contemporary list of the Greek marshes noted that the Trinissa swamp had been drained although there is no indication of a date. "Pinax ton elon tis Ellados," p. 10, 651 Health, Medical Care and Sanitation Malaria, October 1943–July 1946, PAG-4/3.0.12.3.1.0.:8 [S-0527-0729], UN Archives.

152 Subregion "B," For DDT spraying, Region "ABJ," Programs Vol. IV Engineering Malaria Port, PAG-4/3.0.12.2.3.:9 [S-0527-0673], UN Archives; Map "Greece. UNRRA Sanitation Section 'Malaria Control DDT Airspray-Program 1946,' Malaria and Sanitation Greece #22, PAG-4/4.2.:35 [S-0524-0059], UN Archives.

nia, "there are anophelines but no malaria."[153] Skala was one of the first sites where resistance of A. *sacharovi* to DDT was observed and where experiments were conducted in the early 1950s.[154]

After the elimination of malaria, traces of its endemic presence remained in the frequencies of hemoglopinopathies, mostly β-thalassemia and sickle-cell anemia as a token of malaria's selective pressures.[155] In the prefecture-level screening results obtained by the late Nikolaos Skhizas and his coauthors on 15,550 army recruits and published in 1977, the prefecture of Lakonia ranked sixth highest, among 50, for the sickle-cell trait with 2.33 percent, far above the national average of 0.97 percent, and 19th highest for β-thalassemia, with 9.34 percent or slightly above the national average of 8.41 percent.[156] Given the millennia of year round malaria presence in the district, these high percentages, particularly those for the sickle-cell trait, suggest the effects of evolutionary pressures on the inhabitants. However, these figures refer to the entire prefecture; the contribution of the population of Elos to these averages must have been decisive. Whether its population enjoyed the advantage of natural resistance to malaria or not, it appears that they maintained a stable, perhaps millennia-long, residential pattern amid the physical and mental hardship caused by the disease.

Orkhomenos, Copais

The area of Lake Copais was one of the most emblematic malarious regions in Greece. Like most Greek lakes, its shoreline varied over time. It was the subject of drainage and land reclamation projects since antiquity. Millennia of malaria made the area, particularly the village of Petromagoula, one of the foci selected by a group of Greek hematologists and pediatricians in the

---

153 World Health Organization and the Interregional Conference on Malaria for the Eastern Mediterranean and European Regions, *Information*, 8.

154 Livadas and Georgopoulos, *Development of Resistance*; Livadas, "Malaria Vector Resistance"; De Zulueta, "Insecticide Resistance in *Anopheles Sacharovi*"; Hadjinicolaou and Betzios, "Resurgence of *Anopheles Sacharovi*." The A. sacharovi still in the area is contributing to the recent reemergence of *vivax* malaria cases. See Kousoulis et al., "Malaria in Laconia."

155 See chapter 1.

156 Skhizas et al., "Sykhnotis," 201. Khalkidiki and Lesvos, respectively, topped the sickle-cell and β-thalassemia frequency lists (or Arta and Corfu, respectively, from Old Greece).

late 1950s and early 1960s to study the sickle-cell trait and other polymorphisms associated with inherited immunity to malaria.[157]

A hydraulic and sanitary problem in ancient times, the lake and plain of Copais later acquired a place in medical topography in references to Thebes and the "swampy shores of Lake Topolias" in the eighteenth century.[158] Greek statehood added an economic dimension to its management.

Neglect of its maintenance since the demise of Ottoman authority led to a cumulative worsening of the situation each year, which resulted in gradual loss of farmland. As already noted, in Livadeia, out of the twenty ancient drainage conduits, whose traces were still visible in the early 1830s, only one was still working.[159]

One of the first severe epidemic outbreaks, requiring government help, occurred in the summer and autumn of 1834 in this area and was accompanied by a large number of deaths. Toward the end of summer 1834, the War Ministry received cries for help from the provinces of Thebes and Livadeia. By October the situation was perceived as a disaster, one "that is now beginning to become lethal." Unable to deal with the crisis, the only two doctors in the area welcomed the help of additional physicians sent out from Nafplio, the country's capital until December 1834, while the War Ministry supplied medicines for the poor. By late January 1835, the interior minister, Ioannis Kolettis, a doctor himself, considered the fever epidemic to be over but to have affected a large section of the population, including localities previously considered healthy. Kolettis blamed an "atmospheric constitution, which eschews the means of investigation and research of the art; one may also add to this cause the heavy rains and flooding that occurred during the months of last spring."[160]

---

157 Stamatoyannopoulos and Fessas, "Thalassaemia."

158 Finke, Versuch, vol. 1, 122; Hirsch, Handbook, 212–13; Davidson, Geographical Pathology, vol. 1, 238.

159 Thiersch, De l'état actuel, vol. 2, 17. Thiersch's purpose in writing about Copais was to promote the idea of draining the lake to increase national production.

160 I. Kolettis to King Othon, Athens, 21 January/2 February 1835, Sur les médecins envoyés à Thèbes et Lévadie, doc. 013, f. 193, Interior Ministry; also I. Kolettis to King Othon, Nafplio, 28 September/9 October 1834, doc. 003, f. 193, Interior Ministry; I. Kolettis to King Othon, Nafplio, 29 September/10 October 1834, doc. 004, f. 193, Interior Ministry; I. Kolettis to King Othon, Nafplio, 13/25 October 1834, doc. 005, f. 193, Interior Ministry, Othon's administration, GAK. There is evidence that, a few years later, the government tried to promote some drainage or small protective projects. A. Polyzoides to King Othon, Athens, 18 May 1837, "Concernant les travaux pour le lac de Copais," doc 012, f. 232, Interior Ministry, Othon's administration, GAK; the document does not mention fevers or health; G. Glarakis to King Othon, Athens, 18 October 1838, doc 025, f. 232, Interior Ministry, Othon's administration, GAK; the document refers to an order to the inhabitants of Kokkino, above Lake Copais, to block a water passage with rocks. See also Ruisinger, Das griechische Gesundheitswesen, 159–60.

In the 1838–40 survey, the villages around the lake were registered as "unhealthy" due to intermittent fevers and the two hallmarks of endemic fevers, cachexia and splenomegaly (*emphraxeis*, occlusions). Some of the villages, such as Karamousa in the municipality of Khaironia, were occupied only in the winter by Vlach shepherds (*vlakhopoimenes*), who withdrew to the mountains in the spring. The municipality of Orkhomenos also included Petromagoula and had a population of 1,430 inhabitants, who produced cereals, legumes and some vegetables, cotton, and wine. Petromagoula itself was said to be "very dangerous because of the frequent flooding" of the River Kifissos. Thus, "[i]n the summer and autumn, intestinal and intermittent fevers are endemic, occasionally accompanied by nervous and malignant symptoms. Chronic intermittent fevers are common as are chronic inflammations and enlargements of the organs of the abdomen, intestinal diarrheas [and] dysentery, particularly among young children." This brief description is consistent with endemic *vivax* and *falciparum* malaria, that is, with centuries of malaria mortality, evolutionary pressures and selection for the hemoglobinopathies studied in the 1950s and 1960s.

Livadeia, the district capital, was exposed to wintery winds that descended from the barren mountain above it. In the winter, these conditions produced acute inflammation diseases. In the summer, the daytime heat reflected from the mountain, which alternated with the nighttime chill and produced unhealthy conditions, according to the survey. Also in the summer, winds from the swamp swept unhealthy emanations into the town. The summer diseases listed were "gastric, continuous fevers, occasionally acute bowel and the liver inflammations of a nervous nature; children in particular suffered from diarrhea, dysentery, various types of intermittent fevers, especially toward the late summer and early autumn, occasionally accompanied by malignant and nervous symptoms, at times also latent fevers (*larvatae*)."[161]

In the municipality of Akraifnio, Topolia (now Kastro), the village that gave its name to the lake, had a population of 185 individuals, most of whom had developed cachexia. Mouriki had become a transient village of 102 individuals, who came to cultivate its fields from other municipalities rather than settle permanently. The lakeside village of Siggera was occupied by two

---

161 Kalogeropoulos, "Iatrostatistikoi pinakes tis dioikiseos Voiotias."

families, who grew wheat and barley, and were affected by "endemic intermittent fevers, cachexia and chronic inflammations of the abdomen" that were attributed to the proximity to the lake.

The town of Thebes and its surrounding villages, with a population of 2,929 inhabitants, mostly farmers and a few merchants, was situated in a healthy location and suffered sporadic intermittent fevers in the summer. Interestingly, the only resident physician in the entire prefecture of Boeotia, Nikolaos Kalogeropoulos, who conducted the survey, and the only pharmacist, Argyris Nikolaou, both lived in Livadeia. Thebes was served by only three licensed traditional doctors.[162]

By the mid-nineteenth century, firsthand medical observations of the broader area described Boeotia as a region totally subjected to intermittent fevers. Even harvest time brought "no crowds, no rejoicing, no laughter, no songs, and the imprint of malaria lay on all the faces," according to Henri Belle, a French diplomat who toured the region in the early 1870s.[163]

The people mostly grew grain, spoke Albanian, and were perceived as dull and backward. Fevers spread, as it was believed, by winds blowing over the virulent emanations of Lake Copais; they emerged each year in May, turned malignant in early August, peaked in September, and receded in October. Enlarged spleens were universal, which earned the inhabitants the nickname "*bakaniarides*" (big-bellies). Intestinal symptoms were also extremely common and associated with intermittent fevers, according to Titos Papadopoulos, the local physician. Two observations impressed him most: "Many inhabitants with considerably large spleens have never felt the convulsions of intermittent fevers, other than loss of appetite, fatigue, occasional pains—all symptoms that gradually build up a marshland malaise."[164]

Equally striking was the size of some of their spleens, particularly in children. In some cases, they occupied the entire abdomen. Papadopoulos, who singled out the villages of Vagia, Neokhori, and Palaiopanagia, was amazed to see one such child living to become a hard-working, twenty-four-year-old adult.[165] The situation, according to Papadopoulos, was no better in the town of Thebes; it was just as subjected to intermittent fevers as the rest of

---

162 Ibid.
163 Belle, *Trois années en Grèce*, 131.
164 Papadopoulos, "Physiologia," 450.
165 Ibid., 454–55.

the Boeotian plain, but its inhabitants "were beginning to become slightly more civilized. . . . The art of medicine cannot advance, without being preceded by the intervention and performance of superstition,"[166] was his melancholic conclusion.

Following a cotton boom in the 1860s a large number of Livadiots had partially drained swathes of land in the Copaïs plain, which they were now exploiting with rented labor to raise cotton and maize. They had begun on a small scale with very rudimentary means but some had almost tripled their original capital investment in the meantime.[167]

Some twenty years later, contrasting the area to the general improvement of the rest of the country, Stéphanos singled out Copais as the lake par excellence that spread malarial fevers to its surrounding villages and was one of the few remaining locations with serious and extensive malarial cachexia, although the expanse of the affected area was diminishing.[168] He associated the spread of malaria with the cultivation of grain. "The same applies, to a lesser degree, to lakes surrounded by arid soil or devoted primarily to the cultivation of cereals (already harvested by the time of the great increase of malaria), such as Lake Copais, etc., which are the starting points of light breezes that flow all around above a burning terrain."[169] The fact that the fields had already been harvested when malaria spread suggested to Stéphanos that the gentle winds were free to carry the miasma over the "burning soil" of the empty fields.

Copais remained a heavily malarious area even after its drainage, proof that if left incomplete, drainage works could worsen the situation by creating thousands of small pools of stagnant water.[170] After a succession of failed drainage and colonization projects by Greek, French, and British entrepreneurs, and with local farmers constantly encroaching on the receding shoreline, a French company completed the project in 1886. Soon afterward, the exposed peat that had accumulated at the bottom of the lake auto-ignited. The fire burned for several years and reduced the level of the former lake

166 Ibid., 460.
167 Belle, *Trois années en Grèce*, 158–60.
168 Stéphanos, *La Grèce*, 492 and 501.
169 Ibid., 496.
170 Livieratos, "I elonosia," 175–76. Indeed, Kardamatis argued that lakes and swamps distracted lay and medical attention away from smaller water collections, which were a more serious threat to public health. See Kardamatis, *Statistikoi pinakes*, 177.

by some 4 meters, eventually destroying the entire French drainage system. Under a new contract with the Greek government, the British-owned Lake Copais Company took over the assets of the French company in July 1887 and completed the work in September 1892. As a result, farm labor arrived from outside the area, for instance from Zeriki (now Elikonas) and Kyriaki in the municipality of Distomo,[171] to cultivate the land reclaimed from the lake, now an estate of some 243 square kilometers owned and managed by the British company.[172] The 1880s fire though reduced the productivity of the soil and must have also unsettled the habitat of the local *Anopheles* population.[173]

Even after the completion of the Copais drainage project, much of the broader region was still covered by marshes, ensuring that endemic malaria remained a serious problem. In 1901 the two doctors of Skripou, in the municipality of Orkhomenos, reported that, despite the public works in the area such as the widening and deepening of the River Melas and the draining of Lake Copais, they had not observed any significant difference in the occurrence of malaria. That year it was on the increase owing to a rainy spring and remained endemic with a great deal of cachexia. "The worse foci of fevers are the uncultivated areas around the villages of the municipality; those slightly healthier are the more cultivated."[174]

The area had suffered three successive rainy years from 1903 to 1905, "when the humidity was great in the spring and fevers were general (100 percent)." In 1906, thanks to a dry winter and the drought that ensued, fevers were much less prevalent throughout the area. Malignant fevers were generally controlled with quinine.[175]

Owing to the suffering caused by the 1905 epidemic, the Copais Company invited Ronald Ross to recommend antimalarial measures for the relief of its staff, who were managing an estate "of some 60,000 acres [243 square kilometers] of reclaimed lake or swamp."[176] Ross spent a good week,

---

171 Savvas, Kardamatis, and Dasios, "1906," 471.
172 A. C. Whitmee, Secretary, Lake Copais Company, to Ross, 22 December 1905, Ross/89/02/02, London School of Hygiene and Tropical Medicine (LSHTM) Archive.
173 Fatouros, *Limnon periigisis*, 232–33.
174 "Apantiseis ton k. Iatron," 202.
175 The worse hit was the village of Agios Georgios in the municipality of Petra. Savvas, Kardamatis, and Dasios, "1906," 471–72.
176 A. C. Whitmee, Secretary, Lake Copais Company, to Ross, 22 December 1905, Ross/89/02/02, London School of Hygiene and Tropical Medicine (LSHTM) Archive.

from 28 May to 4 June 1906, that is, early in the malaria season, in Moulki (present-day Aliartos), the seat of the company, and studied the area with the help of Kardamatis, who joined him on his visit.[177] Like most foreign visitors, Ross had not anticipated the level of malaria, which he found comparable to the disease in India and Africa. Particularly in Skripou, "almost every child had an enormous spleen due to malaria," as he recalled in his *Memoirs*.[178]

The Copais Company benefited from Ross's recommendations and managed to reduce the amount of the disease among their staff; during the 1908 malaria season the company manager was able to report that the number of mosquitoes and fevers was the smallest in local memory.[179] Beyond its office and residential compound, however, malaria remained a serious threat to the company. Furthermore, in contrast to the company's seat at Moulki, villages further away, for instance along the Melas river, such as Petra and Skripou, where no measures had been applied, had seen no improvement.[180]

Kardamatis returned three years after his first visit, in November 1909, with Daniel Steele, the director of the Copais Company, to conduct a comparative investigation with the data he and Ross had collected in May 1906 and with an additional item on his agenda: to confirm the efficacy of state quinine in malaria control.[181] The two men also inspected the company's sanitization work at the staff residences in Krimbas and the company's offices in nearby Moulki and established that 61 percent of the British and Greek staff members had contracted malaria that year. In May 1906, 24 percent of the company's staff members had been found with enlarged spleens. No protection could shield them from the mosquitoes in the surrounding villages and other places, where their work duties took them.[182] There the

---

177 Envelope with notes of dates Ross's visit to Greece, Ross/89/02/01.

178 Ross, *Memoirs*, 495. Ross used the hellenized name for Skripou, Orkhomenos. Requested to do so, Ross also examined the towns of Thebes and Livadeia, where more British employees resided, for "their suitability for the residence of members of the office staff during the Malaria season." See A. C. Whitmee to Ross, 15 May 1906, Ross/89/02/27; Ross to A. C. Whitmee, 16 May 1906 (copy), Ross/89/02/28 and Results of spleen examinations round Lake Copais, June 1906, Ross/89/02/36. Ross and Kardamatis carried out spleen examinations on 373 people, of whom 100 were children from Thebes, Moulki, Mazi, Orkhomenos, and Livadia (Ross/89/02/41). Kardamatis then proceeded with the blood examinations to Athens. See Kardamatis, *Ai aparkhai tis exygiaseos tou khoriou Moulki*.

179 Excerpt from the manager's report for the year 1908, Lake Copais Company, 1909, Ross/89/02/51 and B. C. McElderry, Lake Copais Company, to the manager of the company, 22 January 1909, Ross/89/02/52.

180 D. Steele, Works Manager, Lake Copais Company, to Ross, 29 June 1909, Ross/89/02/56.

181 Kardamatis, *Ai aparkhai tis exygiaseos tou khoriou Moulki*.

182 Ibid., 43–44. Results of spleen examinations round Lake Copais, June 1906, Ross/89/02/36.

situation appeared unchanged, particularly in two sources of infection: Moulki itself and Skripou.

As Kardamatis revealed, Moulki, a village of 553 inhabitants to the west of the former lake, was victim of its own progress, as the *Anopheles* source now lay in the pools that formed in ditches along the railway track, in the canals that drained the former lake as well as in several small water collections.[183]

By contrast, Skripou, which lay to the north of the lake and was home to 1,124 inhabitants, had been affected neither by the drainage of the lake nor by any protection schemes. At a small distance to its north, the Spring of the Graces (Hariton springs) gave rise to several more springs over a distance of a kilometer along the foot of Mount Akontio. These springs gushed out huge amounts of cool, clear water, even in the midst of droughts, and generated the River Melas and a marsh of around 0.45 square kilometers "full of aquatic plants and reeds with an abundance of vegetable and animal life-forms, fish among them" and *A. superpictus*. The source of endemic malaria lay in this marsh, in the Souvala marsh and in several small collections of stagnant water.[184]

In fact, a comparative blood examination of the schoolchildren below the age of sixteen in Skripou and Moulki revealed that the two villages were equally infected in autumn 1909, as they had been in spring 1906. One in two schoolchildren had been found with equally enlarged spleens in spring 1906 and in autumn 1909, an indication of a long history of malaria.[185] Malaria symptoms though in Moulki had been milder in 1909; a new law a year earlier, introducing the state-controlled importation of quinine from Italy, meant that better-quality quinine was available.[186] On the basis of the blood examinations of the local schoolchildren,[187] Kardamatis saw a general

---

183 Kardamatis, *Ai aparkhai tis exygiaseos tou khoriou Moulki*, 47.

184 Ibid., 45–47. In the interwar years, the RF IHD malariologists noted: "The drainage of the lake has created a big and prosperous looking agricultural area though malaria still exists. Villages, however, are practically all on the hill slopes around about and it may be that they suffer from *superpictus* malaria from small streams that pass in the hills near by rather than from the breeding in the flats." G. K. Strode diary, entry 27 May 1933, RF, RAC.

185 Kardamatis, *Aparkhai exygiaseos tou khoriou Moulki*, 47–48; Kardamatis, *Pragmateia*, 590.

186 Kardamatis, *Aparkhai exygiaseos tou khoriou Moulki*, 54.

187 At the time, as he wrote later, taking "a drop of blood from their dirty little fingers," Ross attracted the interest and, eventually, the affection of "the whole village—priest, headman, innkeeper, mothers, children, dogs, fowls and fleas." Ross, *Memoirs*, 496.

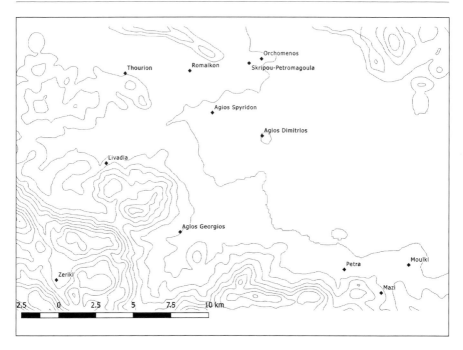

Map 2.4. Copais, 1901–7

reduction of infections between 1906 and 1909, which fell from a rate of 80 to 60 percent in Moulki and from 88 to 44 percent in Skripou. From these reduced figures Kardamatis inferred the beneficial effect of state quinine, rather than of the protective measures taken by the management of the Copais Company. As to the distribution of *Plasmodia* between the two dates, *malariae* and *vivax* malaria prevailed in May[188] and *falciparum* malaria dominated the November infections.[189]

During the First World War, the Orkhomenos area continued to suffer from a spectacular annual average 80 percent malaria morbidity, according to Kardamatis's tables—a level that ranked third among all the municipalities of Old Greece. The municipality of Orkhomenos remained under the influence of the swamps at Dipoti, a swamp of 0.9 square kilometers, at Hariton springs, of 0.45 square kilometers and numerous other smaller

---

188 Respective frequencies were nineteen *malariae*, fourteen *vivax*, and seven *falciparum*.
189 Respective frequencies were fourteen *malariae*, twenty-one *vivax*, fifty-nine *falciparum*, one *malariae* and *falciparum*, two *vivax* and *falciparum*. Kardamatis, *Aparkhai exygiaseos tou khoriou Moulki*, 49–53.

swamps.[190] The municipality of Petra contained swamps at Forteiko (0.85 square kilometers) and other locations, all of which produced a prevalence of 50 percent.[191] The springs, streams, and drainage ditches continued to create *Anopheles* breeding grounds, even at higher altitudes. Kardamatis criticized the drainage project for the priority it had given to land reclamation rather than sanitization.

> An example of such negative results from a malariological perspective are the plains of Rome and our own Lake Copais, where the marshlands have disappeared and the soil was drained [and where] the companies and the state have profited greatly from agriculture; however, public health has not benefited in the least, because malaria is intensely endemic and extensive, for the sole reason that the sanitization works were executed on the basis of the old theories of malaria causation, ignoring the importance of small collections of stagnant water according to current theories.[192]

Kardamatis further noted that in 1923 malaria prevalence among the natives in the entire province of Thebes was 20 percent as opposed to 70 percent among the Asia Minor refugees.[193]

In the 1930s, when the RF team studied malaria in Greece, the disease persisted with spleen rates of 80 percent, owing to *Anopheles* breeding in the drainage ditches of former Lake Copais. Malaria had declined in "intensity" and mortality, but as long as methods of irrigation and drainage were not improved, it remained a serious problem.[194] Moulki, Skripou, and Petromagoula suffered a severe epidemic in September 1930; among the children attending the Moulki school the splenic rate was 84 percent with "enormous spleens" and half the population was ill. Maintenance of the drainage ditches had been interrupted a few months earlier on account of a court dispute between the villagers and the Copais Company.[195] Even on the eve of

---

190 Kardamatis cited Souvala (0.4 square kilometers), an unnamed swamp at Elliniko of 0.06 square kilometers, small collections of water from the Kifissos River, canals, and ditches. Kardamatis, *Statistikoi pinakes*, 126.

191 Ibid., 32, 126, 182, and 197. Kardamatis cited an unnamed swamp of 0.266 square kilometers, at Plaka and Degle bridge (0.003 square kilometers each) and several small water collections. Ibid., 126.

192 Ibid., 248.

193 Ibid., 253.

194 Balfour, "Some Features," 12–13; entry 3092, 9 November 1930, Strode diary 1930, RFA, RAC.

195 [Mikhai Ciucă], Organisation de la lutte antimalarique en Grèce, Geneva, 14 February 1931, pp. 6–8, CH/Malaria/154, Malaria Commission, Health Organisation, League of Nations.

the Second World War, the Malariology Division of the Athens School of Hygiene still recorded an 80 percent splenic rate and a 40 percent parasite index at Skripou, which were among the highest rates in the country.[196]

It is worth noting that like the Copais project, the ambitious drainage and land reclamation projects of the late 1920s in the valleys of Axios and Strymon in Macedonia failed to eliminate malaria. As noted by malariologist Christos Damkas in his 1946 report, drainage created new breeding sites "in drainage ditches with marsh formation, pits from which soil was taken, old dykes etc." Other than drainage no additional antimalarial measures were carried out in these valleys and malaria epidemics continued to break out as previously.[197]

The situation in the Copais plain after liberation from the German occupation was described in an UNRRA report of February 1945. The villages, Skripou and Petromagoula among them, were approximately 100 percent malarious. Cotton plantations in the drained marshland that "require watering every ten days so that the soil is kept permanently humid with collections of water into small pools where the *Anopheles* breeds" were responsible for the failure to reduce malaria morbidity. A shortage of quinine, which resulted in the inefficient distribution of some ten tablets per individual, was also to blame.[198] The UNRRA antimalarial campaign in the Copais area began in May 1945 in Moulki, the seat of the Copais Company, which assumed half the labor cost for the measures, while at the same time requesting UNRRA to provide equipment, DDT, and quinine for its own property and staff.[199] After the 1946 and 1947 campaigns the company director called the effect "little short of miraculous," adding:

---

196 Livadas and Sfangos, *I elonosia en Elladi*, vol. 1, 160.

197 Christos Damkas, "Malaria," p. 560, Health Division, Final Report (November 1946), Greece Mission, Region "EG" (Northern Greece), Health Division Final Report, Greece #38, Region "EG," PAG-4/4.2.:36 [S-0524-0060], UN Archives.

198 Paris Consantinides, Report on the General and Especially on the Health Situation of Levadhia District, 7 February 1945, Provincial 11-17 Levadhia, PAG-4/3.0.12.2.3.:7 [S-0527-0671], UN Archives. Other villages included in this report were Agios Spyridon, Agios Dimitrios, Thourio, Davlia, and Romeiko. Another report noted that 30 percent of the population in Petromagoula were under the age of fourteen, a sign perhaps that it had been "comfortable, well-to-do" before the war. Dorothy MacKay, Child Welfare Specialist to Harry White, Athens, 12 July 1945, Provincial 11-17 Levadhia, PAG-4/3.0.12.2.3.:7 [S-0527-0671], UN Archives.

199 Activities and Programme of Sanitation Section, p. 2 (draft), Sanitation 01-00, PAG-4/3.0.12.2.3.:1 [S-0527-0665], UN Archives; G. L. Daily, Lake Copais Company to Chief of Medical Section, Athens, 28 May 1945, Sanitation 01-50 Malaria, PAG-4/3.0.12.2.3.:1 [S-0527-0665], UN Archives.

Where previously it was common for more than half of the population of the 52 villages bordering on the erstwhile Copaic lake to be down with malarial fever, particularly in the autumn months of August–October, there has hardly been a single case during the past two years. This is strikingly evidenced not only in the more plentiful labor supply thereby made available but also of its more virile quality.[200]

In their research on hemoglobinopathies in Greece mentioned earlier, George Stamatoyannopoulos and Phaedon Fessas found that a large number, 20.2 percent, of the schoolchildren of Petromagoula they examined had heterozygous sickle-cell anemia, "a very high frequency," and that 12.6 percent had thalassemia.[201] These findings indicated that the local population had developed these high frequencies in response to centuries of selective pressures caused by *falciparum* malaria, as suggested by the malaria hypothesis. Prefecture-level data from the 1970s, however, present a less dire picture. In screenings of army recruits the prefecture of Boeotia ranked eighth among fifty for the sickle-cell trait (2.02 percent), and twenty-second for thalassemia (8.58 percent being heterozygous).[202]

An area of heavy malaria endemicity, Copais remained a focus of the disease, true to its legendary image well into the modern era, even after 1892 when the lake was drained.

Petalidi

In the account of his experience with the French Scientific Expedition in the Peloponnese, Bory de Saint-Vincent reported that Petalidi, on the western coast of the Messenian Gulf, was "unhealthy" when he and his companions camped there in September 1828 along with a French military contingent. However, while the intervening hills and mountains were healthy, the western littoral of the peninsula, Navarino, already recorded in Finke's medical geography, and the Gialova lagoon were infinitely more malarious and lethal than the east[203];

---

200 Resident Director, Lake Copais Company, to D. E. Wright, Athens, 24 February 1948, folder 4, box 1, D. E. Wright papers.

201 Stamatoyannopoulos and Fessas, "Thalassaemia," 877.

202 Skhizas et al., "Sykhnotis," 201.

203 Finke, *Versuch*, vol. 3, 96.

the army's cases of fever increased more than tenfold within two weeks of en-tering the western zone during the September rains. To their horror, the French noted that the Egyptian Army, which had preceded them on the same location, had suffered terrible, sudden losses; the French presumed that the Egyptians had died of "malignant fevers."[204]

Even years later, when peace had been restored, the area around Petal-idi, comprising three municipalities, all in the province of Pylia, continued to be sparsely populated and impoverished. At the time of the 1838–40 sur-vey, the municipality of Vias, of which Zaimogli was the principal town, had no more than twelve families and no endemic diseases.[205] Its fertile land was mostly uncultivated and its olive trees had turned wild and awaited grafting. Its small production, consisting of some wheat, barley, maize, oats, cotton, wine, cheese, wool, and animals, was destined for self-consumption rather than for the market. In the neighboring municipality of Voufrasio, the hilly terrain was covered with a forest that supplied shipping timber; its plain, cultivated with grain, cotton, and tobacco, also produced silk, wine, wool, cheese, butter, and animals. The principal town, Vlakhopoulo, with eighty families, lay on a hilltop with trees and vineyards and was reported to be healthy. Only the forty-five families of Veli, a village in a recess, where "the air cannot blow freely," with a small swamp, suffered from malignant inter-mittent and chronic fevers and splenomegaly.[206] Finally, the municipality of Koroni also consisted of hilly and fertile terrain, uncultivated with indig-enous trees suitable for grafting. It was well irrigated and healthy and pro-duced a small amount of wheat, barley, maize, onions, wool, cheese, butter, and animals. Petalidi, the principal town of merely sixty-seven families by the coast, partly lay in a recess and was mildly unhealthy: men suffered from "simple" intermittent fevers, whereas the children had helminthic infections and "abdominal occlusions," perhaps enlarged abdomens. Of the remaining villages,[207] only Polystari, with no more than eighteen families at the foot of a hill, was reported likewise to be unhealthy.

---

204 Bory de Saint-Vincent, *Relation*, vol. 1, 225–27.
205 The remaining villages were Pelekanada, Kourtaki, Daras, Miska (Neromylos) and Karakasili. Galatis, "Iatrostatistikoi pinakes tis dioikiseos Messinias kai tis ypodioikiseos Pylias."
206 The remaining villages were Khatzi, Arnaoutali (Petritsi), Kroustesi (Kharavgi), Khalapreza (Kalokho-ri), Somiri, Soulinari, and Kambai. In ibid.
207 Khaikali (Akhladokhori), Vigla, Kakorama, Pera, Pastrimogli, Paniperi, Polystari, Kastania, Dranga (Mathia), Lefka, Bali (Agia Paraskevi), and Trypes. In ibid.

The relatively light malaria burden of the 1830s may indirectly reflect Mavrogiannis's general mortality estimates for the Peloponnese. Mavrogiannis calculated prefecture deaths per population on the basis of numbers of deaths for 1839 and population figures for 1840. Argolis (1:31.7), Achaia (1:35.8), Ileia (1:44.7), Messinia (1:46.5), and Korinthia (1:47.4) had the worst rates, Trifylia (1:75.7) and Pylia (1:88.8) were clearly in a better condition, while the Peloponnese average was one death for every 52.6 inhabitants.[208]

During the currant boom of the 1870s and 1880s, when currant cultivation spread to the southwestern Peloponnese, the town of Petalidi prospered, helped by its fertile soil and meandering irrigation canals fed from the numerous streams crisscrossing the area, although a river had silted at less than an hour's distance from the town and one-quarter of the surrounding land still remained uncultivated. In the years before the boom, Mount Manglavas, which rose to the west of Petalidi, had been entirely free of malaria. However, when the villagers cleared the forest to cultivate and irrigate the slope, and to take advantage of the high exports prices for currants, the disease advanced to settlements at higher altitudes from the plain below. Subsequently, after the currant trade crashed in the early 1890s, the town and its surrounding area readapted to the new market realities. Meanwhile, by the time of the 1907 survey, malaria had also infected inhabitants in the village of Vlakhopoulo, one of the largest in the region, which was situated at an altitude of 450 meters. Further downhill, at an altitude of about 260 meters, the villages of Kastania, Bali, Polystari, and Panyperi were all seriously affected by malaria in the same year. The reason given in the survey was that peasants used to sleep outdoors to guard their crops.

On average, as many as 80 percent contracted malaria, mostly in September and October, although Petalidi itself, a town of 2,000 inhabitants, usually only suffered from a malaria morbidity of 30 percent. However, in 1905, an epidemic year for most of Greece, the town also experienced 80 percent malaria prevalence. Particularly, though, in the villages Miska and Karakasili nearly all of the inhabitants were chronic malaria cases, perhaps

---

208 Mavrogiannis, "Protai grammai iatrikis topografias," 314; Mavrogiannis, "Protai grammai mias topografias," 539 and 543.

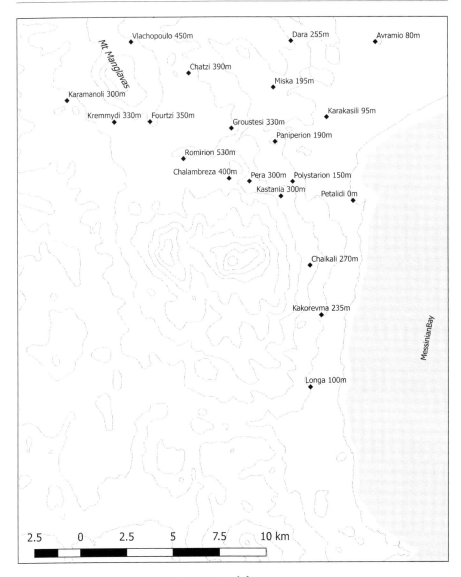

Map 2.5. Petalidi, 1901–7

owing to poor water absorption in the soil. In most villages malaria was well entrenched, varying slightly over the years in prevalence and virulence and with some 50 percent of chronic cases.[209]

---

209 "Apantiseis ton k. Iatron," 233; "1905. Ai peri tis kata topous elonosias pliroforiai ton Iatron," 444; Savvas, Kardamatis, and Dasios, "1906," 582; "1907," 372 and 530–33.

Thus, though economically quite comfortable, by the early twentieth century these peasants carried a heavy and quite constant malaria burden, most of all their children. Spleen examinations on the 190 primary and secondary schoolchildren of Petalidi in October 1907 produced a 37 percent splenic rate; as many as 85 percent of the children reported having contracted malaria that year. The disease seriously affected youths under the age of fifteen, particularly children below the age of five. The local doctor found women to be particularly affected by cachexia and attributed six out of ten deaths indirectly to malaria. "If one observes the local population, he will see that vigour and life are totally lacking," he noted.[210]

Approximately ten years later, the average malaria morbidity rate between 1915 and 1919 for the municipality of Petalidi was calculated at 45 percent, with the landscape much the same, consisting of "many small collections of water, especially in canals and streams."[211] Even after another twenty years of malaria control work, the area of Petalidi in the late 1930s remained heavily and endemically malarious and, according to the data of the Greek Malariology Service, with more *falciparum* than *vivax* malaria, a splenic index of 62 percent and a parasite rate of 37 percent, as shown in the following table.

Year	Splenic index	Parasite index
1937	56%	20%
1938	66%	41%
1939	68%	37%

Table 2.2 Spleen and parasite indices, Petalidi, 1937–39
Source: Livadas and Sfangos, *I elonosia en Elladi*, vol. 1, 162.

Thus, even though recording methods varied between surveys, and, more importantly, nosological entities were not identical from 1838 to 1901, the evidence suggests that in the broader Petalidi area malaria had set in and increased between these two dates, largely owing to increased cultivation, irrigation, and deforestation. A relatively underdeveloped healthy area with

---

210 Gardikas, "Health Policy and Private Care," 135–37; "Apantiseis ton k. Iatron," 234.
211 Kardamatis, *Statistikoi pinakes*, 58 and 137.

no marshes became a zone whose peasants, although not particularly poor, carried a heavy and constant burden of endemic malaria. In fact, the 1915–19 survey only recorded "many small collections, particularly in channels and streams in the locations of Sidirogevanou, Platanaki, Neratza, and Mati."[212]

Late in the period of German occupation, in 1944, a malaria control station was set up in Petalidi for Paris green control work. UNRRA, in collaboration with the Athens School of Hygiene, set up a malaria control station there in 1945, when Petalidi was found to be 100 percent malarious, badly in need of antimalarial drugs, and introduced DDT residual spraying and, later on, aerial spraying.[213]

In the history of Petalidi, the century and a half since statehood was accompanied by economic development but also the spread of malaria.

Sopoto

The area of Sopoto (present-day Aroania) is a case that helps question the commonly held perception that malaria is primarily a disease of the lowlands. While it is true, as Robert Sallares has pointed out, that altitude becomes only a relative source of protection when work sends mountain people to the dangerous fields in the plains, the case of Sopoto demonstrates that the disease can become entrenched in the mountain plateaus and create independent and permanent malaria foci.[214] According to John McNeill, in trying to escape the malarial lowlands in the eighteenth and nineteenth centuries, populations in Epirus, Lucania in Italy, and Anatolia in Turkey moved above the 500 meter threshold, thus increasing the ecological pressure on the fragile mountain environment and contributing to the spread of malaria, which transformed "from a sporadic risk into a true scourge."[215] Such was the case of Sopoto and the entire Kalavryta region.

The broader district of Patras was, in fact, described by Melville Douglas MacKenzie, a member or the League of Nations Commission who visited

212 Ibid., 137.

213 Malaria Control in Eastern Peloponnese, Programs Vol. IV Engineering Malaria Port, PAG-4/3.0.12.2.3.:9 [S-0527-0673], UN Archives; A. Flithet, General Aspect of Villages Visited 1–3 August [1945], Rural Reports Laconia, PAG-4/3.0.12.2.3.:11 [S-0527-0675], UN Archives; Summary monthly report adult control DDT residual spraying, 15 August–15 September 1946, p. 3, Programs Vol. IV Engineering Malaria Port, PAG-4/3.0.12.2.3.:9 [S-0527-0673], UN Archives.

214 Sallares, *Malaria and Rome*, 60.

215 McNeill, *Mosquito Empires*, 350.

the region in February 1929, as follows: "A striking feature of the mountainous country about Patras is the large number of deep-cut ravines and stony beds of mountain torrents which must form at certain times of the year ideal breeding places for mosquitoes."[216]

Sopoto lies in the mountains of the northern Peloponnese, south of Kalavryta, with settlements at altitudes ranging between 500 and 1000 meters above sea level. The physical and social environment differed from the southwestern Peloponnese. It had a shorter and cooler malaria season, thanks to higher altitudes and reduced day lengths, while each settlement lay isolated in its own individual valley that was part of an interconnected network of other valleys and ravines.[217] Sopoto was the principal town of the municipality of Aroania.[218]

On his visit in February 1806, Leake saw an abundance of streams and torrents, vines and maize, gardens and fruit trees. The inhabitants of Sopoto were driven away, not by disease but by the oppression of the notable "Asimaki of Kalavryta, whose worse than Turkish oppression obliges the people to leave the place, so that many houses are empty."[219] In the 1838–40 survey though, Kalavryta, the principal town of the province of Kynaithi, was described as an unhealthy, treeless place occupying a plateau and its adjoining mountain slope. It produced grain, wine, butter, cheese, and wool. The list of prevailing diseases was quite alarming:

[P]neumonia, pleurisy, hepatitis, or liver inflammation, rheumatism, catarrh, diarrhea, dysentery, [and] continuous [*synokhoi*] gastro-choleric and intermittent fevers. These latter fevers are almost always accompanied by gastric or choleric and also nervous symptoms, in the summer and autumn appear with an epidemic character, many of them being malignant. Chloroses, hysterias, and chronic inflammations of the lower abdomen and helminthic fevers among young children.[220]

---

216 League of Nations, Health Organisation, Health Committee, [Villages in District of Patra], 1. Of the sanitary state of the prefecture as a whole, another review noted that it was confronted with malaria and tuberculosis as well as the threat of plague. League of Nations, Health Organisation, Health Committee, *Patras*, 19.

217 See the microecologies offered in Horden and Purcell, *The Corrupting Sea*.

218 The name of the district in the 1838–40 survey was Kynaithi, following the administrative reforms of 1836, but Kalavryta was reintroduced as its official name in 1845 at the time of a new administrative reform.

219 Leake, *Travels in the Morea*, vol. 2, 252–55.

220 Anninos, "Iatrostatistikoi pinakes tis dioikiseos Kynaithis."

As far as intermittent fevers were concerned, their manifestations were in-testinal, choleric, and neurological and are described as often epidemic in nature and malignant, stagnant water collections being blamed as the cause. The general condition of poor health was attributed to the town's lo-cation with its unexpected atmospheric changes, the humidity and mias-matic emanations from stagnant waters, the nearby cultivation of maize, and the general state of filth.[221] The state physician carrying out the sur-vey recommended migration from Kalavryta, which he thought would be a simple matter, "since it has very few inhabitants and it is unlikely that it should ever acquire more on account of the unhealthiness of the climate and its remoteness from commerce." Also, drainage and cultivation of the marshlands and uncultivated lands, prohibition of maize cultivation, cleanliness and better housing and living conditions were required. As for treatment, he prescribed the "anti-inflammatory method for the inflamma-tions [and] antiperiodic for fevers."[222]

By contrast, however, the municipalities of Aroania (2,788 inhabitants), Psofis (2,220 inhabitants), Kleitoria (1,870 inhabitants), and Paos (1,583 in-habitants) were described as mountainous, wooded, and generally healthy with rivers running through them. Specifically Sopoto, the principal town, situated at an altitude of around 900 meters, as well as the remaining vil-lages of the Aroania municipality,[223] produced grain, wine, tobacco, chest-nuts, and butter; they lay among fruit trees and were reported to be healthy with some intermittent fevers in the summer and autumn. Likewise, Livar-tzi, the principal town of the municipality of Psofis, which was situated at an altitude of around 850 meters, was described as relatively healthy with some intermittent fevers, with the remaining villages fully healthy.[224] The municipality of Kleitoria had a summer principal town, Mazi—a healthy place on a mountaintop surrounded by trees—and a winter principal town,

---

221 In his *Mosquito Empires* (p. 205), J. R. McNeill has drawn the connection between maize cultivation and malaria on the basis of evidence from Ethiopia. Indeed, research by a Boston University and Harvard School of Public Health team in that country found that consumption of maize pollen contributed to the successful breeding of anopheles larvae and, thus, to the size of the adult anopheles population. McCann, *Historical Ecology of Malaria in Ethiopia*, loc. 2358 and 2362. For an association with irrigation practices, see chapter 3.

222 Anninos, "Iatrostatistikoi pinakes tis dioikiseos Kynaithis."

223 The remaining villages were Anastasova, Dyskos, Dravolavós, Mostitzi, Kastalia, Kleitor, Tzaroukhli, Agridi, and the Agioi Theodoroi monastery.

224 The remaining villages were Morokhova, Khozova, Lekhouri, Keresova, and Kamenianoi.

Mazeika (since renamed Kleitoria), which was treeless, situated on a hill in the middle of a plateau at an altitude of around 550 meters, and unhealthy. Suffering was more serious in the autumn, a fact suggesting that *falciparum* malaria had already become entrenched. The remaining villages were healthy.[225] Strezova (now Dafni), the principal town of the municipality of Paos, occupied the foot of a wooded mountain and was generally healthy with only rare simple intermittents in the summer, consistent mostly with *vivax* malaria.[226] Therefore, with the exception of Kalavryta, and a limited amount of fevers in the other main towns, the general state of health in the area in the late 1830s appears to have been satisfactory, particularly in the small mountain villages.

By the turn of the century, the region had clearly changed from a sanitary perspective. Like the country in general, the entire region had benefited from the currant market boom of the 1870s and 1880s. Apart from a certain amount of internal migration, the mountain population also participated in the boom as a result of the need for seasonal labor in the vineyards and in the export trade. Grain imports became more affordable thanks to the improved balance of trade generated by currant exports. As a result, the population of Greece benefited overall with a rise in its nutritional standard.[227] The collapse of the currant market in the 1890s, therefore, spelled poverty for the mountain peasantry. Without an outlet in the currant-producing hills and plains of the south- and northwestern Peloponnese, peasant families from the impoverished mountain villages adapted to the new economic circumstances by sending their sons in large numbers as migrants to America.[228]

Meanwhile, malaria appears to have developed into a serious problem for the entire region. Writing in the early 1880s on the basis of information from local doctors, Stéphanos identified the "elevated basins of Kalavryta" as a location of epidemics of "pernicious fevers" signifying that *falciparum* malaria had become prominent in the disease mix.[229] From at least 1896, further to the northwest of Sopoto, in the plateau of Soudena, and later on

---

225 The remaining villages were Kani, Karnesi, Vrostena, Kastriá, Plaktyrou, and Arpounas.

226 The remaining villages were Nasia, Vosini, Skoupi.

227 Kalafatis, *Agrotiki pisti kai oikonomikos metaskhimatismo*, vol. 1, 130–33; Petmezas, "Agrotiki oikonomia," 110; Franghiadis, "Peasant Agriculture and Export Trade," 37.

228 Franghiadis, "Peasant Agriculture and Export Trade," 291–94.

229 Stéphanos, *La Grèce*, 499; Kardamatis, *Pragmateia*, 55.

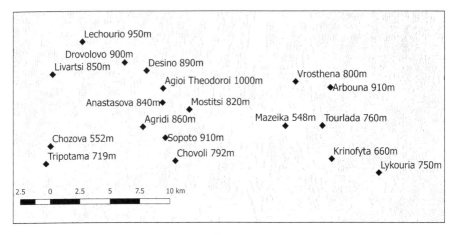

Map 2.6. Sopoto, 1901–7

in Strezova to the southeast as well, the government spent considerable state funds on drainage works consistently every year.[230]

The local physician, Spilios Arvanitis, had set up practice in Sopoto in the more prosperous days of 1889. At that time, the town was at least healthier than most of the surrounding villages, where malaria had become endemic and, thus, attractive to medical practice. Nearby, in the village of Agridi, at a distance of 20 minutes to the northwest of the town, there was a small marsh, whereas near Lekhoni, at one hour and 15 minutes distance from Sopoto, in the same direction, there was another large marsh. While Sopoto and the villages of Desino and Drovolovo were the healthiest in the area, the village of Mostitzi and the area around Tripotama, which, as the name suggests, stood at the confluence of three rivers, were the most heavily infected. The heavy spring rains in 1901, though, and intense summer

---

230 Government funds for drainage works in Soudena and Strezova, 1896–1904

Year	Location	Funds (in drachmas)
1896	Soudena	10,700.50
1897	Soudena	5,392
1898	Soudena	4,267
1899	Soudena	2,258
1900	Soudena	2,500
1901	Soudena	1,005.27
1902	Strezova	2,650
1903	Strezova	1,890.93
1904	Soudena	6,863

From "Ta mekhri 1906." Figures before 1896 are only nationwide annual totals and do not show distribution by location.

heat set off an epidemic in the town of Sopoto which infected 75 percent of its inhabitants.[231]

In the following years, however, even in 1905, the year of a nationwide epidemic, malaria prevalence fell back to its normal 30 percent rate. In contrast, 80 percent of the residents of the nearby heavily malarious town of Mazeika, which normally had a morbidity of 40–50 percent, fell ill in the same year; children under the age of fourteen were hit hardest, particularly with brain seizures. Although that year the villages surrounding Mazeika fared marginally better, with approximately half their inhabitants ill with malaria, their mortality figures were higher because the sick failed to reach a doctor in time. Again children under fourteen suffered the most. The accounts are consistent with the presence of both *vivax* and *falciparum* malaria with fevers peaking twice during the malaria season: in June and in late September. Like Mazeika, in the village of Livartzi, located in a deforested mountain environment, two-thirds of the population fell ill in 1905, twice as many as in a normal year, a large proportion of whom had "enormously enlarged spleens," a hallmark of endemic malaria. In Tripotama, in particular, malaria hit almost the entire population of seventy families. The brunt was borne by children aged between two and ten. On the other hand, in 1905 Lykouria, a village insulated in its own valley, recorded a malaria prevalence of a mere 15 percent, which was higher, however, than previous years.

In 1906, after the nationwide epidemic of the previous year, a heavily rainy season lasted until mid-June and was succeeded by a scorching summer heat. Sopoto experienced a worse malaria epidemic than 1905, with 75 percent of its inhabitants falling ill once again. All villages were affected, but Agridi and Anastasova, both near marshes, were worst hit. Mazeika, on its plateau of extensive swamps, was again by far more malarious than its surrounding villages, whose inhabitants contracted the disease when they descended to the plateau to cultivate their fields and spend the nights in huts. In the town around 70 percent fell ill, a rate slightly lower than the year before, but somewhat worse than in previous years. Malaria, therefore, hit mostly the townspeople, those living along the river network and those who had property in the plateau. Interestingly, malaria traveled from the

---

231 "Apantiseis ton k. Iatron," 217; "1905." 433–35; Savvas, Kardamatis, and Dasios, "1906," 535; "1907," 314 and 530–31.

Mazeika plateau to places like Dimitsana in Gortynia in the bloodstream of returning traders.[232] Overall, in the district of Kalavryta 1906 was considered worse than the previous year with more than half the population of around 45,000 (according to the 1896 census[233]) having contracted "all types" of malaria.[234]

After a heavily malarious year in 1906 for the entire area, the following year brought some respite: except for Mazeika, 1907 was a drier year all round. Morbidity figures returned to average levels in the area of Sopoto, with some communities, such as Sopoto itself, Agridi, and Khovoli, suffering more than others.[235] In the Mazeika region, which attracted much rain in the winter and spring of 1907, the valley remained just as malarious as in the preceding years, the town itself experiencing an 85 percent malaria prevalence, making it almost twice as heavily affected as the surrounding communities, owing to a stream that ran close to the town. As a result of an ill-advised attempt to fill the stream, the flooded area had tripled in size. Villagers with properties in the Mazeika plateau continued to place themselves at additional risk.

In October 1907, at the end of the malaria season, the physicians of Sopoto and Mazeika conducted a malaria investigation of spleen rates at the local primary and secondary schools and took the testimony of the children themselves. The use of a similar methodology in Petalidi would suggest that perhaps the local doctors acted upon recommendations sent out by the Anti-Malaria League in Athens. Both investigations confirmed the doctors' observations: that the town of Mazeika and the villages around Sopoto were more heavily malarious than the town of Sopoto itself.

The observations are consistent with the highly fragmented mountain landscape of insulated valleys and often the differentiation between a main town, on the one hand, and small villages scattered around, below or above

---

232 Savvas, Kardamatis, and Dasios, "1906," 541.

233 Royaume de Grèce and Ministère de l'Intérieur, *Resultats statistiques*, 13.

234 In Lykouria, also, malaria in 1906 was considerably worse than the previous year, at around 50 percent. In the town of Strezova, about 20 percent of its 2,000 inhabitants fell ill with malaria, while the surrounding villages had similar amounts, except for Tzaroukhli, where around 90 percent were recorded with malaria. The municipality of Psofis also suffered a severe malaria season that year; rains lasting until mid-June and the ensuing scorching heat led to a very malarious summer with 75 percent of the inhabitants falling ill with malaria, worse than the previous years, particularly for the villagers of Tripotama and Khozova, which lay by the rivers. In Savvas, Kardamatis, and Dasios, "1906," 539.

235 In Livartzi also, morbidity returned to average levels.

it, on the other, a topography that could explain the uneven surge and fall in intensity of malaria morbidity from one year to the next and the coexistence of patterns of endemic and epidemic malaria.

Ten years later, when Kardamatis was compiling his statistical tables of average malaria frequencies between 1915 and 1919, the region around Sopoto had not changed much. Mazeika and its surrounding villages in particular, which had an average malaria prevalence of 70 percent, ranked among the most malarious in the country south of Macedonia.[236] There were no large lakes in the region, but a considerable number of marshes and swamps.[237]

Twenty years later, the situation remained equally alarming. The Greek Malariological Service data for the years 1937–39 reported an 86 percent splenic rate and a 45 percent parasite index in the Strezova region.[238]

After the Second World War, early UNRRA plans for malaria control in the Kalavryta region included drainage, reforestation, and flood measures.[239] Much, however, depended on funds, supplies, and communications. The whole area was not easily accessible to DDT spraying teams. In May 1946, the local newspaper, *Foni Kalavryton* (Voice of Kalavryta), declared that local schoolchildren, already weakened by wartime hardship, needed supplies of quinine, particularly those in malarious regions such as Mazeika.[240] That summer, however, the Kalavryta area, including Mazeika as well as Araxos

---

236 The corresponding malaria prevalence for the municipality of Aroania, i.e., Sopoto and surrounding villages, was 55 percent; Psofis, that is, Livartzi and villages, 50 percent; likewise, Lefkasia with Lykouria, 50 percent, and Paos with Strezova, 25 percent. Kardamatis, *Statistikoi pinakes*, 198, 227.

237 In the municipality of Aroania (Sopoto), there was Leivadi or Longos (0.2 square kilometers), a swamp of unknown extent by the River Aroanios, a small swamp by the village of Agridi and small collections of water by the village of Tripotama. In the municipality of Kleitoria (Mazeika), there was the swamp named Tsapourna (0.5 square kilometers), and others called Loutses (0.4 square kilometers), Mylos Petmeza (0.1 square kilometers), and Fefeika (0.1 square kilometers). In the municipality of Lefkasia (Lykouria), there were small swamps by the villages of Krinofyta, Lykoiura, Fyleika, Kalyvia, and Rethi, totaling in extent 0.008 square kilometers and swamps in the valley created by the Ladonas, Aroanios, and Tragos rivers, over an area of 2 square kilometers. In the municipality of Paos, there were the swamps of Xironisia, Mouzi and Platanos, totaling 0.1 square kilometers, Metokhi Varka (0.1 square kilometers), Anginara (0.1 square kilometers), and Nisi Angeli (0.07 square kilometers). In the municipality of Psofis, there was the Lekhouritikos (0.25 square kilometers) and Versitziotikos (0.15 square kilometers) marshes and swamps created by the Aroanios and Erymanthos rivers and the Xirias ravine. In ibid., 35 and 131–32.

238 Information from the Greek Malariological Service data for 1937–1939, published in, Zeiss, *Seuchen-Atlas*, Maps VII/4 and VII/4a.

239 K. Robicek to Regional Director, Patras, 5 April 1945, Malaria, PAG4/3.0.12.2.3.:22 [5027-0686], UN Archives.

240 Excerpt from *Foni Kalavryton*, 12 May 1946, Malaria, PAG-4/3.0.12.2.3.:22 [S-0527-0686], UN Archives.

airfield and village, received the benefit of DDT aerial spraying in a joint effort by UNRRA and the British Army.[241]

In a fragmented environment such as the mountains, valleys, and streams of Sopoto, the Mazeika, and Kalavryta area averages mask the complexity of the local epidemiology reflected in the early-twentieth-century surveys of the Anti-Malaria League.

Gerli, Farsala

The town of Gerli, present-day Armenio, in Thessaly and its surrounding communities are interesting because of their shifting hydrological environment. In the early twentieth century they were also the scene of agrarian unrest of landless farmers. Harvests attracted even more farm laborers from remote parts of the country. The low-lying communities and Gerli itself lay along the unstable edge of Karla, a shallow lake whose contours oscillated as a result of flooding and droughts. The local doctor, Alkiviadis Pallis, described it as a swamp when it filled with rainwater, a lake when it filled with floodwater from the River Pineios, or an arid expanse in years of drought. Besides the lake in its various shapes, cultural factors such as the improper disposal of household wastewater turned the village streets into *Anopheles* breeding sites.[242] Years later, in January 1946, this type of hydrology caused Gregory S. Benetatos, the UNRRA regional sanitary engineer for Thessaly, to call Lake Karla "the spottiest place in Thessaly."[243]

When Pallis first set up practice there in 1895, malaria affected every local family, including his own. After two epidemic years of residence, malaria drove him away. He moved back to Gerli with his family in 1899 after the lake had dried out and a normal state of health had returned, which, in Pallis's perception, was a 30 percent morbidity level.[244] In 1904, however, the lake filled up again with river floodwater as a result of precipitation in the

---

241 J. W. Shipp to S. E. Fontaine, D. E. Wright, and others, Patras, 1 October 1946, Malaria, PAG-4/3.0.12.2.3.:22 [S-0527-0686], UNNRA.

242 Savvas, Kardamatis, and Dasios, "1906," 627.

243 G. S. Benetatos to N. Trayfors, 1 January 1946. Monthly Report, p. 1, 657 Sanitary Reports, August 1945–September 1946, PAG-4/3.0.12.3.1.0.:8 [S-0527-0729], UN Archives. A contemporary list of the Greek marshes included Karla as a lake, but left the expanse column blank. "Pinax ton elon tis Ellados," p. 3, 651 Health, Medical Care and Sanitation Malaria, October 1943–July 1946, PAG-4/3.0.12.3.1.0.:8 [S-0527-0729], UN Archives. See also Fatouros, *Limnon periigisis*, 136.

244 "Apantiseis ton k. Iatron," 253–54.

Pindus mountain range, hundreds of kilometers to the northwest. For two years, about 80 percent of the locals in and around Gerli suffered.[245] Then, after a dry winter in 1906, the size of Lake Karla shrank as did the manifestation of malaria, which fell to milder endemic levels of 30 percent.

The doctor in neighboring Alifaklar (present-day Kalamaki) across the lake, Ioannis Livanidis, who had set up practice there in 1904 and also covered the nearby hillside communities, gave a similar account of the lake's history of flooding and droughts. In Alifaklar, however, unlike Gerli, after a common bad year in 1904, when all but a few adults fell ill, in 1905 malaria prevalence fell to average levels of 50 percent, with "infants and children" hit in particular.[246] The doctor drew a distinction between the town and the low lying villages on one hand, and the hillside communities on the other. The former of which were less hit, contrary to what one might expect and for which he had no explanation. One can only speculate as to how this may have occurred: perhaps because of self-medication with quinine and the absence of diagnostic means for detecting symptomless endemic malaria, the local doctor may have underestimated its incidence. More likely, however, villagers from higher altitudes who worked as farmhands in the plain enjoyed less protection against malaria symptoms owing to a lower degree of immunity, much like the "infants and children" in the plain.[247]

Regarding immunity among mountain villagers in general, M. A. Barber and J. B. Rice, malariologist and entomologist, respectively, with the RF, remarked in a 1933 report: "Any decrease in immunity due to diminished infection is an important matter since it leaves a population more vulnerable.... [V]illages situated in the mountains at some distance from large breeding places of *elutus* or *superpictus* had a low parasite and spleen rate in 1932, which will probably continue low so long as [A]nopheles remain relatively few."[248]

Before the outbreak of the Second World War, in 1939, the Malariology Service measured a splenic index of 90 percent and a parasite index of 27 percent in nearby Kileler, a small village of 494 inhabitants according to the

---

245 "1905," 453.
246 Ibid., 454.
247 Kardamatis's wartime survey is unclear about malaria prevalence around Lake Karla, associating it with 25 percent morbidity on the Armenio, or Gerli, side and 60 percent on the southern side. Kardamatis, *Statistikoi pinakes*, 145.
248 Barber and Rice, "Malaria Studies in Greece: The Infection Rate," 19, folder 18, 749 I, RF 1.1, RFA.

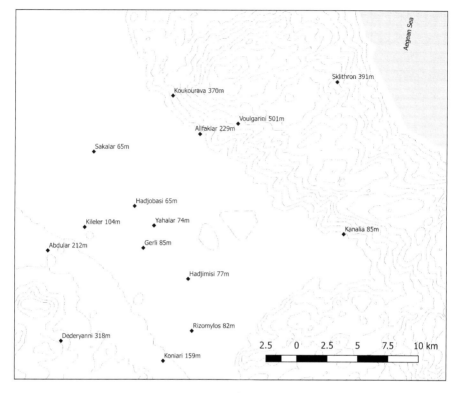

Map 2.7. Gerli, 1901–7

1928 census. These diverging percentages suggest a relatively light year in a seriously endemic location.[249]

After the Second World War, Gerli (or Armenio), with a population of 737 inhabitants in 133 dwellings, received its first DDT spraying on 30 August 1945.[250]

Fanari, Karditsa

As Balfour had stated, malaria in Greece was more frequent in areas within 250 meters of sea level.[251] The case of Fanari illustrates the advantage of higher ground to escape the brunt of malaria in a generally dry but heav-

---

249 At the time the name of the village had been changed to Kypseli. Livadas and Sfangos, *I elonosia en Elladi*, vol. 1, 156.

250 1945 DDT Residual spray, January 1946, Monthly report, 651 Health, Medical Care and Sanitation Malaria, October 1943–July 1946, PAG-4/3.0.12.3.1.0.:8 [S-0527-0729], UN Archives.

251 Balfour, "Malaria Studies in Greece," 329.

ily malarious plain. Located at the western edge of the rolling plain of Karditsa in Thessaly at a slight elevation from the plain, 450 meters above sea level, in the northeastern end of the Agrafa range,[252] Fanari, with a population of 2,000 inhabitants, was the largest and healthiest community in the region. The local doctor, Nikolaos Zoumbos, resided there and also practiced medicine in eleven surrounding villages within a 10-kilometer radius, totaling a population of 15,000 potential patients. Fanari and Kanalia (350 meters above sea level), both located at some slight elevation from the Thessalian plain, were healthier than the other villages of the group. In 1905, the malaria epidemic appears to have overstretched the doctor's ability to treat the poor farmers in the plain and even lacked detailed information about conditions in all but the two more fortunate communities. Fanari and Kanalia suffered a 20 percent malaria morbidity and nineteen malaria deaths. As for the villages in the plain, Zoumbos gave a vague estimate that "40, not to say 50 percent" of the local population came down with malaria, a rate higher than in previous years and highest among children between the ages of three and fifteen. A drought in the following year considerably reduced overall malaria prevalence. Gralista, another one of Zoumbos's villages, was even spared completely thanks to its elevated position of 640 meters. By 1907, with the crisis over, his villages returned to lower morbidity rates.[253]

With regard to this area, Kardamatis's note in the 1924 publication of his 1915–19 survey only mentions "many small water collections in the plain" and an annual average malaria prevalence of 15 percent with no reference to marshes. Yet, the wider Karditsa hinterland had its share of marshes and rice fields, producing malaria morbidity levels as high as 75 percent around the marsh of Karditsomagoula, which extended over an area of 15 square kilometers, perhaps the principal source of malaria in the region.[254]

---

252 In his 1931 recommendations on malaria control in Greece, M. Ciucă proposed a study "of local conditions, in particular of the numerous malarious zones located at the sea front and at the foot of mountains" expecting insights in the use of "natural barriers of this kind that obstruct the long-range flight of Anopheles." [M. Ciucă], Organisation de la lutte antimalarique en Grèce, Geneva, 14 February 1931, p. 11, CH/Malaria/154, Malaria Commission, Health Organisation, League of Nations.

253 "1905," 460; Savvas, Kardamatis, and Dasios, "1906," 616; "1907," 484. Also, Gardikas, "Health Policy and Private Care," 134–35.

254 Kardamatis, Statistikoi pinakes, 147.

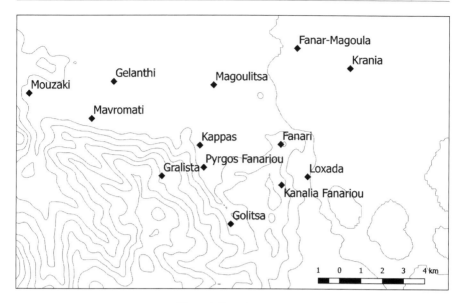

Map 2.8. Fanari, 1901–7

After the war, in the summer and autumn of 1945 the district benefited from UNRRA's DDT spraying program. Loxada, for instance, with a population of 362 inhabitants, was first sprayed on 1 October.[255] Following the parliamentary elections of 31 March 1946, at a time when the political alignments leading up to the Civil War were being drawn, Fanari became a DDT spraying station for the region and, thus, a center for employment opportunities, presumably with the backing of the right-wing government in Athens. It was not long before the fate of the malaria program in the entire regions of Larissa and Karditsa lay in the hands of armed bands on both sides of the Civil War.[256]

Interestingly, hematologists George Stamatoyannopoulos and Phaedon Fessas selected the area of Karditsa as one of five locations, which included Petromagoula near Lake Copais mentioned earlier, to study the hemoglobin polymorphisms which are related to the evolutionary pressures of malaria. They examined a sample of 428 boys from the Karditsa high school and divided them into three groups, representing three categories of elevation and

255 1945 DDT Residual spray, January 1946, Monthly report, 651 Health, Medical Care and Sanitation Malaria October 1943–July 1946, PAG-4/3.0.12.3.1.0.:8 [S-0527-0729], UN Archives.
256 Frederick West to Chief of Mission, Volos, 29 July 1946, Malaria Control Program, PAG-4/3.0.12.0.0.:4 [S-0527-0534], UN Archives; [illegible signature], Malaria Inspector, to Prefect of Karditsa, Karditsa, 28 May 1946, Malaria Control Program, PAG-4/3.0.12.0.0.:4 [S-0527-0534], UN Archives.

reflecting corresponding degrees of malaria endemicity, namely lowlands of 100–300 meters altitude that were highly malarious and semimountainous, areas of 301–800 meters altitude with medium endemicity, and highlands with an elevation above 801 meters, which were malaria-free. In areas below 300 meters, they discovered a positive correlation with the presence of β-thalassemia and G6PD deficiency among the population, a token of a history of centuries of endemic malaria. With a frequency of 19.7 percent, the amount of β-thalassemia encountered in the sample from the lowland zone was "one of the highest frequencies observed in Greece until now."[257] This correlation was also corroborated by the prefecture-level findings of Nikolaos Skhizas and his coauthors. In their sample of army recruits, Karditsa ranked seventh with a 2.04 percent frequency of sickle-cell anemia, far above the 0.97 percent national average, and third with an 18.15 percent frequency of β-thalassemia, which was also far above the national average of 8.41 percent.[258]

These six epidemiological profiles illustrate the great complexity and variety of the landscapes defining them. Perhaps their most striking common feature in all but the most heavily endemic areas is the great degree of instability most areas had acquired by the late nineteenth century. This is expressed in the painful shifts between mild endemicity and epidemic outbreaks. It is reasonable to suspect that these shifts must have incurred instability in the levels of immunity in the population and changes in the age at which some degree of acquired immunity became established.

MAPPING THE SMALL SCALE

The case of Euboea represents an interesting, ground-level exploration of an island with a variety of landscapes and degrees of isolation from the mainland. The island appears to have been overlooked by antimalarial policies except for a few pockets of interest to specific powerful groups.

In January 1946, Ernest V. Adames, a British sanitary officer with UNRRA, began a detailed preliminary survey of Euboea to prepare for the next season's antimalarial measures, particularly aerial spraying, on the ba-

---

257 Stamatoyannopoulos and Fessas, "Thalassaemia," 876.
258 Skhizas et al., "Sykhnotis," 201.

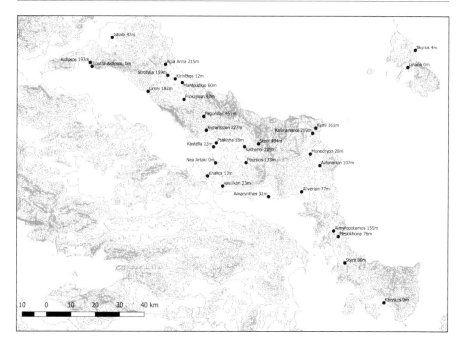

Map 2.9. Euboea, 1946

sis of his own observations and information collected from town and village authorities.[259] His records and a set of thirty-seven hand-drawn maps enable a close inspection of the natural environment around the towns and villages of Euboea in the immediate aftermath of the Second World War.

He began on 2 January 1946 in Aliveri, at the time a town of 3,400 inhabitants. In more than a century of independent statehood, it had never been subjected to malaria control work and therefore had a malaria morbidity of 50 percent. The main risk factor was its proximity to Lake Dystos, about 7 kilometers to its southeast, and a great deal of flooding south of the town whenever it rained. In 1945, field welfare worker Jean Williams reported that the villages near the "evil-looking swamp" had an enormous death rate

259 D. E. Wright to J. P. de Vries, Athens, 3 November 1945, Malaria ABJ, Sanitation 01-50, PAG-4/3.0.12.2.3.:1 [S-0527-0665], UN Archives; W. B. Uderski to Petroleum Pool, [Athens], 20 July 1945, Malaria ABJ, Sanitation 01-50, PAG-4/3.0.12.2.3.:1 [S-0527-0665], UN Archives. Interestingly, in his interwar activities in Greece, Wright had included mapmaking and map reading in his brief training program for malaria inspectors. General outline of the program for the division of sanitary engineering as planned for the Athens Centre of Hygiene by Daniel E. Wright, p. 7, Conference on rural health centres, Budapest, 27–30 October 1930, CH 937 Geneva, 23 October 1930 (vol. 317), League of Nations Health Organisation.

due to malaria, a lake swarming with millions of mosquitoes, and that everyday for 10 months of year a new person became sick.[260]

A week later Adames studied Vasiliko, a town of 2,500 inhabitants close to Khalkis, which had never seen any malaria control work either. Several of its inhabitants had suffered from malaria, the main source being a large pool of wastewater in the town itself and a breeding site by the sea, 2 kilometers southward at Lefkandi. In Amarynthos, similar in size and located between Lefkandi and Aliveri, the wells in the town had been the main source of malaria. They had been treated with petroleum by the inhabitants themselves.

Further north, the small village of Prokopi, with a population of some 650 inhabitants, was heavily malarious but had never been subjected to malaria control work. Not only had the entire population fallen ill with malaria in 1945, but half the school population as well as the village were infested with lice. The village had a rich supply of water, with mosquito breeding sites flanking the pipes, wells, springs, and churchyards.[261]

The next day, Adames studied Nea Artaki, a town of 3,200 inhabitants, inhabited mostly by refugees from Asia Minor. There was a substantial amount of malaria, but there the last malaria control work was carried out by the Athens School of Hygiene in 1935. The source of malaria lay to the north of the town, in the seaside marshes. Psakhna, a town of 4,000 inhabitants, was his next stop, on January 23. He found some malaria there, but no malaria control work had ever been carried out. Although a drainage scheme had begun in 1935/36, it was later abandoned; a swamp to the south of the town and the overflow from wells in the town itself were still the sources of malaria. He then proceeded to Kathenoi, a village of 850 inhabitants at an elevation of 209 meters. Though no control work had ever been carried out, it was relatively healthy with an *Anopheles* source in a stream half a kilometer to its east.

In early February, Adames surveyed Kyparissi, a small village of 230 inhabitants at an altitude of 227 meters. Eighty percent of the villagers had

260 Jean Williams to Miss Diers, Provincial 11-30 Euboea, PAG-4/3.0.12.2.3.:8 [S-0527-0672], UN Archives. Similarly, another report noted that, while the general malaria prevalence was about 25 percent, villages around the lake were 100 percent malarious. Regional Medical Officer to Dr. Low, 12 June 1945, Provincial 11-30 Euboea, PAG-4/3.0.12.2.3.:8 [S-0527-0672], UN Archives.

261 In recommending serious surveying and spraying, Adames added on January 21: "The fact that Mr. Noel Baker MP is at times in residence here might add weight to any recommendations put forward for improving sanitary conditions." His wife had in fact contributed some relief to four extremely poor nearby villages. Col. Dodge, Notes of visit to Euboea [May, 1945], Provincial 11-30 Euboea, PAG-4/3.0.12.2.3.:8 [S-0527-0672], UN Archives.

contracted malaria in 1945 and the source appeared to be a swamp to its south, which also posed a threat to a nearby village, Koumaritsa. Like other villages in Euboea, Kyparissi had never received any control work.

Pagondas, further north, a small and poor village of 200 lice-stricken inhabitants at an altitude of 451 meters, suffered 75 percent malaria morbidity in 1945, lost one child to the disease and had never received any control work. A swamp between the village and a stream was the source of *Anopheles*. The village had a school building but no teacher.

He found Kastella, a small town of 1,000 inhabitants closer to the sea, to have had 40 percent malaria the previous year, with its source of *Anopheles* in the large swamp on the coast to its southwest. In 1937/38 the Agriculture Ministry started a drainage program, which it never finished. A few days later, on February 10, Adames surveyed Pournos, a village of a mere 280 inhabitants at an elevation of 133 meters. Some malaria had been reported in 1945, along with its *Anopheles* source in the River Lilas and its streams that encircled the village. No previous control work had been done there either.

Toward the end of February, Adames moved north to the town of Agia Anna. With a population of 1,700 it was located at an altitude of 215 meters and had never received any malaria control work. Half the population had contracted malaria in 1945. Branding it as a "known danger spot," Adames identified the *Anopheles* sources: "Marshy ground to east (coastal belt). Small streams (3) passing through the village. Wine presses used as rain water storage tanks during summer."

In early March, he surveyed Steni, a town of 1,400 inhabitants located some 500 meters above sea level, which had received no previous malaria control work. In 1945, it had some 100 cases of malaria and the *Anopheles* source lay in the nearby river and streams. Its high mortality from tuberculosis was due to imported cases, as it was being used as a sanatorium in the summer.

The mining town of Mantoudi, with a population of 2,250, was surrounded by a large swamp on its northern side in the plain between the town and the sea, which also infected all nearby villages. In 1945, 80 percent had fallen ill and 20 people had died from malaria, which was considered to be the root cause behind "all deaths." The Athens School of Hygiene had done some malaria control work there before the war and so had the Italians in 1943 with Paris green and oil.

Khalkis, the main city of Euboea with a population of 19,776 in 1940, which Adames surveyed on 12 March 1946, had a few malaria cases in 1945 and had received some control work by the Athens School of Hygiene before the war. Swamps were noted on the map at a fair distance from the city in three places: north of Nea Artaki, to the south of the city closer to Vasiliko, and also across the channel on the mainland opposite the city.

Toward the end of the same month, on 27 March, Adames surveyed Karystos, in the south of the island. Also a mining town by the sea, it had a population of 3,035 inhabitants. Although it had been relatively malaria-free in 1945, between 1941 and 1944 it suffered 95 percent malaria morbidity. In 1943, the Athens School of Hygiene had carried out some malaria control work, which remained unfinished. A river delta and irrigation channels to the west of the town and small streams to its east caused the problem. The local doctor attributed the impressive drop in malaria morbidity to UNRRA intervention; in 1945 the administration had indeed distributed large quantities of Atabrine, the synthetic antimalarial drug, to the population.

Styra, a village of 850 inhabitants to the north of Karystos, was surveyed next, on 1 April. With 20 percent malaria the previous year, it had the typical stream passing through it and no prior malaria control work. The following day, Adames surveyed the small village of Almyropotamos, 550 meters above sea level with 155 inhabitants. Never the subject of malaria control work, it had suffered 75 percent malaria morbidity in the previous year. Deaths were usually due to "pneumonia following malaria debility." A river and its delta were causing all this unhealthiness. Nearby Mesokhoria, with a population of 1,070, was a healthy small town, free of malaria and equipped with a clinic.

In mid-April, Adames surveyed Kalimerianoi, a town of 1,100 inhabitants at an altitude of 210 meters, which he also described as a healthy, "clean and tidy village." Nearby Kymi, a town of 4,200 inhabitants at 161 meters above sea level, reported very few cases, and those it had were said to be imported. On 27 April he surveyed Avlonari, a town of 1,600 situated 107 meters above sea level, which was also located on the cooler, eastern side of the island. It had very few cases, no past malaria control work, and some suspected *Anopheles* present in late April. To its north, the village of Monodryo, with 875 poor inhabitants, suffered 75 percent malaria in 1945, many deaths from malnutrition and had never received any malaria control work. It was surrounded by a river and streams, which appeared to be *Anopheles* breeding grounds.

The main town of the island of Skyros, surveyed on 29 April, had a population of 3,438. Highly malarious, in 1945 it suffered a 60 to 70 percent morbidity rate and lost six or seven children to the disease. Most deaths were attributed to malaria debility, tuberculosis, and heart disease. There was a permanent stream flowing through the town and a large marsh about 7 kilometers to the north, in the very fields where the locals went to work. In 1939, the Athens School of Hygiene had tried to control the *Anopheles*, reported to be *superpictus*, with petrol. Skyros was seen as a tourist destination in need of malaria control, relatively easy to achieve because, according to Adames, it was a "self-contained small island." Linaria, on the western side of the island, only had 185 residents but 75 percent of them had contracted malaria in 1945. The community itself had carried out some petroleum control work that year to prevent *Anopheles* from breeding in the stream and pools within the village. Beyond the village, there was an extensive marsh and rivers to its north and at the locations of Palaiokastro further north and Sarkofay further southeast.

On his return from Skyros, Adames surveyed the village of Kirinthos on 22 May. With 530 residents, it was surrounded by two marshes and a river and was highly malarious. In 1945 it had 75 percent malaria morbidity, while during the war the Italians had performed some control work there. The following day, he surveyed the northern end of the island, that is, the town of Aidipsos and its spa resort, Loutra Aidipsou, and Istiaia. The town of Aidipsos had a population of 1,450, reported no malaria incidence and, with a population of *Anopheles sacharovi* and *superpictus* breeding in the nearby marshes, was kept under constant control from 1936 by the Athens School of Hygiene with Paris green and diesel oil.[262] The same applied to the spa resort, Loutra Aidipsou, which had 1,700 residents. By late May, Adames noted *sacharovi* in swamps and *superpictus* in streams but no malaria thanks to the annual application with Paris green and diesel oil since 1938. On the other hand, Istiaia, a large town of 5,000 inhabitants, had suffered 60 percent malaria morbidity and three deaths from malaria in 1945. The local ma-

---

262 Livadas and Sfangos, *I elonosia en Elladi*, vol. 2, 87–99. Contrary to *A. sacharovi*, which prefers brackish, slightly saline waters in marshes and low-lying stagnant waters, *A. superpictus* likes streams, brooks, springs, and rock pools in the hills. Balfour, "Some Features," 18–19; Wenyon, "Malaria in Macedonia," 37–37. For a typical *superpictus* landscape, see Appendix II.

laria inspection officer had spent the previous month larviciding a wooded terrain with diesel, in an area unsuitable for aerial spraying.

Returning south, Adames surveyed Limni, a town of 3,251 inhabitants 182 meters above sea level. It had suffered a 75 percent malaria morbidity in the previous year. Before the war, there had been some oiling of storage tanks but nothing more. They and the River Sipias were thought to be mosquito breeding sites. Adames ended his survey in early June in Strofylia, a small village of 675 residents some 160 meters above sea level, never controlled for malaria with a morbidity of 50 percent in 1945, suffering from the stream to its west. Owing to the lack of soap among the poor villagers, lice were common.[263]

The uneven distribution of health and disease, filth, poverty, and privilege emerge quite clearly from this single-handed, unique, five-month sanitary inspection work.

The Malaria Season

Greece was a country of interrupted, seasonal malaria transmission with a dwindling reservoir of endemic or stable malaria, a situation that fueled frequent localized and irregular nationwide epidemics. Climate variability contributed to the instability of the disease. Apart from seasonal instability, climatological irregularities from one year to the next were of particular interest to malaria epidemiology. The malaria season in Greece displayed features that were directly associated with place. The erratic effect of climate on malaria prevalence, however, was not only the result of geographic fragmentation. Variations in weather patterns between years created an unpredictable malaria season nationwide. As in the case of instability within the year, rainfall was likewise the most important source of instability in malaria across years.

The country lies between latitudes 41° 44' 53" and 34° 47' 56" NE, with Macedonia and Thrace, the territories ceded to Greece in 1913 and 1920, respectively, lying north of latitude 39° 48' N. According to interwar climatological data, it occupied the zone between the 14.5°C annual isotherm in western Macedonia and the 19.5°C annual isotherm that ran through the

---

263 Sanitary Surveys ABJ, Sanitation 01-20, PAG-4/3.0.12.2.3.:1 [S-0527-0665], UN Archives.

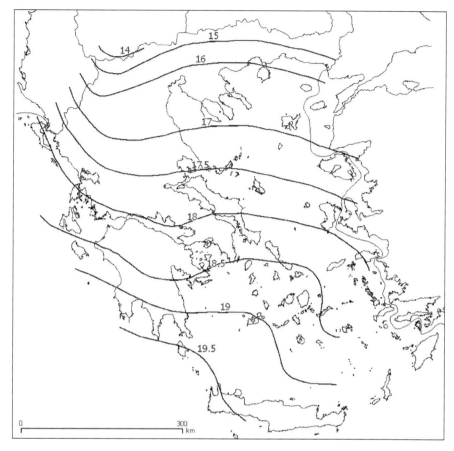

Map 2.10. Annual isotherms of Greece

Source: Mariolopoulos, *To klima tis Ellados.*

southern Peloponnese, Kythira, and Crete; in other words, a latitude of almost 7° corresponded to a 5°C shift of annual isotherms.

In January, however, the maximum range of isotherms reached 9°C.[264] Latitude range also influences local day length differences between seasons, which vary between approximately 10 hours 30 minutes and 15 hours 30 minutes of daylight in southern Crete and 10 hours 20 minutes and 16 hours 20 minutes in Thrace in the north of the country. Day length, in turn, affects temperatures.[265] Prevailing winds and mountain layout affect the onset of

---

264 Mariolopoulos, *To klima tis Ellados,* 40 and 52–54.
265 Ibid., 42–43.

summer earlier in the south and east and later, mostly in June, in the north and west. Mean temperatures were generally higher in the autumn than in the spring by 3 to 4°C in the south and in the islands and by 2 to 3°C in the north.[266]

Atmospheric temperature is important both in the life cycle of the *Plasmodia* and in the longevity of the female mosquito. *Vivax* transmissions cease at temperatures below 16°C. At the same temperature, *P. vivax* completes its cycle inside the mosquito and is ready to be injected into a human much earlier than *P. falciparum*, which requires temperatures above 20°C.[267] Ambient temperature and other climatic conditions are also determining factors of the size of the *Anopheles* population and the longevity of its members. Atmospheric temperature also controls whether and to what extent *Anopheles* hibernate, thus shortening their infective life span and affording humans a short reprieve from their bites. In the tropics, for instance, their life extends to between two and three weeks, whereas in the temperate zone they may live for months, helped also by hibernation. Their longevity, an important factor in malaria transmission, is adversely affected at a mean temperature higher than 35°C and humidity below 50 percent.[268] Therefore, isotherms define the range within which malaria occurs.

In the old, or pre-1950, climatological regime in Greece, the effect of latitude on temperature was greater in the winter months. Thus spring and the advent of the malaria season would arrive earlier in the south, where the transmission season would therefore be considerably longer. The effect of altitude, on the other hand, became more significant with the advent of summer. As a result, the start of the transmission season in the mountains would follow that of the plains below.[269]

Nonetheless, the effects of latitude on the spread of malaria are difficult to assess as many other factors were at play in the country's different regions. In this context, the question whether the northern Greek lands were

---

266 Ibid., 48, 50.

267 Macdonald, *The Epidemiology and Control of Malaria*, 11; Sinden and Gilles, "The Malaria Parasite," 12 and 25–28.

268 Service and Townson, "The *Anopheles* Vector," 68.

269 Mariolopoulos, *To klima tis Ellados*, 62. On the differences in rainfall variability in Greece between the pre- and post-1950 regime, see Hatzianastassiou et al., "Spatial and Temporal Variation." Sallares noted with regard to the Alban hills south of Rome, that the line separating cereal cultivation from viticulture, a crop that required intensive attention, ran along the altitude below which malaria began. Sallares, *Malaria and Rome*, 244.

more or less malarious than the south occupied malariologists in the inter-war years. Were the plains in Macedonia and Thrace in the cooler north of the country less malarious than the warmer low-lying areas of Crete or the southern Peloponnese, for instance? Did the local *Anopheles* enjoy a shorter season in the north than in the south? Furthermore, to what degree may the exceptional morbidity and mortality levels encountered among the Allied armies in the First World War and the Asia Minor refugees in the 1920s be attributed to short-term wartime disturbances and demographic displacement? Or could the difference be due to the economic backward-ness of the new regions?

After the wartime experience of the Allies, and especially owing to the suffering of the refugees settled there after the defeat of Greece in Asia Minor in 1922, these northern lands acquired the reputation as the most heav-ily malaria-infested regions in the country. Yet, evidence collected during the war does not corroborate the view that the northern regions had always suffered higher levels of malaria morbidity and mortality. Between 1913 and 1919, that is, before the major influx of the refugees from Asia Minor and their distribution throughout the country, Ioannis Kardamatis carried out his sixth nationwide malaria morbidity survey, in which he did not include the foreign army units stationed in northern Greece during the war. In con-trast to subsequent perceptions regarding the distribution of malaria, Kar-damatis concluded that southern Greece was, indeed, considerably more

Sterea Ellas and Euboea	47.02
Thessaly and Arta	32.55
Ionian Islands	100.12
Cyclades	46.31
Peloponnese	44.08
Aegean islands	64.88
Crete	41.93
Macedonia	31.93
Epirus	30.83
Western Thrace	24.20
National average	39.54

Table 2.3. Population density by square kilometers, 1920

malarious than the new lands of northern Greece. He isolated two factors, none of which included climatology, to explain the difference: namely population density and hydrology. Old Greece had a higher population density than New Greece.[270]

Also, despite the fact that New Greece had larger and more marshes, it was the extensive prevalence of small pools over most of the south that presented a more serious health malaria hazard.[271]

	Population	Average malaria morbidity, 1915–19 %*
Old Greece	2,835,008	31.02
New Greece	2,127,796	23.95
Total	4,962,804	27.99

Table 2.4. Malaria morbidity in Old and New Greece
during the First World War
Source: Kardamatis, *Statistikoi pinakes.*
* The percentages have been recalculated from the raw data.

As for malaria among the allied troops in Macedonia, C. M. Wenyon (1878–1948), who studied the spread of malaria among the British units there, attributed the epidemic outbreaks to military movements in areas previously only slightly malarious rather than to their extensive swamps.[272] If, therefore, malaria prevalence in cooler northern Greece varied in response to historical circumstances in comparison to the south, to which one may also add the region's economic backwardness,[273] clearly differences in latitude and its effect on climate were not the only determining factors. Likewise, no simple effect of latitude on morbidity or mortality figures for 1905 and 1915–19 in southern Greece or on changes that might have occurred between the two periods are visible in the following tables.[274]

---

270 République Hellénique, Ministère de l'Économie Nationale, Statistique Générale de la Grèce, *Recensement*, xv.
271 Kardamatis, *Statistikoi pinakes*, 177.
272 Wenyon, "Malaria in Macedonia," 5–6.
273 This subject is taken up in chapter 3.
274 1905 was an epidemic year and, therefore, cannot serve as a basis for comparison with the five-year averages of 1915–19.

Region	Recorded Population*	Sick	Deaths	Morbidity (%)	Case mortality (‰)	Gross mortality (‰)
Peloponnese	205,799	102,035	483	49.58	4.7	2.3
Central Greece	96,358	50,455	451	52.36	8.9	4.7
Thessaly	56,658	41,951	139	74.04	3.3	2.5
Ionian Islands	34,634	9210	75	26.59	8.1	2.2
Euboea	21,974	6152	25	28	4.1	1.1
Saronic Islands	21,943	4710	14	21.46	3	0.6
Aegean Islands	10,702	4396	60	41.08	13.6	5.6
Total	448,068	218,909	1247	48.86	5.7	2.8
12 largest cities	369,573	77,821	331	21.06	4.3	0.9
Grand total	817,641	296,730	1578	36.29	5.3	1.9

Table 2.5. Regional malaria morbidity and mortality in 1905

Source: Kardamatis, "I elonosia en Elladi kata to 1905."

* Population not included in the survey: 1,616,165.

Rural Thessaly appears to have had 50 percent more malaria than rural Peloponnese, which in turn had just as much as rural Central Greece. Overall, mainland Greece suffered more than the islands.

Region	Morbidity, 1905 (%)	Morbidity, 1915–19 (%)
Peloponnese	41.23	37.22
Central Greece	21.88	28.75
Euboea	28	36.41
Thessaly	84.22	38.98
Ionian Islands	16.84	14.02
Saronic Islands	21.46	20.34
Aegean Islands	41.08	10.14

Table 2.6. Regional differences in malaria morbidity between 1905 and 1915–19

Again, differences in latitude are not visible in the morbidity rates, whereas morbidity in mainland Greece hovered around 35 percent. These figures need to be treated with reservation, since the 1905 data was based on less than half the population. However, it is safe to infer that the evidence does not support the thesis of an overall reduction in malaria morbidity between 1905 and the wartime years in southern, or Old Greece, but that there was a marked difference in morbidity rates between mainland Greece on the one hand and the smaller islands on the other.[275]

Table 2.5 summarizes the figures collected from the 102 physicians' responses to the 1905 questionnaire and from national mortality statistics of the country's largest cities regarding the 1905 nationwide epidemic. On the basis of this partial data, Kardamatis extrapolated that 960,048 Greeks out of a total population of 2,433,806, or 39.45 percent, contracted malaria in the 1905 epidemic, of whom 5,916, or 6.2 per thousand, died, suggesting a gross mortality rate of 2.43. In table 2.6 regional figures also take into account the 1905 data from the urban centers and therefore differ from those of table 2.5.

More important than latitude, however, was the great degree of geographical fragmentation of the land and the interplay of land with the sea, which gave the Greek climate its most distinctive feature of steep, unevenly distributed temperature shifts. In the words of Elias Mariolopoulos, professor of climatology at the University of Athens, "the distribution of temperatures presents so many and such a variety of irregularities in this small country, as in few places on earth."[276]

Under the pre-1950 climatological regime, mean temperatures were generally warmer by 0.5°C in the Ionian Islands in comparison to the eastern Greek coast, although summer arrived earlier in the east than in the west of the country.[277] An important rearrangement of temperature distributions occurred in May, when three localized heat zones emerged, each measuring a mean temperature of 20.5°C, which made these zones suitable for *falciparum* transmission: one over the Peloponnese and Central Greece (Sterea Ellas), one over central Macedonia and a third one over Crete. By June though, these zones had become one.[278] In July, the 28°C isotherm corresponded to the area of Central Greece and Thessaly and to the southern Peloponnese, with Crete considerably cooler by two degrees and Thrace by another two degrees. August presented a similar pattern, being only half a degree cooler.[279]

---

275 Kardamatis, "I elonosia en Elladi kata to 1905," 190–91.
276 Mariolopoulos, *To klima tis Ellados*, 52 and 70. In the classical literature on the Mediterranean, Fernand Braudel, in *The Mediterranean*, vol. 1, 27–28, comments on climate variability in the mountainous Mediterranean lands. For a vivid account on the extreme variability of winds on the island of Corfu, see Hennen, *Sketches*, 154–60 and 239–41; in his words, "a person must have resided there, to be at all able to describe or even to imagine them." Yet, according to Hennen, the climate of Cephalonia was even more variable. Hennen, *Sketches*, 264.
277 Mariolopoulos, *To klima tis Ellados*, 48 and 53.
278 Ibid., 56 and 58.
279 Ibid., 59.

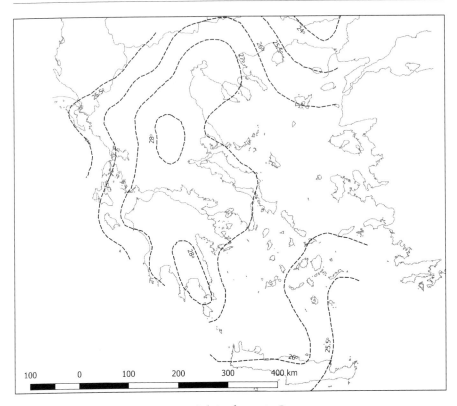

Map 2.11. July isotherms in Greece
Source: Mariolopoulos and Livathinos, *Atlas climatique de la Grèce.*

In September, the isotherm shift that occurred in May was reversed with temperatures dropping faster in the north of the country and more gently in Crete. By October, western Thrace lay on the 17°C isotherm and southern Peloponnese, Kythira, and southern Crete on the 21.5°C isotherm. By November, the temperatures pattern had assumed a clear distribution by latitude with a difference of 7°C between central Macedonia (11°C isotherm), when even *vivax* malaria transmission would normally have ceased, and Crete (18°C isotherm). Thus, latitude affected mean temperatures in the winter months, while localized heat zones generally affected mean temperature distribution in the months between May and August, that is, during the greater part of the malaria transmission season.[280]

---

280 Ibid., 60–62. The winter months isotherms indicate that temperatures prevented malaria transmission. In January the country lay between the 4° isotherm in western Thrace and Macedonia and the 13° isotherm that ran through the southeast Aegena and across Crete; in February, between 1.5° in Thrace and 13° south

As a measure of climate variability, air temperature could range annually over 23°C in western Macedonia, the spread narrowing as one moved further south and east, to over 12.7°C in the southeastern Aegean Islands.[281]

Altitude also affected temperatures, depending on the season. On the basis of data collected between 1900 and 1929, the average impact of a difference of 100 meters was estimated at 0.6°C. According to other estimates, this difference was 0.8°C in the east and 0.6°C in the west of the country. However, some plains, such as that of Lake Copais, suffered from temperature inversions, which Mariolopoulos saw as the reason why most settlements in Greece were located on mountain slopes rather than in plains or valleys.[282]

Annual rainfall was generally greater in western Greece.[283] However, the seasonal rainfall distribution was also highly irregular with a large degree of local variability. In January it was mostly determined by the layout of mountain ranges of the mainland.[284] There was a significant reduction in the amount of rain in April in most of the country with the exception of Epirus, and certain locations in the Peloponnese, while rainfall increased in Macedonia and Thrace. The summer drought began in mid-May with the exception of central Macedonia and Thessaly, where there was a secondary rise in rainfall. In May, mostly after it had significantly determined the level of malaria prevalence of the year, overall rainfall distribution assumed a latitudinal pattern.[285] Latitude, according to Mariolopoulos, was the principal factor affecting the climate of Greece, with landmass distribution, terrain, sea surface, and air currents also contributing.[286] Indeed, the comparisons made by Greek physicians between Old and New Greece reflect their interest in the effect of latitude on climate, mostly rainfall and temperature, as a determinant of malaria prevalence. However, as noted above, their observations produced a far more complex picture.

of Thira and across central Crete; in March, between 7° in western Thrace and 14° from Thira, Naxos, along the northwestern coast of Crete, Kythira, the coast of Lakonia, Messinia, and Zakynthos; in April, between 11° north of western Thrace and 17°, sufficient to permit *vivax* malaria transmission, from the northeast Aegean, south of Thira through western Crete. Mariolopoulos, *To klima tis Ellados*, 54–56.

281 Ibid., 67–68.

282 Ibid., 82–84.

283 The average annual rainfall in Athens and Central Greece was around 40 cm, in western Greece it could be up to 76 cm, occasionally reaching 127 cm in Epirus. Often the Peloponnese, Attica, and Central Greece received no rain between June and September, while in Macedonia rainfall was more evenly distributed throughout year. M. C. Balfour, "Some Features," 4.

284 Mariolopoulos, *To klima tis Ellados*, 170.

285 Ibid., 172–73.

286 Ibid., 300.

M. C. Balfour narrowed down the contribution of rainfall to malaria prevalence to its monthly distribution rather than its total annual amount. "The winter rains and the snow, which falls on the mountains, are the foundation upon which the following malaria season develops." Then in April and May, variation from normal rainfall in either direction "is reflected in the anophelism of the year."[287]

With regard to the degree of instability of malaria in the temperate zone, George Macdonald's epidemiological observations are particularly relevant to the irregular climatological context, the fragmented geography of the Greek lands, and their immunological repercussions. In classifying the regular annual malaria outbreaks in the temperate and subtropical zone countries as "a periodic epidemic," he pointed to their stable rather than unstable character "both in time and degree." This seasonal outbreak normally occurred "a month or so after the mean daily temperature first exceeds 15C." Other factors however, less regular than temperature, such as variations in rainfall from one year to the next, could contribute to an increase in mosquito breeding sites and a degree of instability in *Anopheles* reproduction and, therefore, cause unstable disease outbreaks. In such cases "the scale of the annual epidemic may vary very much from year to year" and would result in an initial phase of *vivax* and, a few weeks later, of *falciparum* malaria, which would culminate in increased deaths in the summer and autumn. A community enjoying a level of immunity from recent encounters with malaria would receive "a fresh stimulus" to its communal immunity that would protect it from the effects of a serious epidemic, even in unfavorable environmental circumstances. Thus, instability was relative to the factors that influenced transmission in a particular locality, for instance by reintroducing infecting *Plasmodia* or *Anopheles*, by increasing "[A]nopheles density, biting habit or longevity, or by disturbing the immunity of the population." In Macdonald's words, "in some places minor causes are effective precipitants of epidemics whilst in others only the grossest changes produce any visible effect."[288]

---

287 Balfour, "Some Features," 4. On a visit to Serres in 1935, Wilson G. Smillie, a member of the board of scientific directors of the RF, observed that more studies on the effect of microclimate on the *Anopheles* population with the help of a climatologist would be necessary. Wilson G. Smillie to the President and Board of Trustees, Report of a brief visit to the Activities of the International Health Division in the Balkan States, 4 July to 2 September 1935, p. 5, folder 3794, box 559, 1935, RG 2 General Corr. Stacks, RFA.
288 Macdonald, *The Epidemiology and Control of Malaria*, 48–49.

Under such irregular circumstances, prediction, and therefore climatic data collection, became vital. Early travelers and foreign medical officers read medical geographies and topographies before visiting the country and, in turn, produced their own accounts. Finke and other medical authors warned travelers to Greece of the dangers of autumn.[289] Experience and the climatological component of the broader field of early-nineteenth-century medical geography must have taught British topographer W. M. Leake, for instance, to avoid the warm months and not travel in the Peloponnese after May.[290] Leake also specifically warned of the risks of the summer and autumn climate in Patras. He wrote:

> The excessive heat and the marshy tract to the southward and westward of the town still create dangerous fevers and dysenteries in summer and autumn, so that with the exception perhaps of Anápli and Corinth, Patra is still the most unhealthy town in the Moréa. It is the prevailing opinion that the fevers are chiefly owing to the wind from Mount Voidhiá [Panakhaiko or Vodias], which, say the people of Patra, is unwholesome, because it is heavy. ... Patra has proved fatal to a great number of new settlers, particularly to the French, who, about forty years ago, had several mercantile houses there.[291]

During Leake's stay in Ioannina, further north, where malaria attacks would have been known to begin later in the season, a late June visitor, the "celebrated Roman artist Lusieri," noted the gnats and the marshes surrounding the stagnant lake and initially considered an early departure:

> [S]o much was he alarmed at those which his Italian opinions led him to consider as infallible symptoms of malaria. But the picturesque beauties of the place had such a powerful attraction for him that he was induced to hazard a longer visit, until his fears having been calmed by my own experience, and that of the Ioannites in general, he prolonged his stay for six weeks.[292]

The warm season became associated with malaria fevers. John Davy, a British military physician based on the Ionian Islands, was puzzled by "the ir-

---

289 Finke, *Versuch*, vol. 1, 115–17; Lombard, *Traité*, vol. 3, 277–78.
290 There are no entries in his travel account after the end of May. Leake, *Travels in the Morea*.
291 Leake, *Travels in the Morea*, vol. 2, 142–43.
292 Leake, *Travels in Northern Greece*, vol. 4, 160–61. The artist was the Italian landscape painter Giovanni Battista Lusieri (1755–1821). For a detailed account of travelers' encounters with fevers in the Greek lands before independence, see Skhizas and Skampardonis, "I elonosia stin arkhaia Ellada."

regularity of its occurrence, and this even in situations where it occasionally operates with extraordinary intensity and violence." Calling on his experience in Ceylon, whose environment, he believed, was comparable to that of Zante (Zakynthos) and Lefkada, he was "not aware of a single circumstance, excepting one, which with propriety can be called a common one, always existing where there is malaria, or where there are fevers attributable to it, and this is warmth, or a certain temperature many degrees above the freezing point; its exact limit is not easily defined."[293] Raymond Faure, a French authority on intermittent fevers, argued that it was the heat that actually caused them and cited his experience with the French expeditionary force in the Peloponnese in 1829.[294] John Hennen also remarked of the warm season in Corfu:

> There is scarcely a square mile in the island free from [exhalations]. . . . Every shower of rain that falls, if succeeded by heat, at whatever season of the year, is productive of miasmata; but August and the beginning of September are the periods in which these exhalations are produced in the greatest abundance; during those months, the town and its environs are constantly covered with fog in the mornings, but to a much less extent than the more distant villages; hence the town is, beyond comparison, more healthy than the country. A wet summer is invariably followed by an unhealthy autumn, which is felt by all classes of inhabitants throughout the island; but especially by those who expose themselves after sun-set.[295]

Lefkada was, for the British, the most unpredictable of all the islands, according to Hennen. The commander there could not decide on a healthy village for his troops, "those which were free from disease one year, proving pestiferous the succeeding, and vice versa."[296]

The seasonal nature of the disease in Greece is clear in the 1838 medico-statistical survey, in which physicians drew a broad distinction between winter fevers due to respiratory infections (*flogistikoi pyretoi*), on the one hand, and, on the other hand, spring, summer, and autumn intermittent fevers (*dialeipontes pyretoi*), the term by which contemporary physicians

---

293 Davy, *Notes and Observations*, vol. 2, 244–45.
294 Faure, *Des fièvres intermittentes et continues*, vol. 1, 41–43 and 61–62.
295 Hennen, *Sketches*, 161.
296 Ibid., 366.

mostly understood malaria. In some heavily malarious communities, in the Kalamata area for instance, the survey points to the prevalence of malignant estivo-autumnal fevers, clearly *falciparum* malaria.[297]

The first statistical research carried out on the records of the Astykliniki, the Athens University outpatient clinic, for the years 1860–70 by Georgios Karamitsas points to a doubling of cases diagnosed as intermittent fevers between June and July and a peak, in which it doubled again, in August and September.[298]

January	290
February	294
March	388
April	382
May	509
June	600
July	1,150
August	2,229
September	2,103
October	1,300
November	679
December	449
N = 10373	

Table 2.7. Monthly cases of intermittent fevers recorded in the Astykliniki, 1860–70

Source: Stéphanos, *La Grèce*, 497; Karamitsas, "Peri elodon i eleiogenon nosimaton," vol. 2, 734. The figures have been recalculated by the author.

On the basis of 43,562 cases diagnosed with malaria in Athens hospitals, Kardamatis calculated their monthly distribution emphasizing, however, that primary cases began in May and appeared until the first week in December; cases appearing between that date and early spring were relapses. His larger sample produced a modified distribution with a peak in August and September.[299]

---

297 Galatis, "Iatrostatistikoi pinakes tis dioikiseos Messinias kai tis ypodioikiseos Pylias."

298 References to months in the Greek sources prior to March 1923 have been preserved in the Julian calendar, which corresponds to some two weeks later—twelve days in the nineteenth and thirteen days in the twentieth century—according to the Gregorian calendar. For more on the Astykliniki, see Gavroglou, Karamanolakis, and Barkoula, *To Panepistimio*, 304–6.

299 Kardamatis, *Pragmateia*, 503.

Month	Cases	Percentage
January	1706	3.91
February	1283	2.71
March	1711	3.92
April	1777	4.07
May	2271	5.21
June	3299	7.59
July	5311	12.19
August	7122	16.34
September	7095	16.26
October	5722	13.13
November	3850	8.99
December	2415	5.54
N = 43,562		

Table 2.8. Monthly distribution of 43,562 malaria cases

Source: Kardamatis, *Pragmateia*, 503.

On the basis of demographic data for 1864–78, Clôn Stéphanos showed that July and October had the highest proportion of annual deaths (1.84/1,000 and 1.83/1,000 inhabitants, respectively), whereas the general annual mortality rate was 20.7/1,000 inhabitants or a monthly average of 1.72/1,000. As with Hippocrates in antiquity, autumn with its 5.41 deaths per 1,000 inhabitants (monthly average 1.8/1,000) remained the most unhealthy season, particularly the month of October; May and June had the least deaths (1.56/1,000 and 1.47/1,000 inhabitants, respectively).[300] Stéphanos associated regional differences in mortality with monthly differences in malaria incidence and concluded that only the October rise in mortality was directly attributable to malaria, summer rates being influenced particularly by infant mortality, most notably in Athens. These, in turn, were largely due to gastrointestinal diseases which, like many of his colleagues, he believed were in some way related to pernicious fevers. However, malaria morbidity, which was on the rise by August, also contributed to November mortality, Stéphanos believed, indirectly through its effect on respiratory infections of migrants returning from the mountains to the

---

300 Stéphanos, *La Grèce*, 455 and 457–60.

plains. Deaths in November largely coincided with the locations that had demonstrated a rise in mortality also in August. With respect to this delay, Stéphanos correlated "the greater rise in autumn mortality," on the one hand, with "the rise of summer temperatures," on the other, and suggested the likelihood that humans may become adversely sensitive to "atmospheric influences following a certain time lapse after a period of a great increase of malarial miasma."[301]

In the days of miasmatic theory, the onset of hot weather was perceived to coincide with a number of factors that were thought to cause intermittent fevers, while the onset of cold weather could result in complications for those already weakened by malaria. Peasants working the fields in the daytime heat and sleeping outdoors at night exposed themselves to malaria; consuming fruit that was abundantly available but caused "dietary disorders" was also perceived as encouraging malaria, which began with gastrointestinal symptoms; these, in turn, were thought to develop cerebral phenomena.[302] Late September rains "feed malaria," while in the cooler weather people caught colds that brought latent cases of malaria into the open. Endemic malaria lasted until October or November, "depending on location." As the period of endemic malaria came to an end, rain and cold northern winds set in that caused respiratory infections, which further weakened sufferers from "the malarial miasma."[303] Henri Clermond Lombard in his study of medical climatology based his analysis on records of British hospital malaria admittances in the Ionian Islands, which peaked in July and August and also associated malaria with hot weather. Like Stéphanos, he noted that mortality peaked in the autumn with 42.6 percent of all deaths occurring during that season, probably on account of "remittent and typhoid fevers" that were designated as "quinine fevers, just as seen in Rome, Algeria and the entire Orient."[304]

Miasmatic theory did not search for specific causes. In this context, winds became a versatile explanatory tool for uncovering immediate origins of morbidity. As Konstantinos Mavrogiannis wrote in 1840, for in-

---

301 Ibid., 460–65; Lombard, *Traité*, vol. 3, 277. In the case of Athens death statistics, Lombard estimated that in many deaths attributed to gastrointestinal diseases malaria should be acknowledged as the principal cause of death.

302 Stéphanos, *La Grèce*, 491.

303 Ibid., 492.

304 Lombard, *Traité*, vol. 3, 278–79. The terms "remittent" and "intermittent" fevers were not used interchangeably by physicians but were both perceived as results of "marsh miasmata" and causes of "great mortality, and obstinate visceral obstructions among the survivors." See Hennen, *Sketches*, 336.

stance, winds were particularly important for disseminating exhalations, and thus explained the high malaria burden of Corinth. Like many of his contemporaries, he believed that "we should not lose hope for the future improvement of the climate of Corinth, despite the fact that the closest, immediate, independent causes of the aforementioned fevers elude all means of observation. It is true that miasmas reveal themselves in their effects, never in their essence or their composition, which are unknown. We may, however, determine the indirect causes of endemicity, and turn the salutary public health measures in that direction."[305] Consistently with this belief, Mavrogiannis advised building the new town on the site of the ancient city, facing north.[306]

Hennen's description of Cephalonia is enlightening about the explanatory power of summer winds in miasmatic theory. "Now, it is obvious," he observed, "that all these winds must convey the miasmata of marshes to the town of Argostoli, which is encircled by them on all sides. When they blow over the adjacent lagoon of Cutavo, they come with undiminished power upon the town. When they blow from the more remote marsh of Livadi, although the distance is such as to neutralize the effects of the exhalations from that unwholesome spot in a very considerable degree before they reach Argostoli, yet the continued action of the wind must naturally convey a portion of these vapours to the town, especially when in its course it sweeps along the mountains that bound the harbor on its northeastern shore, and collects in its progress the malarious vapours which arise from every ravine, and from the bed of every winter torrent that indents their precipitous sides."[307]

In his review of the sanitary conditions of Greece, Stéphanos added winds to the factors that, despite the country's achievements in reducing the number of foci, spread the annual malarial miasmas to mountain villages and islands, particularly after calm weather, when miasmas were allowed to "condense." Then, when spread by a gentle wind or sea breeze, they generated epidemics, which struck the less-accustomed populations of the cooler, humid mountain slopes. "It is believed that, in a cold and damp atmosphere, even the smallest amount of malaria acts in a most in-

305 Mavrogiannis, "Paratiriseis epi ton klimaton tis Ellados," 349.
306 Ibid., 352.
307 Hennen, Sketches, 264–65.

tense manner, whereas the manifestation of a once latent malarial infection is made easier."[308] Until the end of the nineteenth century, the inhabitants of Livadeia feared the winds blowing from the direction of Lake Copais for the same reason.[309]

The likelihood of conflating diseases with one another in the context of miasmatic theory required doctors to consider the time of year. Most notably, remittent fevers could easily become misdiagnosed for typhoid fever and the reverse. Still within the miasmatic paradigm, Karamitsas taught that often distinguishing between the two was virtually impossible, unless they overlapped with endemic intermittent fevers in the right season. Furthermore, according to Karamitsas's teaching, if both remittent and typhoid fevers were endemic, "typhoid fevers are more frequent than remittent fevers, which become more widespread only when an epidemic of intermittent fevers prevails."[310]

By 1890, Italian malariologists had identified the human parasites for *vivax, malariae,* and *falciparum* malaria. It had, therefore, become necessary to also examine their frequency and seasonal patterns. Shortly thereafter, in the early twentieth century, the questionnaires of Kardamatis and the Anti-Malaria League began by including items on weather conditions, and months of outbreak, peak, and decline. While Greek physicians seemed to agree that the peak of the malaria season occurred mainly in August and September, their timing of its outbreak varied enormously, ranging from March to September. Even allowing for semantic ambiguities about the meaning of an outbreak, a range of six months is hard to discount completely.

Kardamatis, however, advanced his search even further; on the basis of his blood sample analysis of 4,851 cases collected between 1900 and 1910, he found that 60 percent of these cases had been *falciparum* infections. Moreover, he correlated his findings with mean monthly temperatures in Athens.[311]

---

308 Stéphanos, *La Grèce,* 495–96.
309 Karamitsas, "Peri elodon i eleiogenon nosimaton," vol. 2, 733.
310 Ibid., vol. 2, 784.
311 Kardamatis, "Peri tis par'imin sykhnotitos ton eloparasiton," 63. Kardamatis's analysis extends over eleven years and does not present an annual breakdown. Twenty-one mixed infections are not represented in the graph. Kardamatis, *Pragmateia,* 152–53. Much to his surprise, on his visit to the highly malarious Copais area in early June 1906, Ronald Ross found half the children already suffering from malaria. Jones, Ross, and Ellett, *Malaria,* 11.

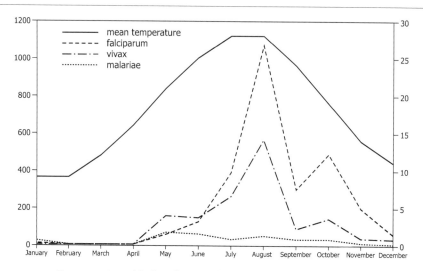

Figure 2.1. Monthly distribution of malaria cases by mean monthly
temperatures in Athens, 1900–10

Source: Kardamatis, "Peri tis par'imin sykhnotitos ton eloparasiton."

Wenyon observed slightly different infection patterns among the British troops in Macedonia, primarily because of the predominance of *vivax* over *falciparum* malaria. The distribution of *Plasmodium* parasites identified among the 29,594 British troops in Thessaloniki admitted for malaria during 1916, the first year spent on the Macedonian Front, varied by month with *falciparum* malaria increasing sharply in the autumn, as shown in the following table.

Month	Benign Tertian	Sub-Tertian	Quartan
June	88.46	11.54	0.00
July	81.07	18.93	0.64
August	89.03	10.33	0.64
September	60.74	38.85	0.41
October	44.07	54.90	1.03
November	25.87	73.32	0.81

Table 2.9. Monthly percentages of malaria among British troops,
June–November 1916

Source: "Report on the incidence of malaria in the Salonika army in 1916; on the measures taken for its prevention; and on the measures proposed for its prevention during 1917," WO32/5112, TNA. The term "sub-tertian" was used for "malignant tertian." The apparent discrepancy between the British and Greek monthly data could be explained by the use of different calendars that were almost two weeks, or thirteen days, apart in the twentieth century. The Julian calendar was in use in Greece until February 1923.

On the basis of around 40,000 positive blood film examinations collected by the army laboratories in 1917 and 1918, Wenyon showed that, among the troops on the Macedonian Front, the prevalence of *vivax* (or benign tertian) malaria was greater than that of *falciparum* (or malignant tertian) malaria and that the numbers of *vivax* cases rose and fell before those of the *falciparum* cases, as shown in figure 2.2.

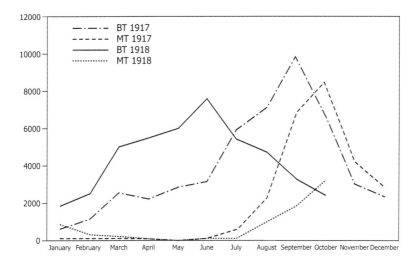

Figure 2.2. The British Army in Macedonia: Monthly malaria admissions, 1917–18
Source: Wenyon, "Malaria in Macedonia."
BT=Benign tertian, MT=Malignant tertian

At end of 1917, the frequency of both *vivax* and *falciparum* malaria cases was practically equal. Thereafter, the gradual fall and practical disappearance of *falciparum* cases led to an increase in the relative proportion of *vivax*, so that between March and May well over 98 percent of positive films of hospitalized malaria patients were for *vivax* malaria. From May onward, practically all *falciparum* cases were primary, whereas a considerable proportion of *vivax* cases were relapses of infections of the previous year.[312]

Having witnessed primary *falciparum* cases as early as the beginning of May, Wenyon questioned the view that outside temperature was the cause

---

312 Wenyon, "Malaria in Macedonia," 47–49. Wenyon remarked that, owing to its severity requiring that patients be hospitalized, *falciparum* malaria was overrepresented in these hospital figures.

for its the late appearance. Rather, by relapses and recrudescence, *vivax* cases carried the infection over to the following year. "With malignant malaria, on the other hand, though the individual attack may be more severe, the cases are more amenable to quinine treatment and there is little tendency for one season's case to persist," he wrote, noting however that the effect of quinine on *vivax* cases was to kill their gametocytes and render them less infective. His prediction was a long-term one, namely "that it should be easier to eradicate *P. falciparum* from a population than *P. vivax*. The former ... is more severe while it lasts but has a natural tendency to disappear before the next malaria season."[313]

These seasonal patterns of malaria incidence corresponded to the observations regarding summer heat made by individual doctors practicing in the Greek countryside, as one, Dionysios Markopoulos, reported from Petalidi in 1907:

> In the region in question malaria fevers appeared as usual in the beginning of June at a temperature of 23°–25°C. At that time 10–15 percent of the peasantry was infected, mostly with quotidian fever. Around early July, 30 percent of those residing in the countryside were infected, while in the town there were few cases; the temperature was 35°C. In early August, 50–60 percent of those in the countryside were infected; temperatures were 20°C. Fevers peaked in the first ten days of September, with almost everyone in the countryside being infected, certainly 80–90 percent of them, and 20–25 percent of those in the town; the same intensity persisted almost until mid-October, when the temperature dropped to 12°C and it rained for the first time (when speaking of fevers, I do not include chronic cases).[314]

Scientific findings were also consistent with the experience of the villagers of Elos, within the limited confines of the lower Evrotas valley. As noted above, they witnessed a similar progression of the malaria season, with the first adult mosquitoes emerging in late May from the flood waters of the Vassilopotamos and Phorvas rivers, followed by the first malaria cases in early June in Vriniko at a time when mosquitoes had not yet appeared in Vlakhiotis, some 3.5 kilometers further inland, and when harvesters, already in

---

313 Wenyon, "Malaria in Macedonia," 49–50.
314 "1907," 191–92.

the plain since late April, were returning home to the malaria-free villages of Mount Parnon.[315]

Thus, within a broad range of variability, the seasonal distribution of the two most common malarial infections followed the general pattern: *vivax* springtime recurrences were followed by *vivax* primary infections in the early summer, while *falciparum* malaria peaked in late summer or autumn, when most of the malaria deaths occurred.

Seasonal migration of transhumant shepherds, a topic treated in the following chapter, removed them from the malarious lowlands during the dangerous months.[316] However, the departure from the plains of a significant proportion of animals that would have otherwise fed the hungry *Anopheles* left the lowland populations even more exposed to mosquito bites, as suggested by Robert Sallares with regard to the Pontine marshes.[317] Autumn rains though and the return of grazing animals was not without further hardship. November rains in Lake Copaïs before its drainage also entailed an advancing shoreline and, therefore, a seasonal loss of farmland.[318]

With the *Anopheles* mosquito part of the explanatory mechanism after 1898, scientists paid greater attention than before to the effects of environmental factors, most notably rainfall, on the abundance of *Anopheles*, or anophelism.

Geographical fragmentation, in turn, could be seen at play on local differences in rainfall irregularity. It is of interest to our understanding of malaria in Greece that a study on the twentieth-century history of malaria transmission in Africa draws the conclusion that "areas of highly variable, episodic climate suitability (the southwestern Congo basin and northwestern Tanzania) were also driven by fluctuations in rainfall rather than temperature" and calls for "refinements in maps and models of precipitation patterns."[319] As early as 1946, M. A. Barber noted that "the curve of malaria prevalence from year to year varies more in Macedonia than in Africa, much depending on the annual rainfall. We experienced one long period in Macedonia, 1932–35 inclusive, during which summer rains were below normal and the number of *Anopheles* and the amount of malaria of many villages greatly di-

---

315 Triantaphyllakos and Oeconomou, *Le paludisme*, 11.
316 Franghiadis, "Peasant Agriculture and Export Trade," 76n1.
317 Sallares, *Malaria and Rome*, 239.
318 Belle, *Trois années en Grèce*, 139.
319 Small, Goetz, and Hay, "Climatic Suitability," 15344.

minished. The diminution of malaria and of anophelism during these years seemed to be due wholly to lack of rain; for certain control villages situated in the vicinity of more permanent breeding places showed little decline."[320] Indeed, writing in 1908, Kardamatis warned that all nationwide epidemics had been preceded by an exceptionally rainy spring. Therefore, he devised a suitable motto to imprint the fact on the minds of his audiences and included questions on rainfall in the Anti-Malaria League surveys.[321]

The following graph draws from schoolchildren data from untreated villages and towns published by the Malariology Division of the Athens School of Hygiene. It reflects the consistently high parasite and splenic indices in western Greece (Epirus and Aitoloakarnania), where the levels of annual rainfall were also high, and the erratic behavior of these indices in the Peloponnese, where rainfall was highly variable.[322]

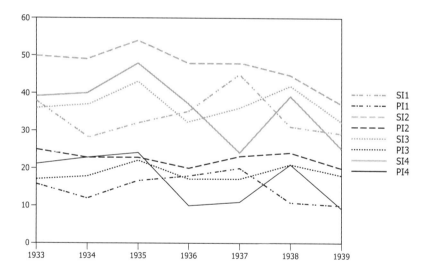

Figure 2.3. Splenic and parasite indices, 1933–39
Source: Livadas and Sfangos, *I elonosia en Elladi*, vol. 1, 138–39.
SI=Splenic index, PI=Parasite index, 1=Macedonia and Thrace, 2=Epirus and Aitolo-
acarnania, 3=Central Greece and Thessaly, 4=Peloponnese

In their attempts to predict the likelihood of an exceptionally epidemic year, some malaria experts and army physicians calculated that malaria epidem-

---

320 Barber, *A Malariologist in Many Lands*, 85.
321 For instance, Kardamatis, "Ai Athinai," 53, and Kardamatis, *Pragmateia*, 27, 49–50.
322 Livadaras and Sfangos, *I elonosia en Elladi*, vol. 1, 138–39.

ics in Greece occurred every five or six years.[323] These predictions were actually confirmed as often as they were not, so that others used a more flexible range of intervals between epidemics: "epidemic outbreaks are observed periodically [in Vovoda] every two to five years, as in most of the country," noted Grigorios Livadas and his coauthors.[324] However, the surveys conducted from 1933 by the Malariology Division of the Athens School of Hygiene demonstrated that endemicity was more stable in small villages with greater variability from year to year in larger villages and towns.[325] In describing such fluctuations, Balfour reported that 1930 had been, in most of the country, a year of low endemicity; 1931, preceded by a winter of heavy rains and snow until late March even in the lowlands, developed an epidemic season, followed by three years of a progressive decline in transmission, followed by a general increase in 1935.[326] Ermoupolis hospital admittances also suggest an irregular pattern; between 1834 and 1850 "fevers,"a general term that included no fewer than fifteen subcategories, fluctuated between a peak of 65 percent in 1835 and a low of 34 percent in 1838.[327]

Often an epidemic that broke out in one year would, in fact, extend into the following, as untreated cases would increase the reservoir of gametocyte carriers still infective at the beginning of the second year, which would then develop a slightly milder epidemic, primarily of *vivax*, that would nonetheless place a strain on an already worn-down community.[328] However, with an eventual return to normality, a great deal of the acquired immunity would be lost, leaving the population at risk of renewed physical and mental hardship in a few years' time. Indeed, as demonstrated above, from the midnineteenth century a considerable number of formerly endemic areas had begun to benefit from the development of agriculture without, however, becoming fully malaria-free. With their populations no longer immune, these areas remained exposed to erratic fever epidemics and suffering.

Interestingly, an epidemic year presented a rise in the relative increase of *falciparum* malaria. In the cases examined over a four-year period (1930–

323 For the Ionian Islands, for instance, see Hennen *Sketches*, 336, who drew on the experience of the locals as well as on "the observations of the Venetian, Russian, French and English residents."

324 Livadas, Kanellakis, and Valaoras, "Paratiriseis," 5.

325 Dimissas, *Engkheiridion*, 108–10.

326 Balfour, "Some Features," 4.

327 Leivadaras, "To proto nosokomeio," 60–68.

328 Also, Wenyon, "Malaria in Macedonia," 49–50.

33) in several villages around Aigio, Balfour found that, while the numbers of *vivax* and *malariae* infections remained almost stable, the source of fluctuation lay in the *falciparum* infections, which more than doubled. During an epidemic, therefore, it was essential to provide free quinine to the indigent, not merely to alleviate suffering but principally to prevent deaths.[329] The consumption of quinine, in turn, was probably at least partly responsible for the surge mostly in *falciparum* in comparison to *vivax* cases, given that quinine is effective against *vivax* but not *falciparum* gametocytes.[330]

As already suggested in Kardamatis's research and the early-twentieth-century surveys, instability significantly affected the start and duration of an epidemic, depending on the effect of local conditions on the lifecycle of the *Anopheles*. For instance, an early and successful *Anopheles* hatch among a human population of gametocyte carriers due to relapses from the previous year would lead to an early outbreak in the year in question. On other occasions, a fresh population arriving at a location toward the end of the malaria season would generate a late outbreak of primary infections. Such had been the case in 1936 at the Larissa garrison, where a group of recruits arrived from Athens in late October. The first malaria cases appeared among these nonimmune recruits in early November with the last of the primary infections occurring on November 23.[331]

As explained by Macdonald, the most important factor contributing to the level of infection is the intensity of transmission, which was largely determined by the biting frequency of *Anopheles*.[332] In the Greek lands, this factor was also extremely variable and depended largely on seasonal variability, which, in turn was also irregular. In Macedonia, for instance, ac-

---

329 Balfour, "Malaria Studies in Greece," 309–12.

330 Warrell, Watkins, and Winstanley, "Treatment and Prevention of Malaria," 269. Indeed, in experiments conducted at the Macedonian Front in 1918, Wenyon had already observed that "quinine has a greater influence in benign tertian cases in rendering them noninfective to mosquitoes than in malignant tertian cases; in other words, the gametocytes of *P. vivax* are more susceptible to quinine than those of *P. falciparum*. Both these factors would tend toward the more rapid dissemination of *P. falciparum*. Furthermore, the malignant tertian malaria in man develops more rapidly toward a large infection and produces in a shorter time a greater number of gametocytes than the benign tertian malaria. It is not uncommon to encounter individuals in whose blood very large numbers of crescents are present without there being any acute symptoms. In benign tertian cases such large numbers of gametocytes are not seen and gametocytes, when present in any number are generally associated with sufficient asexual forms of the parasite to make the individual acutely ill." See Wenyon, "Malaria in Macedonia," 49–50. The fact that quinine did not kill *falciparum* gametocytes had been known since 1900.

331 Manoussakis, *To elonosiakon provlima*, 34.

332 Macdonald, *The Epidemiology and Control of Malaria*, 18–19 and 25–26.

cording to Wenyon, *A. maculipennis*, a term that, at the time of his writing, also included *A. sacharovi*, was active in the plains and valleys between May and November, while *A. superpictus* was active in the hills between July and October. The longer malaria season in the plains and valleys, thus, according to Wenyon, would explain why "the number of infected mosquitoes in the valley would always be higher, owing to their longer exposure to infection."[333] In fact, the distinction between the two *Anopheles* species became clear to malariologists in Greece in late 1932 or early 1933 when the RF scientists were in contact with L. W. Hackett over his recent findings. In January 1933, Barber wrote to Balfour from his station in Kavalla: "You probably have seen the new egg figs. of Dr. Hackett."[334]

The first generation of *A. maculipennis* and *sacharovi* generally emerged in April, reached their highest density in June or July and, in certain areas, became rare after July, or, in favorable locations or years, could remain in high densities until August. In contrast, *A. superpictus* first appeared in June and usually reached its highest density in August and September. Climate patterns could favor the early appearance of one or the other species. It was, in fact, characteristic of malaria epidemiology in Greece and, moreover, a factor of its instability, that one year could be favorable for *A. sacharovi* while another for *A. superpictus*. "A year in which both species are abundant," noted Balfour, "is apt to be an epidemic year, and a long sustained period of morbidity results."[335]

If abundance of rainfall generally favored the proliferation of *Anopheles*, *A. superpictus* could be an exception and benefit from dry summers. If reduced, the flow of stream water, the environment in which it hatched and spent the larval stage of its life, would protect its eggs and larvae from being washed away. Indeed, on his visit to Greece in 1945, Fred L. Soper, the RF malariologist and public health expert, noted of *A. superpictus* and its contribution to the 1942 epidemic that "in years of exceptional drought and high summer temperatures [it] becomes very dangerous and can produce severe

---

333 Wenyon, "Malaria in Macedonia," 41. *A. maculipennis*, the least anthropophilic of all three *Anopheles* species, favors clear, fresh, and still water and was often found in the plains in coexistence with *A. sacharovi*, and in low-lying valleys, marshes, ditches, and irrigation channels. Barber and Rice, "Malaria Studies in Greece: The Infection Rate."

334 M. A. Barber to M. C. Balfour, Kavalla, 24 January 1933 [incorrectly marked 1932], folder 13 749 I (Malaria) 1928–1933, box no. 2 folder nos. 12-18, Projects Series 749 Greece, RG 1.1, RAC.

335 Balfour, "Some Features," 7.

malaria outbreaks." Furthermore, he considered this as "an explanation of why *superpictus* is so much more dangerous in southern Greece and Cyprus, where the summer rainfall is low."[336] In other words, rainy springs indicated an abundance of *A. maculipennis* and *sacharovi* and a dry summer promised thriving *A. superpictus* populations and a protracted and severe malaria epidemic.[337] The same could, indeed, also be true, and equally dangerous, for water flows that were intercepted, diverted, and tamed to run watermills and irrigate gardens.[338]

The following instances from the hills surrounding the highly malarious Thessaly plain illustrate the complex influence of climate on a range of interconnected factors that affected mosquito abundance. They show hydrology playing a major part in the succession between the two more anthropophilic of the local *Anopheles* species, *A. sacharovi* and *A. superpictus*, and indicate how this succession could affect local malaria epidemiology. In several Thessalian villages, such as Paliouri, south of Karditsa, the streams and torrents descending from the surrounding hills gave rise to makeshift irrigation networks used by the villagers to water their gardens and fields and run their mills. The networks would overflow and generate marshes full of *Anopheles* species, *sacharovi* and *maculipennis* in May and June and *superpictus* later on, in the same locations. According to Emmanouil Manoussakis, an army physician, agricultural areas home to *superpictus* usually had a malaria prevalence of 15 to 50 percent, depending on their distance from the mosquito breeding sites and on the date in the season when *superpictus* managed to become the dominant species. In other words, given that infections generally began in May, the severity of a malaria season, according to Manoussakis, depended not so much on its total duration as on the capacity of *superpictus*, the latecomer among the three species, to sustain the chain of infection from *A. sacharovi* and *maculipennis* and keep it constant without a breach in continued transmission.

In this process hydrology was critical. Least affected were the villages where the volume of the water flow from the streams and torrents was reduced only late in the season, thus the *A. superpictus* would be late in be-

---

336 F. L. Soper's diary 1944–1946, p. 9, entry 27 September 1945 [diary starts new page numeration on 1 August 1945], box 58, RF 12.1, RAC.

337 Christos Damkas, "Chapter X: Malaria," p. 568, History, Region EG, Health Division Final Report, folder Greece #38, box PAG-4/4.2.:36, [S-0524-0060], UN Archives.

338 Dimissas, "Eisigisis epi tis epidimiologias tis elonosias en Makedonia kai Thraki," 25.

coming the dominant species. Indeed, in areas wherever *A. superpictus* became dominant after August, where, additionally, there were no longer any *sacharovi* sites that would prolong the summer malaria infections, the belated development of *superpictus* would be of little significance; it would be of a short duration among a human population with a light malaria burden, which would not seriously infect the *superpictus*. In contrast, villages close to streams and torrents whose flow was reduced early and, additionally, were near marshes full of *sacharovi*, would suffer a malaria prevalence almost as bad, as if they had been in the immediate vicinity of swamps. Indeed, *A. superpictus* would continue the infection where *sacharovi* had left off. Deadliest of all were those torrents and streams descending from low, treeless hills to the plain that housed both species and formed rocky as well as muddy pools, the so-called *kolymbes*. Such highly malarious formations could be found in the Tsambaslar and Mousalar torrents, both near Larissa, Tsagli (present-day Eretria), close to Farsala, the torrent of Velestino near Volos, Rodosiva near Elassona, and Khalamvrezi (Kedros) in Karditsa.[339]

The effect of rainfall on water content in organic materials also played a role in malaria prevalence. At the village of Ambelonas (formerly Kazaklar), north of Larissa, there was an abundance of pools full of village effluvia and other organic matter. These waters became unsuitable for *Anopheles* but not for common, or *Culex,* mosquitoes, particularly in periods of drought. Successive days of rain, however, as was the case in mid-September 1937, diluted and cleared the water to such an extent that *A. sacharovi* was able to reproduce there. Thus, an extreme meteorological shift between the summer drought and autumn rainfall had made Ambelonas the home alternately to two different kinds of mosquitoes, one harmless in the summer that was succeeded by an efficient malaria vector, in September, when the pools had cleared.[340]

Likewise, a sudden change in local conditions—for instance a drought in a neighboring village or the departure of sheep flock, increased anophelism, with gusts of wind transporting *Anopheles* from nearby, coinciding with a large number of gametocyte carriers from a previous epidemic—could lead to a renewed epidemic outbreak. Manoussakis observed such an

---

339 Manoussakis, *To elonosiakon provlima*, 312–14.
340 Ibid., 125–26.

incident in Thessaly after ten days of persistent rain in mid-October 1937. Wind-blown *Anopheles* fed on, and were infected by, a population suffering at the time from relapses from an earlier malaria epidemic. A small epidemic of primary infections first emerged in November. By early December, however, the number of malaria cases had exceeded the infections of the entire summer.[341]

CONCLUSION

In 1924, in a letter to Ludwik Rajchman, the director of the Health Organisation of the League of Nations, Lewis Hackett opposed the simple approach to malaria control that was limited to treating human carriers of malaria.[342] For Hackett "malaria is not one problem . . . but must be broken up into thousands of constituent problems before it can be solved. *Divide et Impera*; for one of these local problems differs from every other. There may be a method of choice in each individual case, but there is no single formula for solving them all."[343] While Hackett saw the division as one of quinine treatment versus antilarval measures, Nicolaas Swellengrebel wished to reformulate the divide between the "American" and the "European" camp, or, in his words "the misleading division between antilarvists and quininists" as one between "the modern and historical school or antimalarians and rural sanitarians." Swellengrebel believed in "a preventive organisation taking account of the total nosology of the country . . . by the methods successfully adopted in many countries before the advent of the modern era, but applied by the light of modern science."[344] Furthermore, the lessons drawn by the missions of the League of Nations Malaria Commission to Greece in 1924, 1929, and 1930, also pointed to the "importance of factors of variability in endemic malaria for the outbreak of waves of lethal epidemics, both among the refugees and among the aboriginal population."[345]

---

341 Ibid., 207–8.

342 This was also the approach adopted by the Greek medical authorities; see chapter 4.

343 Lewis Hackett to Ludwik Rajchman, Rome, 3 November 1924, 33609, 28002, 12B R873, League of Nations Archives.

344 N. Swellengrebel to L. Rajchman, Amsterdam, 21 March 1928, 63935, 28002, 12B, League of Nations Archives. See also, Evans, "European Malaria Policy in the 1920s and 1930s"; Sallares, Bouwman, and Anderung, "The Spread of Malaria," 311–12.

345 [M. Ciucă], "Organisation de la lutte antimalarique en Grèce", Geneva, 14 February 1931, p. 2, CH/Malaria/154, Malaria Commission, Health Organisation, League of Nations.

After the Second World War, the UNRRA men, equipped with DDT, which they believed had revolutionized malaria control, saw in Greece's landscape fragmentation an opportunity rather than a challenge, as midway in the long Greek summer, a "progressive drying-up of watercourses and higher placed swamps whose levels recede, tending to concentrate the breeding grounds" facilitated natural control rather than spraying.[346] At the same time, the clustered nature of Greek settlement patterns promised to function in favor of DDT spraying: "in Greece the houses are not scattered all over the country, but are grouped together in small villages. This made DDT house spraying easier." Similarly, "the many small isolated mosquito breeding spots near villages," such as springs supplying water to mountain villages but which also bred *A. superpictus* in their run-off water, lent themselves to DDT focal spraying. With DDT doing the killing, malaria control in a contained milieu ceased to be the labor-intensive, herculean enterprise it had been in the days of Paris greening. For lowland villages, however, under attack from *A. sacharovi* and *A. maculipennis*, where the distribution of the enemy was diffused over "large swamps, lakes and rice fields," aerial spraying presented a uniquely economical option.[347] Thus, in its very modernity the arrival of DDT also eroded and undermined the fragmentation of the Greek landscape.

In fact, it no longer made sense even to carry out another nationwide malaria survey. On the basis of his interwar experience of the country, planning the DDT campaign confidentially in Cairo in the early UNRRA days in April 1944, Daniel E. Wright protested that "literally hundreds of malaria surveys have been made in Greece."[348] In May 1945, as he was drawing public attention to UNRRA's malaria campaign in Greece, which he described

---

346 Vine, "Malaria Control"; J.M. Vine, "Malaria control on a national scale—Greece, 1946," pp. 4–5, Malaria and Sanitation, folder Greece #22, box 35, PAG-4/4.2.:35 [S-0524-0059], UN Archives. Evidence of such decreased acreage of sprayed swampland in June and July 1946 in Thessaly, in Francis Hennessy, "Historical Survey, UNRRA Health Division, F Region," 28 November 1946, pp. 16–17, Greece #60, Historical Report, Region F, PAG-4/4/2/:38 [S-0524-0062], UN Archives.

347 Gordon E. Smith, "Preliminary Report on the Uses of DDT in Greece, 1946," pp. 2–3, Greece #22, Malaria and Sanitation, PAG-4/4.2.:35 [S-0524-0059], UN Archives.

348 W. E. Brown and Laird Archer to James A. Crabtree, Cairo, 28 April 1944, Greece, Organisation and Plan, Health Division, File no. 150 (1), HQ Balkan Mission, Balkan Mission, Central Registry Series, PAG-4/3.0.2.0.3.0.:14 [S-0527-0278], UN Archives. Wright told the UNRRA staff in Greece that between 1930 and 1931, the Rockefeller Foundation men had visited 8,000 out of the 11,000 villages of Greece. D. E. Wright, "Malaria control in Greece," 18 December 1945, Talks to UNRRA staff by UNRRA officials, PAG-4/3.0.12.0.1.:5 [S-0527-0539], UN Archives.

as "the greatest anti-malaria offensive ever practiced in Europe," he told Alekos Angelopoulos, a war correspondent at the International News Service, that Greece was "an open book from the survey viewpoint."[349]

This is an overstatement, to which it is not hard to find exceptions, all of them, however, are confined to surveys of local conditions. At the end of the war, for instance, Phokion Kopanaris, general secretary of the Ministry of Health, invited the US Navy 404 Epidemiological Unit to carry out a malaria survey of the Greek islands.[350] Wright himself, while still in Cairo, called for setting up local malaria and mosquito squads which would carry out "careful surveys of all areas in their territories for possible breeding places for anopheline and *Aedes* mosquitoes."[351] Beyond the purview of the Sanitary Section, the Health Division of UNRRA in Greece conducted horizontal surveys, such as that covering the villages of Evrytania in September and October 1945, as a result of the hardships inflicted by the German Army. Along with other medical problems, the survey also revealed the extent of malaria in these mountain communities.[352] Welfare Division officers conducted a survey of Euboea that also included medical matters, malaria among them, in May and June 1945.[353]

The point raised by James Webb on the "scientific modernity" of the global eradication campaign and the demise of local epidemiological studies could also apply to the assumptions of the DDT campaign. In Webb's words: "The complexities of the local ecologies were sidelined by this belief in universal science, in particular by the delivery of a brilliant, unitary mathematical model of malarial dynamics by George Macdonald."[354] The fragmented environment affecting the erratic manifestation of malaria consisted not only of the heterogeneous landscape of physical properties and social particularities but also of Greece's great annual and seasonal climate variability.

---

349 Daily News Digest, nos. 1-100 (29 March–27 July 1945), *UNRRA Daily News Digest*, No. 30, Athens, 2 May 1945, pp. 3–4, PAG-4/3.0.12.0.1.:1 [S-0527-0535], UN Archives.

350 PAG-4/(3,4,5), UN Archives.

351 These ideas were detailed in his "Plan for medical care program for Greece by Health Division, UNRRA, during the military phase," 5 August 1944, pp. 6–7, W/01 (2) Health, PAG-4/3.0.12.2.0.:1 [S-0527-0641], UN Archives.

352 See Provincial 11-24 Evrytania, PAG-4/3.0.12.2.3.:8 [S-0527-0672], UN Archives.

353 See Provincial 11-30 Euboea, PAG-4/3.0.12.2.3.:8 [S-0527-0672], UN Archives.

354 Webb, *Humanity's Burden*, 169.

CHAPTER III

MALARIA IN PEACE AND WAR

Malaria responds differently to times of peace and times of war. This chapter considers the effect on malaria of regular, peacetime human activities, that is, agriculture, colonization, industry and urban development, and the impact of war on malaria epidemiology.

RURAL MALARIA

In his wartime survey, Ioannis Kardamatis drew a distinction between lakes and swamps on the one hand, to which he attributed an average malaria morbidity of 48 percent among the populations at risk, and small water collections on the other, which were responsible for a morbidity rate of between 50 and 90 percent among the populations at risk. For this far more serious condition, he blamed the man-made mosquito breeding sites that resulted from pretty much any outdoor rural activity. "Ditches opened up to delimit or protect private land from animals or to drain it," he warned,

> ditches on either side of railway lines, water collection pools (commonly known as *loutses* or *báres*), irrigation channels, rainwater tanks, all kinds of tanks (in oil presses, vineyards, etc.), fountains, reservoirs, wells, barriers between seaside swamps and the sea, meadows, roadside protective ditches, rice fields, small streams, vineyard irrigation, fields and landed estates when flooded, the treatment of flax and rushes, construction works, the operation of industrial plants, particularly potteries, brick and tile works, and various other sources of livelihood and social needs.[1]

---

1   Kardamatis, *Statistikoi pinakes*, 247. On the recent literature, see also Packard, *The Making of a Tropical Disease*, 11; Coluzzi, "Malaria and the Afrotropical Ecosystems," 223–27.

Kardamatis's two categories may have been useful as analytical tools to assess relative risk. In everyday practice, however, particularly with carriers traveling between town and country, exposure to one of these two environments was not always unequivocal. The analysis that follows looks into how diverse productive activities accommodated, shaped and exploited natural environments shared with *Anopheles*. As Margaret Humphreys has pointed out with regard to malaria, "location was everything, and it was tied to economic conditions as well."[2]

Agriculture

Megali Vrysis: An Extremely Difficult Case

In mid-July 1907, Kardamatis, with two colleagues from Lamia, visited Megali Vrysis, an estate in Fthiotis belonging to the Merlin family. The Merlins also had property in Corfu and were related to the wealthy Corfiot Theotokis family. The Megali Vrysis estate came into the public eye in April 1907, when Georgios Theotokis's government was accused of planning to include Megali Vrysis in a bill on the drainage of swamps; one opposition newspaper denounced the prime minister for planning to spend public money to triple the value of his relatives' property.[3]

The estate lay less than 4 kilometers east of Lamia on the road to Stylida; only about half was under cultivation, while the rest was covered by a marsh extending over an expanse of about 6 square kilometers in the winter and about 4.5 square kilometers in the summer. This marsh communicated with two more marshes: Mavromandyla and Avlaki. Besides rainwater, the marsh received clear fresh water all year round from two abundant springs.[4] At the time, Kardamatis believed he had found *A. maculipennis* dominating exclusively in the estate. As already noted, however, in the interwar years, Lewis Hackett in Rome, puzzled by the absence of malaria at locations with *Anopheles*, found out that, in fact, what had previously been thought of as one *Anopheles* species, *A. maculipennis*, was indeed a com-

---

2 Humphreys, *Malaria*, 55.
3 Charles William Louis Merlin was director of the Ionian Bank and British consul in Piraeus in the nineteenth century. See "Ta filika telmata"; I thank Helen Gardikas Katsiadakis for bringing this article to my attention.
4 Kardamatis, "Ekthesis peri tis en to Fthiotiko pedio elonosias," 26.

plex of several species, some of which were harmless. However, among the members of the complex was *A. elutus*, an alternative name for *A. sacharovi*. The most dangerous species for humans in Greece, it preferred brackish waters. Some of the other members of the *maculipennis* complex were, in fact, refractory to *Plasmodia*.[5] The estate most probably was preponderantly home to *A. sacharovi*.[6]

The Megali Vrysis estate was home to about 100–120 individuals,[7] namely its tenants, two millers, the leaseholder of the estatae, and their families. A few years earlier, in 1903, the landowner had constructed a small village of twenty-five two-room houses for some of the tenants and the leaseholder about a kilometer away from a spring, near the Stylida railway station. Everyone else lived by the marsh.

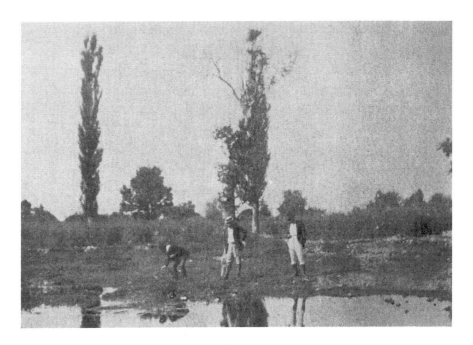

Figure 3.1. The Megali Vrysis
Source: Kardamatis, *Pragmateia*, 561.

5   Fantini, "Anophelism without Malaria"; Hackett, *Malaria in Europe*, 28–46.
6   Livadas and Sfangos, *I elonosia en Elladi*, 2: 103; Hadjinicolaou and Betzios, "Resurgence of *Anopheles Sacharovi*." After a close study of the location, Grigorios Livadas concluded that "its malaria problem is extremely difficult." For photographs from Kardamatis's visit to the Megali Vrysis estate, see Kardamatis, *Pragmateia*, 561–62.
7   Savvas and Kardamatis, "Apantiseis dimarkhon," 534–35.

Kardamatis counted about 200–300 *Anopheles* on average in merely one corner in each of the newly constructed houses and estimated that each home contained more than 2,000 *Anopheles*, "not counting those under the beds, tables, closets, the ceiling, and other locations where mosquitoes spend the day." Despite his long experience, Kardamatis had never seen anything like the situation in Megali Vrysis. He then examined spleens and blood plates on his portable microscope and found mixed infections of all three types of malaria parasites in all fifty of the cases examined, except for fifty-five-year-old Stavros Triantaphyllou and his sixteen-year-old son Konstantinos, who had never come down with malaria nor had ever taken quinine; evidently the two men were protected by natural immunity. Clearly, Kardamatis's account of an entire community infected with malaria by mid-July is consistent with hyperendemicity.[8] One of the Lamia doctors had suggested that in 1906 perhaps everyone on the estate was ill with malaria.[9]

How did the serious sanitary conditions in Megali Vrysis affect the surrounding region? Could the dangerous marsh on the Megali Vrysis estate influence morbidity in the town of Lamia, which lay beyond the normal flight range of 1 to 2 kilometers of female *Anopheles*? Kardamatis formulated an interesting hypothesis: in Lamia there existed a settlement of some 600 Gypsies; considered to be "cheaper and more suitable laborers for all kinds of work in the marshes, they were preferred over anyone else." Besides supplementary seasonal field work, therefore, this cheap labor force was employed in heavy work such as drainage, clearing, digging canals, and in the collection of reeds growing in the marshes. Such activities further exposed them to malaria, for which Gypsies were not protected by any kind of immunity, as Kardamatis had observed all over Greece. They returned to their settlement in Lamia with the *Plasmodia* of Megali Vrysis in their bloodstream to infect the local mosquito population and ignite a fresh cycle of human infections.[10]

---

8   Snow and Gilles, "The Epidemiology of Malaria," 89.

9   Savvas, Kardamatis, and Dasios, "1906," 482. The photo of one of the malarious children displaying his enlarged spleen can be seen in Kardamatis, *Pragmateia*, 305.

10 Underprivileged social groups often incurred increased risk of malaria. Take, for example, the impoverished widowed women in Mani, who found themselves at the lower end of the social scale. Each June they became gleaners, or *stakhomazokhtres*, in the harvested fields and exposed themselves to a high risk of malaria; Dikaios Vagiakakos, personal communication (March 2006).

The story of Megali Vrysis suddenly ends here. Kardamatis was compelled to abandon Lamia without testing his hypothesis, summoned by a new crisis: a heavy epidemic outbreak of malaria among Eastern Rumelian refugees who had settled in Almyros, in the department of Magnisia in Thessaly, during their first summer of displacement, to which I shall return later in this chapter.[11]

In the early twentieth century, the banks of the River Sperkheios and the Megali Vrysis estate were the two most serious foci of endemic malaria left in the Fthiotis plain. The entire region, however, had a long history of fevers, social unrest, and tensions among seminomadic shepherds, peasants, and landlords. A frontier region with the Ottoman Empire, its mountainous hinterland was home to intensive brigandage, which the state managed to bring under control after a nationwide clampdown that followed the Dilessi murders in 1871.[12]

Reflecting on the nosological history of the plain, one physician complained in 1882: "Unfortunately, in Fthiotis complete peace and security have never prevailed." Coastal Fthiotis, which was, moreover, in the hands of absentee landowners, was a treeless and "particularly swampy country, with plants that thrive in lakes and marshes, such as reed, willows, wickers and the like." Megali Vrysis was one such coastal landscape where the fresh swamp water mixed with the sea waves.[13]

Throughout the plain men and women of the lowlands mostly lived in huts and cottages; they were weak and suffered from cachexia and often "monstrously" enlarged spleens. After the winter snow and heavy spring rains were followed by flooding and intense summer heat, epidemics erupted in 1858 and 1859. A particularly serious epidemic occurred in 1864 after a very wet winter and spring. Another milder epidemic broke out four years later and yet another severe one in August 1870, following the unprec-

---

11 Kardamatis, "Peri tis en to Fthiotiko pedio elonosias," 25–29. In April 1907, an article in the press warned against settling the refugees in the malarious plain of Almyros. Politis, "To agrotikon zitima," 5. See p. 177 in this book.

12 For a comprehensive history of the social and environmental tensions over land usage and ownership in the Sperkheios valley, focusing on the Imirbey estate, present-day Anthili, see Louloudis, "Georgikos eksynkhronismos," 107 and 372. On brigandage in Central Greece, see Koliopoulos, *Listes*, 163–65 and 245–51, for instance.

13 Rizopoulos, "Nosologiki katastasis tis eparkhias Fthiotidos," 499–502. Similar landscapes were also located in Akhinos, Stylida, Agia Triada, and the springs at Thermopylae. Absenteeism and brigandage were two factors of neglect also stressed by Henri Belle with regard to the Copais plain, before its drainage. See Belle, *Trois années en Grèce*, 133.

edented flooding of the Sperkheios over the entire plain, "which resembled a lake, in which the lowland villages appeared as islets." To conclude the misery, the river burst its banks in late May and destroyed the crops.[14]

The turmoil that followed the end of the Russo-Turkish War of 1877–78 and Greek expectations of territorial gains generated a temporary reemergence of brigands and irregular border fighters. Nonetheless, the progress in agriculture begun in the early 1870s continued and many waterlogged areas gave way to farming. In addition to safety from brigandage, milder weather also stimulated the expansion of agriculture; as a result, the size of the large swamps of the plain was reduced, landowners now took an interest in their estates and reinforced the banks of the Sperkheios to protect their properties from flooding. This must have reduced the amount of anophelism.[15] Still, a number of villages in the coastal zone closest to the marshes with a total population of about 30,000 inhabitants remained at increased risk of intermittent fevers.[16] Endemic fevers and marshland malaise were so extensive that malaria was often symptomless, detectable, according to the local physician D. Rizopoulos, only through "careful examination" and treated by large doses of quinine sulphate. The locals called this marshland malaise latent temperature (*kryfothermi*) or temperature (*thermi*) of the bones. The most serious foci of endemic fevers were Megali Vrysis, with a population of fifty or sixty families, and Moskhokhori, with some eighty to a hundred families, which lay south of the eastern-flowing river.[17]

Despite some improvement due to progress in agriculture and minor drainage, for Kardamatis, the overall situation in the entire plain remained extremely serious. Besides the two zones of hyperendemic malaria, namely the river banks and Megali Vrysis, epidemic outbreaks of malaria erupted in most of the plain, from small foci varying in origin.[18]

---

14 Rizopoulos, "Nosologiki katastasis tis eparkhias Fthiotidos," 519–20; Stéphanos, *La Grèce*, 500. On the 1858 epidemic in Fthiotis, see also "Peri dimosias ygeias apo 1 Oktovriou 1858 mekhri protis Ianouariou 1859," 431.

15 Rizopoulos, "Nosologiki katastasis tis eparkhias Fthiotidos," 506. Evidently, writing in 1882, Rizopoulos was unaware of the mosquito's role in malaria transmission.

16 Ibid., 509. These towns and villages were Lamia, Stylida, Akhinos, Avlaki, Agia Marina, Megali Vrysis, Saramousakli (Roditsa), Imirbei (Anthili), Alamana, Komma, Moskhokhori, Smixades, Amouri, Lianokladi, Kastri, Khalili (Mesopotamia), and Arakhni.

17 Ibid., 511.

18 Stéphanos, *La Grèce*, 500; Kardamatis, "Ekthesis peri tis en to Fthiotiko pedio elonosias," 19–20; "Apantiseis ton k. Iatron," 203.

In the broader area, as in many parts of Greece, occasional drainage works in the Sperkheios basin were undertaken with the collaboration of the local inhabitants, mostly without expert technical advice. Indeed, very few physicians were aware of the risks inherent in land development projects; "so far, the most dangerous marshes, at least in our country, are man-made," noted a physician from the Ionian Islands before the First World War, recommending that rural doctors inform authorities as well as the population of the associated dangers.[19] For instance, in the Peloponnese, not far from Tripoli, a significant amount of malaria was limited to a small area in the village of Kapareli in Tegea and its mills by Lake Taka, after the lake had been drained in the summer of 1905.[20] Emmanouil Manoussakis, the army malariologist, also believed that large drainage schemes undertaken by state or other authorities created the most numerous malarious sites.[21] By the time Manoussakis was writing his treatise, international experience had demonstrated that "in many well-populated and highly cultivated areas it is not an exaggeration to say that most of the places where mosquitoes breed are the result of man's interference with natural drainage."[22] Worse still, quoting R. C. Connor, Hackett added: "'man-made foci of mosquito breeding can be attributed to the negligence and carelessness of construction engineers. After insanitary conditions have been created by them it is usually a difficult problem to get them to spend the money necessary to correct them.'" He sternly added: "Until construction engineers develop a conscience with regard to malaria, they must be regarded by the health officer as one of the most dangerous and difficult of his malaria hazards."[23]

According to Kardamatis's wartime survey, Lamia was plagued by an average morbidity of 60 percent within the broader highly malarious Sperkheios valley.[24] The town acquired a short-lived state Antimalarial Service station in 1930, which performed blood examinations and found 75 percent positive cases and a large amount of malaria imported from the plain to villages at altitudes between 600 and 800 meters among shepherds who

19 Alvanitis, "Peri profylaxeon apo tis fymatioseos kai tis elonosias," 140.
20 "1905," 430.
21 Manoussakis, To elonosiakon provlima, 240. For a biography of Emmanouil Manoussakis, see Papadimitriou, Emmanuel Manoussakis.
22 Hackett, Malaria in Europe, 269–70.
23 Ibid., 270.
24 Kardamatis, Statistikoi pinakes, 127.

visited Ypati regularly in the autumn.[25] The main activity, though, of the La-mia station was to distribute quinine to local schoolchildren through their teachers. In hyperendemic locations, such as Megali Vrysis, where the Ro-manian physician Mihai Ciucă, at the time the secretary of the League of Nations Malaria Commission, who was visiting Greece in 1930 at the gov-ernment's request, found a spleen rate of 75 percent, the Antimalarial Ser-vice doctors themselves issued quinine directly to the inhabitants, princi-pally women and children, on a daily basis. In fact, a delegation of Megali Vrysis women came before Ciucă and his team to protest against the assis-tant physician, "who woke them up in the morning to make them swallow their quinine" to ensure compliance.[26]

Acknowledging the serious malaria situation in the broader region, the RF IHD team in Greece set up an observation station in the Sperkheios valley in 1934, based in the spa resort of Ypati.[27] With the support of local hotels, this station developed into "the most important center of malaria study" in Greece, according to Grigorios Livadas.[28] The center put to the test several control measures and thus received international attention.[29] A state malaria control station was reestablished in the town of Lamia in 1938 to serve the entire region of Central Greece and mainly carried out larva control with Paris green and gambusia fish. It appears that drainage projects around the town of Lamia never went beyond the planning stage.[30] Thus, "as malaria control today is about 85 percent drainage (perhaps too much so),"[31] according to one interwar malariologist visiting Greece, the situation in the Lamia area was still serious when Greece entered the Second World War.

25 Société des Nations, Organisation d'Hygiène, Commission du Paludisme, M. Ciucă, "Organisation de la lutte antimalarique en Grèce," Geneva, 14 February 1931, pp. 11, 17, CH/Malaria/154; Kopanaris, *I dimosia ygeia en Elladi*, 204–5.

26 Société des Nations, Organisation d'Hygiène, Commission du Paludisme, M. Ciucă, "Organisation de la lutte antimalarique en Grèce," Geneva, 14 February 1931, p. 22, CH/Malaria/154. League of Nations, Health Organisation, Malaria Commission, "Ten years of activity of the Commission," Geneva, 1 March 1934, p. 8, C.H./Mal./212.

27 Greece—annual report 1938 pp. 31–34, folder 2937, box 243, Series 700, RG 5.3, RF, RAC.

28 Livadas and Sfangos, *I elonosia en Elladi*, vol. 2, 66.

29 W. S. Sweet, "Diary of a European trip" 1938, entry 6 May 1938, 100 I, folder 511 Swe-1, box 51, Series 100, RG 1, RF, RAC.

30 Livadas and Sfangos, *I elonosia en Elladi*, vol. 2, 101–7. Malaria control with gambusia fish became so successful and popular, that children would enjoy distributing the fish they collected from the local hatcheries in the lakes of Langadas, Giannitsa, Kastoria, Drama, Serres, Philippi, and Lamia. Dimissas, *Engkheiridion*, 140.

31 Brian R. Dyer, "Inspection of malaria control work in the U.S., Europe, Cyprus, Ceylon and India" [Nov.–Dec. 1937], p. 3, Dye-1, folder 474, box 48, Series 100 I, RG 1, RAC.

During the war, the drainage system in the Sperkheios valley, set up in the interwar years under the supervision of the RF IHD, fell into disrepair. The valley flooded again and the Germans began a repair project which they left incomplete. In December 1944, antimalarial medication was being distributed mostly by the local health department of the National Liberation Front (EAM), which was leftist in sympathies, and, to a much lesser extent, by a British-controlled regional distribution committee.[32] In August 1945, when a comprehensive recovery plan was drawn up by the UNRRA staff, the valley still lay flooded, full of *Anopheles* mosquitoes.[33] In the coastal zone, where 80–100 percent of the village population were reported to be suffering from malaria, consumption of Atabrine was "enormous." "Nearly all the population has had malaria, so that with every fresh illness (such as the present mild epidemic of flu) the drug is given to prevent the appearance of a malarial relapse."[34]

In this context of extreme hardship, the twenty houses at Megali Vrysis received their first DDT spraying from UNRRA in 1945,[35] while the whole Lamia plain was sprayed intensely with DDT between 1946 and 1959. In 1957, Lamia housed one of the country's three malaria research stations.[36] Furthermore, extensive drainage work conducted after the end of the war had provided thousands of acres for agriculture and diverted streams for irrigation; as a result *A. maculipennis* and *A. superpictus* vanished, leaving *A. sacharovi*, the most dangerous malaria vector in Greece, as the principal species in "enormous density" and just as anthropophilic as in the past, having in the meantime developed resistance to DDT.[37] In 1970, Megali Vrysis had a gambusia fish hatchery.[38]

32 Lt. Col. Dodge to Maj. Hopkins, Lamia, 10 December 1944, Phthiotis, Provincial 11-23, PAG-4/3.0.12.2.3.:8 [S-0527-0672], UN Archives.

33 Vernon P. Crockett to K. G. Dodge, 22 August 1945, Sanitation 01-00, PAG-4/3.0.12.2.3.:1 [S-0527-0665], UN Archives.

34 Dr. Low, Report "Lamia Valley," Lamia, 22 April 1945, Phthiotis, Provincial 11-23, PAG/4-3.0.12.2.3.:8 [S-0527-0672], UN Archives. During the war children under eight had received milk from the International Red Cross distribution networks; those over twelve were "put to hard work" while those between eight and twelve "seem to have suffered most from stunted growth and general nutrition." Worse off were the children of Stylida, who were "anemic looking." The synthetic antimalarial drug Atabrine that also went by the name of Mepacrine was developed by Bayer in 1932 but the Allies succeeded in producing large quantities for their own wartime needs. Greenwood, "Conflicts of Interest," 864–65.

35 Mick Bartholomeos to Vernon P. Crockett, Lamia [1945], Malaria ABH, Sanitation 01-50, PAG-4/3.0.12.2.3.:1 [S-0527-0665], UN Archives.

36 The other two were established in Skala and Serres. Vassiliou, "Politics, Public Health, and Development," 288.

37 Hadjinicolaou and Betzios, "Biological Studies on *Anopheles Sacharovi*."

38 Hadjinicolaou and Betzios, "Gambusia Fish."

The story of Megali Vrysis epitomizes many of the malaria-related issues observed throughout Greece, such as the tension between endemic and epidemic malaria and between town and countryside, the ambivalent interrelation between malaria and agriculture and its relation to landowners and minority ethnic groups; its relation to landscapes was affected by the inroad of technological innovation and management.

Irrigation and Grazing

Farming methods, particularly primitive irrigation practices, were responsible for the spread of malaria. Some of the heavily malarious plains in the Peloponnese were used in the winter as pasture lands by nonlocal peasants. For instance, in the early nineteenth century, the peasants from Tripolitsa brought their cattle to Elos to graze. Buffaloes were used by farmers for tilling the hard soil, specifically in Nafplio, Gastouni, and Nisi near Kalamata.[39]

John Hennen offers a distressing account of an irrigated garden in Zakynthos, around 1822, whose management cost the lives of several of its owners:

> In a country house, beautifully but treacherously situated, on the western side of this ravine, where it expands into a basin, the Fort Adjutant, Lieutenant Miles, of the 8th regiment, took up his abode. On each side of his house a mountain stream ran down into the main channel; one of these was dammed up for horticultural and domestic purposes, and supplied a tank which lay immediately below the house. Above, the Castle Hill arose abruptly; and around, the olives grew so thickly as almost to touch the walls. In this habitation the mistress, her child, her maid, and three male servants, were violently attacked with autumnal remittent fever, the genuine product of malaria. The master was also unwell, but not to such an extent as materially to affect his health: of the other individuals, all died with the exception of one male servant, who, after repeated struggles with the disease and its consequences, died from a third attack of visceral disease, accompanied with dropsy. Though the spot which I have now described is the largest in size of any in the neighbourhood of the town, yet the clay hills which nearly surround it, and on which the castle is built, abound in many smaller gullies of a

---

39   Leake, *Travels in the Morea*, vol. 1, 197.

similar character, and, from the retentive nature of the soil, a constant source of malarious vapour is presented to the action of the summer sun.[40]

Around the same time, in 1828 and 1829, a British visitor to Greece saw the peasants of the Peloponnese grow maize with no regard to the effects of stagnant water on health and noted: "The unhealthiness of the Morea is not solely attributable to the want of cultivation, but also to a bad system of irrigation; for when it is necessary to inundate land for the growth of Indian corn, the water is so ill conducted, that it is allowed to become stagnant, and in consequence it invariably occurs, that wherever this species of wheat is cultivated the vicinity is subject to malaria and its terrible effects."[41]

Not far from Athens, on the rural northeastern side of Attica, the villagers of Marathon secured the irrigation of their vegetable plots from water mills upstream that received it in abundance from the Oinoi gorge. The overflow joined the rain and spring water to sustain two marshes, Vrexiza and Kato Souli, which caused an enormous malaria burden in the surrounding villages and marble quarries, as noted in 1906.[42]

Some eleven years later, in 1917, the French doctors of the Armée d'Orient made the following observation in the Jelova valley of the Pisoderi region in Macedonia, recently acquired by Greece:

The River Jélova runs through prairies almost all the year round; generally, the fields of maize lie on the plateaux. The river pastures are flooded less by the river, which rarely overflows its banks in the summer, than by the villagers, who use a barbaric, but the least tiring, procedure of irrigation by dams and by changing the water course without draining. The other causes of unhealthiness relate to the trampling of the flooded fields by cattle and ponies, to mill races and, more generally, to the absence of any kind of channeling for the flow of rain or spring water. If the sloughs that result from one of the causes mentioned above are frequent, the marshes are rare: we have not come across but one between Trnovo and Roula.[43]

---

40 Hennen, *Sketches*, 309–10.
41 Alcock, *Travels in Russia, Persia, Turkey and Greece*, 184–85.
42 Anastasopoulos, Kapanidis, and Dimitriou, "Ai elodeis nosoi en to dimo Marathonos kata to 1906," 278–79 and 284.
43 Delamare and Robin, "Carte du paludisme des confins albano-macédoniens," 496–97. Similar behavior is also suggested in Stéphanos, *La Grèce*, 495.

Drainage works may have been effective, but, like similar schemes in Thessaly, Central Greece and Epirus, they were interrupted on several occasions when the economic crisis of the 1930s hit Greece. Lack of maintenance, as in the case of Copais, left the drained area with a persistent malaria problem, largely due to poorly maintained irrigation and drainage canals. Even so, in the words of M. C. Balfour: "If agricultural drainage does not entirely remedy a problem, it will, in many cases, make possible the application of other measures," adding that in 1935 there was an increase in "minor drainage" projects with positive effects.[44]

In the plain of Marathon, where Daniel E. Wright, the RF sanitary engineer, had drained the swamp by 1936, the refugee settlers of Nea Makri cultivated cotton in the reclaimed land, but "there is very little fall in the ditches"; since the work of maintenance and supervision fell on the government, the result of the drainage was doubtful.[45] In some instances, irrigation requirements even prevented the execution of small sanitary drainage works. In the autumn of 1945, a resident in a malarious village of Evrytania in Central Greece explained to an UNRRA medical officer that the locals were not inclined to drain the mosquito breeding sites surrounding, or even located in the center of, their villages "as they are vital for irrigation of the fields."[46]

In the dry plain of Thessaly, it was common practice for the peasants to collect rainwater in ditches and deep ponds, the so-called *báres*, close to the village and there to bath their cattle, buffaloes, and horses.[47] Some rocky and arid locations acquired a malaria problem as peasants collected water in cisterns and used it for personal consumption, for their animals and oil presses.[48]

In the interwar years, there is evidence that communal irrigation rights that were sanctioned by established usage prohibited the management of wa-

---

44 Balfour, "Some Features," 12–13. J. R. McNeill has pointed out the epidemiological perils of irrigation in connection to contemporary irrigation schemes in Egypt, and the role of these schemes in spreading the deadly malaria epidemic of 1942. "The same was true almost wherever irrigation expanded, excepting the richer, better-organized societies." McNeill, *Something New*, 205.

45 Excerpts from W. A. Sawyer's diary notes, entry 22 May 1936, folder 14 749 I (Malaria) 1934–1938, box no. 2, Projects Series 749 Greece, RG 1.1, RAC.

46 L. F. Miller, 16 October 1945, Evrytania, Provincial 11-14, PAG-4/3.0.12.2.3.:8 [S-0527-0672], UN Archives.

47 Savvas, Kardamatis, and Dasios, "1906," 625. Often these bathing ponds close to human habitation were a secondary usage originally resulting from excavations to obtain clay for bricks. Savvas, Kardamatis, and Dasios, "1906," 631.

48 Savvas and Kardamatis, "Apantiseis dimarkhon," 528.

ter courses. A court decision, for example, ruled against directing into the River Enipeas the water from the Laspokhoritis, a stream in Farsala, that put seven villages with a total population of 15,000 inhabitants at risk of malaria and death, "because the water supply moves two mills and must by law pass through all these seven villages, and because buffalo herds graze on its marshy banks."[49] Likewise in eastern Macedonia, in the village of Khrysoupoli, where 75 percent of the children had enlarged spleens and deaths exceeded births, the League of Nations experts found waterholes "everywhere" and buffaloes wallowing in these perfect mosquito breeding sites.[50] In fact, this situation was the norm throughout the country; Daniel E. Wright saw "in practically every instance, large shallow wells for irrigation purposes, pot holes in yards, irrigation ditches and blocked drains. This condition exists in and around villages where the doctor's examination of school children showed from 40–80 percent spleen enlargement."[51] Thus, it would appear that in the mindset of the Greek peasantry, marshland drainage works were welcome projects, for which they were occasionally ready to contribute their own labor. Small water collections, streams and pools, however, which they often integrated into their production methods, were quite another matter.[52]

In the spring, highland grazing lands attracted the seminomadic Vlach shepherds away from the malarious plains, where they normally spent the winter. This direction of seasonal transhumance protected them from malaria to such a reliable degree that in the 1930s the RF researchers in the Kavalla station inferred that in Greece malaria was not transmitted in the winter partly on the basis of microbiological examinations of this ethnic group.[53] However, low-lying marginal swampland also provided pastures, as in the case of the Almyros grazing fields mentioned below,[54] where the prospect of malarious fevers thwarted an attempt by Vlach shepherds to settle on land granted by the government.

Cattle and flock grazing habits appear to have produced seasonal shifts in the prevailing species of *Anopheles*. In the Tyrnavos and Ambelonas

---

49 Manoussakis, *To elonosiakon provlima*, x.
50 League of Nations, Health Organisation, Health Committee, *I The Prefecture of Cavalla*, 8.
51 D. E. Wright to F. F. Russell, Athens, 30 May 1930, folder 25 (Health Services) 1929–1936, 1939, box 3, 749 K, 1.1, RAC.
52 See also Kardamatis, *Statistikoi pinakes*, 177 and 247.
53 Barber, *A Malariologist in Many Lands*, 89.
54 See p. 178 in this book.

marshes, north of Larissa in Thessaly, after harvest time in July, the prevailing species were the zoophilic *A. bifurcatus* and *A. algeriensis*; they replaced *A. sacharovi* and *A. maculipennis* that fed on both humans and animals. The replacement occurred when the shepherds brought their flock to drink from the marsh along with the flock-feeding mosquitoes. Meanwhile, the summer heat limited the flight range of the other two species to a radius closer to human habitation in the nearby villages. Later in the season, in cooler weather, when the villagers returned to the marsh and built huts to guard the produce of their vegetable gardens, *A. sacharovi* and *A. maculipennis* came back to feed on humans.[55]

The forbidding environment of Araxos, west of the city of Patras, was another landscape suitable for grazing. The survey of 1838 recorded only three families permanently settled there, while a small number of tent dwellers descended from the surrounding villages in the winter to graze their cattle.[56] Even after the Second World War, the Araxos swamps were occupied by "primitive native villages" of mud and wood housing "with shallow wells as water sources, and tallow candles their only form of light at night." The inhabitants made a marginal living from some agriculture and coastal fishing. In one village, eight out of ten inhabitants were suffering from malaria. The author of the account, P. S. Robinson, a British air force medical officer, believed he "easily understood why this region has not progressed as rapidly as other better known parts of Greece."[57]

Drainage and Wastelands

Occasional, if unsuccessful, attempts to tame swamplands and bring them under cultivation through small-scale drainage projects ended up by creating wastelands. Close to the western coast of Corfu, seven miles north-

---

55 Manoussakis, *To elonosiakon provlima*, 124–25.

56 Anninos, "Iatrostatistikoi pinakes tis dioikiseos Akhaïas."

57 P. S. Robinson, "Malaria control at Araxos," Malaria and Sanitation Greece #22, PAG-4/4.2.:35 [S-0524-0059], UN Archives. The Araxos villages were Paralimni (now Araxos), Mesa Paralimni, Karavostasi, Lakkopetra, Agios Georgios, Limnokhori, and Kalamaki. R. L. Prichard, Office of Regional Sanitary Engineer, UNRRA, Region C, Patras, Greece, "Summary of activities in Sanitation Division for month of July," 1 August 1945, Sanitation Water Survey, PAG-4/3.0.12.2.3.:21 [S-0527-0685], UN Archives. The desolate landscape resembled the Pontine Marshes, where the only human activities were woodcutting, charcoal burning, fishing, shepherding and buffalo herding, cultivation of a small amount of wheat, and "rough pasturage." Snowden, *The Conquest of Malaria*, 147.

west of the city, in an area that today is a drained badland, the extensive marshland around the lake in the Ropa valley underwent a fair amount of change over time, however tenuous this change may have been. By the time the British occupied the island, in 1814, its edges had come to produce "rich crops of corn, rice and grapes" in the summer and in the winter attracted hunters of the water fowl to which the lake gave refuge. Particularly in the autumn, though, the surrounding villages suffered a heavy burden of intermittent fevers. All the year round, however, it remained a source of fever for its naive visitors.[58] The British discontinued rice culture to protect the region from malaria.[59]

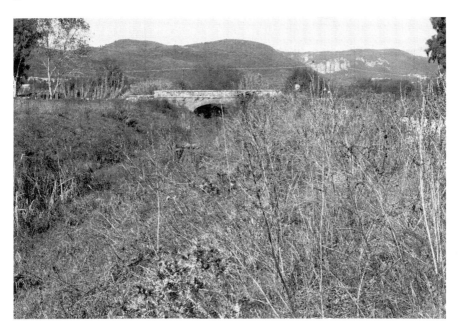

Figure 3.2. Ropa Valley, drainage works.
Photograph by the author.

The agricultural value imputed to the land was such that repeated attempts to drain the swamp were undertaken by private individuals during the nineteenth century. Such attempts involved, for instance, the Theotokis family as well as funds from the Napoleon Zambelis estate, which financed the

58 Hennen, *Sketches*, 146–47. On the effect of steeping flax on fevers in Zakynthos, see Hennen, *Sketches*, 319.
59 Davy, *Notes and Observations*, vol. 1, 358.

construction of an extensive network of drainage canals or *tagies*, still visible today, but had only limited success.[60] In 1906 a local doctor blamed the early outbreak of fever in March on the seasonal digging of vineyards.[61] Indeed, for the League of Nations Commission that surveyed Greece in 1929, the Ropa valley, which was in the course of returning to its prior flooded condition, was typical of drainage projects planned exclusively with cultivation rather than sanitization in mind.[62]

After the Second World War, the channels from the earlier, forty-year-old drainage project of the Ropa valley fell into a state of disrepair, causing it to flood after mid-April. A part of the plain belonging to the Kerkyra Papermill Company contained a large number of springs and was particularly swampy. The UNRRA sanitary engineer surveying the area believed that a comprehensive land reclamation solution would be far too expensive; under the circumstances, he recommended DDT spraying.[63]

The long-time exposure of the local population to malaria was expressed in the high frequencies of hemoglobinopathies, revealed in the research of Stamatoyannopoulos and Fessas. They examined a total of 1,122 individuals and found considerable frequencies of β-thalassemia (13.5 percent) and G6PD deficiency (6.22 percent) in the villages around the Ropa valley, specifically Sokraki, Ano and Kato Korakiana, Skripero, Agios Markos, Doukades, and Kanakades.[64] Skhizas and his coauthors, likewise, found frequencies of β-thalassemia in the army recruits from the prefecture of Corfu to be 18.68 percent, far above the national average of 8.41 percent, making it second only in ranking after the island of Lesvos.[65]

The water shortage on high grounds drove some other Corfiots to the dangerous lowlands. The 750 villagers of Ano (or Upper) Peritheia, which

---

60 Livieratos, "I elonosia," 176–77; Zavitsianos, "I iatriki," 220; League of Nations, Health Organisation, Health Committee, *Visite à l'île de Corfou*, 23–28.

61 Savvas, Kardamatis, and Dasios, "1906," 609.

62 League of Nations, Health Organisation, Health Committee, *Explanatory Memorandum*, 59.

63 [Illegible signature, sanitary engineer], "Ekthesis epi ton anangaion exygiantikon ergon Nomou Kerkyras," Ioannina, 10 August 1946, I Malaria, water, house refuse, supplies, general, 172 F. Sanitation April 1945–November 1946, PAG-4/3.0.12.2.3.:36 [S-0527-0700], UN Archives. The swamp of Vdelaria had already been drained in the summer of 1945, most likely on the basis of a preexisting drainage system. Howard W. Chapman to D. E. Wright, [Ioannina] 11 December 1945, c) Sanitation Funds—Various January 1945–October 1946, HL/23 Sanitary Control, PAG-4/3.0.12.2.3.:36 [S-0527-0700], UN Archives.

64 Stamatoyannopoulos and Fessas, "Thalassaemia," 877.

65 Skhizas et al., "Sykhnotis," 203.

was located at 435 meters above sea level, where water was not adequate, used to move to Kato (or Lower) Peritheia, by Lake Antinioti, in the months when this latter location no longer had mosquitoes. After the Second World War, the lake, today a nature reserve, covered and expanse of about 1.5 square kilometers and was separated from the sea by a narrow strip of land. For these villagers, the UNRRA antimalarial campaign in 1946 signaled the possibility of a safe and permanent relocation to the lower site.[66]

Fishing

The use of freshwater resources generated conflicting interests, most notably with regard to farming and fishing practices. Fisheries were state property[67] and their management added further complexity to the landscape.

The lagoon at the northern end of the Gulf of Navarino, or Pylos, was still serving as a fishery when Kardamatis visited the location in August 1920. In the summer, the lagoon, known as the Divari or Daliani,[68] occupied an area from 2 to 4 square kilometers, but in the winter it ran into the marsh to its north and east; together, they covered an expanse of 20 to 25 square kilometers. To its south, the lagoon had a narrow exit to the gulf through the dunes, the only remaining exit of three preexisting openings, the so-called Bouka, which the fishermen shut off from the sea in the autumn to trap fish inside the fishery. In doing so, they flooded "thousands of *stremmata* of cultivable" land. Thereafter, in the winter months, the salinity of the water changed. The main source of freshwater lay to the east of the lagoon; besides the rainwater from the surrounding hills, there were several springs within an area of 100 by 200 meters, the most important one being the Tyflomitis, and also the floodwater of the Xirolangado torrent. Floodwater from a tributary of the River Gialova, which ran into the gulf, also fed the lagoon. According to Kardamatis's account, even in the summertime the Gialova had sufficient water to power some eight watermills.

---

66 [Illegible signature, sanitary engineer], "Ekthesis epi ton anangaion exygiantikon ergon Nomou Kerkyras," Ioannina, 10 August 1946, I Malaria, water, house refuse, supplies, general, 172 F. Sanitation April 1945–November 1946, PAG-4/3.0.12.2.3.:36 [S-0527-0700], UN Archives; Filotis, "Limno-thalassa." See also Fatouros, *Limnon periigisis*, 296; Savvas, Kardamatis, and Dasios, "1906," 605.

67 See chapter 2, on Elos and Araxos.

68 Fatouros, *Limnon periigisis*, 279.

At the time of Kardamatis's visit, during the first ten days of August, the salinity of the lagoon was, owing to the summer heat and according to his own measurements, at its peak, making it a hostile environment for *Anopheles*. However, he found the fishermen's homes full of *A. maculipennis*. In the light, however, of subsequent advances in entomology, they were more likely *A. sacharovi*.[69] He assumed that they must have originated in the nearby marsh, also the source of the same species of mosquitoes found in all the villages between Gialova and Ligoudista (present-day Khora).

When, however, in the autumn the fishermen shut off the flow of seawater into the lagoon, the rain- and floodwater it received throughout the winter months lowered its salinity level and, at the same time, increased its expanse four- or fivefold; the lagoon and the marsh thus became a unified stretch of shallow, brackish water. Kardamatis concluded that by springtime the location had become an ideal mosquito breeding site, that consisted in the marsh, the lagoon and the adjoining pools that sprung up in late spring and early summer, ready to infect the population in the area.

Kardamatis specifically singled out the villages of Gialova (population 85), Petrokhori (175), Romanos (217), and Osmanaga (571, present-day Koryfasi), as most exposed to endemic malaria, with their populations presenting "a pitiful sight," with anemia, enlarged spleens, "hydremia," and cachexia. The lagoon, however, further affected the health of farmers from a broader range of villages, who "descend in the summer with their entire households" and reside on their low-lying properties, "until they have gathered their crop (currants, etc.)." Additionally, because the state currant warehouse was located in Gialova, a "lamentable mistake" in his view, malaria also struck town dwellers, such as the currant merchants from Navarino (present-day Pylos) on business trips to Gialova.[70] Even though the population paid a heavy price for the activities connected with the fishery, Kardamatis's recommendation to put an end to the lagoon was problematic. An attempt to drain it in the 1950s failed.[71] Even in 1970, the density of *A. sacharovi* was "quite heavy" and resulted in strong complaints from the locals.[72]

---

69   See p. 152 in this book.
70   Kardamatis, "Peri tou para tin Pylon ikhthyotrofeiou, exetazomenou apo ygieinis apopseos."
71   Today the area is a natural reserve.
72   Hadjinicolaou and Betzios, "Gambusia Fish," 5–6.

Interestingly, in the very same month of Kardamatis's visit, but in 1839, long before viticulture and the currant boom transformed the area in the 1870s, E. Galatis, the state doctor responsible for the 1838–40 survey in Messinia and Pylia, made the following observations on the same location: "By the sea there is a fishery, which forms a swamp that appears to attack the health of the inhabitants, when there is a wind from the south; however, this does not occur often." Galatis went on to recommend planting trees as barriers to the insalubrious wind, particularly south of the village of Osmanaga.[73]

Some ten years earlier, according to his 1828 account of the lagoon, Bory de Saint-Vincent focuses on the beauty of the scenery and the horrible remains of war and does not speak of fevers. He describes, however, a method of trapping fish in a circle of *"pallisades de roseaux."*[74] If the fishing techniques had indeed changed since the time of Bory de Saint Vincent's visit, and fishermen had since learned to manipulate the degree of salinity, one may suspect that the malaria situation must have deteriorated considerably.[75]

Similar fishery-management methods were documented at Lake Moustos, in the eastern Peloponnese. In the 1838 survey, it was described as an unhealthy place with malignant intermittent fevers, suitable only for winter residence, with many marshes and a partially drained lake, the work of Bavarian engineers.[76] In the 1870s, however, according to Clôn Stéphanos, the lake was one of the few remaining foci of endemic malaria.[77]

In 1936 the fishery was apparently no longer being worked communally by the locals, but had been leased out. Despite the fact that the terms of its exploitation differed from those in Gialova, the fish-farming practices appear similar. The prefecture's financial officer accused the leaseholder of artificially increasing the area of the fishery by destroying the levees that protected the surrounding fields from flooding and, in the process, increas-

73 Galatis, "Iatrostatistikoi pinakes tis dioikiseos Messinias kai tis ypodioikiseos Pylias."
74 Bory de Saint-Vincent, *Relation*, vol. 1, 227–31.
75 Regarding fishing conditions in Ottoman Elos, Leake described it as a summer activity of the villagers in Dourali, Tsasi, and Vriniko: "in the winter the fish are disturbed by the violence of the wind and by the salt water, which is blown it into the lake over the sandy beach which separates it from the sea." Leake, *Travels in the Morea*, vol. 1, 196–97. However, an Ottoman decree issued before August 1500, suggests that, in the fifteenth century, the Christians of the Morea waited for the rains and turbulent seas to catch fish in the fisheries. The state then claimed half the catch. Alexander, *Toward a History of Post-Byzantine Greece*, 30 and 356. In the early nineteenth century, the Gialova fishery was, likewise, state property and was farmed by the governor of Neokastro (Navarino). See Leake, *Travels in the Morea*, vol. 1, 412.
76 Foteinos, "Iatrostatistikoi pinakes tis dioikiseos Mantineias"; Fatouros, *Limnon periigisis*, 281.
77 Stéphanos, *La Grèce*, 501.

ing the *Anopheles* breeding grounds at the expense of the health of the local population.[78]

The exploitation by fishermen of particular physical features of the marshland environment are well illustrated in a malariologist's account of the lagoon south of the town of Giannitsa in western Macedonia, which was 90 percent malarious in 1929[79]:

> At approximately 3 kilometers south of Giannitsa begins a large permanent lagoon, albeit with variable shores, surrounded by muddy marshland, shallow (1 to 2 meters deep), rich in fish. The muddy terrain around the lagoon is crisscrossed by artificially excavated canals, 2 to 4 meters wide, and about a kilometer long. These canals, which lie at a distance of about 2 kilometers from each other, all converge toward the lagoon, into which they terminate; they are meant to be traveled by fishermen's barges that reach the lake through the muddy marshland which surrounds it. On the side of Giannitsa there are only five or six. Along the lake there are many cottages and huts. Around 500 families of fishermen use them. However, since July the quantity of mosquitoes is such that they must give up spending the night there.[80]

In other words, notwithstanding hostile surface hydrology such as shallow lakes and swamps, the individualistic Greek peasant devised methods to utilize often scarce water resources and integrate these resources into his production techniques without regard to public health risks.

Migration and Labor

With regard to the effect of population movements on malaria endemicity in mid-twentieth-century Africa, Socrates Litsios has noted the difficulty in assessing endemicity, owing to the complexity of the factors involved, as "with more and more people 'on the move,' it would be necessary to examine their recent movements (as S. R. Christophers did in 1924 in India), as well

---

78 Fatouros, *Limnon periigisis*, 281.
79 League of Nations, Health Organisation, Health Committee, *Health and Hospital Survey*, 13.
80 League of Nations, Health Organisation C.H./Malaria/23, G. Pittaluga, "Observations sur le paludisme en Macédoine grecque," Geneva, 26 September 1924, p. 7. For a collection of early-twentieth-century photographs online, see the site of the Museum of the Macedonian Struggle at www.imma.edu.gr/imma/dbs/Artifacts/index.html?start=100.

as their treatment history, to develop a meaningful picture of endemicity, a task no control programme has the resources to undertake."[81]

In the case of Greece, internal migration at varying distances was extremely common. For one, the balance between the deficient economies of the mountain and island regions, which compensated for this deficiency by sending out seasonal laborers to the more fertile regions in the plains or plateaux at harvest time, when the plains became deficient in agricultural hands, was of particularly critical importance to malaria epidemiology. This exchange occurred, for instance, in June and July, when the grain was being brought in, which coincided with the transmission peak of *vivax* malaria, or in August and September, when grapes and currants were being harvested and *falciparum* malaria reached its peak in most areas of Greece. Often, the peasants on the move were the proprietors themselves who chose to live at higher elevations. Residents from the mountain village of Soudena, where malaria had become endemic, were continually infected in the heavily malarious municipality of Dymion in the marshy northwestern coast of the prefecture of Akhaia, where they owned currant vineyards and spent the months from December to June.[82] In the hillside village of Kiourka, not far from Athens, "those who spend the entire year in the village hardly ever catch malarial fevers, whereas those who sojourn in the low-lying riverside places to harvest their fields, thresh their grain, guard their flock, and pick their grapes are almost all attacked by the disease."[83] Mostly, however, infections involved the poorer peasants, who traveled to supplement their income with seasonal work. Furthermore, there is an abundance of evidence that shows peasants engaged in the dangerous habit of sleeping outdoors at harvest time to guard their crops.[84]

According to evidence from UNRRA officials, the mountainous, landlocked district of Evrytania imported most of its malaria from people working in the lowlands, around Messolonghi and Lamia.[85] The same practice persisted throughout Greece. The case of the seasonal migrants of Mazi, in the province of Kalavryta, already mentioned in chapter 2, was a pattern re-

---

81 Litsios, *The Tomorrow of Malaria*, 128.
82 "1905," 435.
83 Anastasopoulos, Kapanidis, and Dimitriou, "Ai elodeis nosoi en to dimo Marathonos kata to 1906," 279.
84 For instance, in the villages of Marathon. Ibid.
85 "Report on the Incidence of Malaria" [1946], Malaria ABJ, Sanitation 01-50, PAG-4/3.0.12.2.3.:1 [S-0527-0665], UN Archives.

peated all over the country. Residents who left for seasonal work brought malaria back to their native Tripoli, for instance, where benign intermittent fevers, or *vivax* malaria, affected no more than 5 percent of the "lower class, mostly among individuals who traveled for work in the malarious municipality of Mantineia, particularly the village of Tsipiana, where malarial fevers are endemic."[86]

In the north of the country, in Ottoman times, nonimmune groups of rural workers who traveled over a week with their families from Mount Orvilo near the current Bulgarian border, for the harvest on the Agios Pavlos estate on the Kassandra peninsula suffered heavy losses from malaria.[87] Furthermore, in the interwar years, the increased mortality figures among men in the mountain town of Arnaia in Khalkidiki may be largely attributed to the travels of these nonimmune mountain dwellers to areas of high malaria morbidity during the dangerous summer months. Thus, carpenters, loggers, workers, and muleteers left Arnaia, which, according to Kardamatis's wartime figures, suffered from 5 percent malaria morbidity, for Mount Pangaion east of the Serres plain, where their mules transported water for the irrigation of the tobacco plants. They also traveled around the peninsula to sell the output of the Arnaia looms to Nigrita as wage laborers, while the carpenters found employment at the military defense works in Sidirokastro for three to four months after August, during the most dangerous months.[88]

The Ionian Islands, however, were a case in themselves and were particularly vulnerable to imported malaria. Ruled by Venice for centuries before its defeat by the French in 1797, the island economy was obliged to produce marketable crops, i.e., olives and currants, for the Republic. With the exception of Cephalonia, the islands had no subsistence farming or diversity in agriculture, or polyculture, that would have protected the peasants against famine. Deficiency in grain was, therefore, systemic. Thus, even before the 1820s, when the Greek revolution put a temporarily check on the practice, the peasantry of Zakynthos were

---

86 "1905," 430.

87 Nicolaidy, *Les Turcs*, vol. 2, 66–67.

88 In the 1928 census, the number of women in Arnaia exceeded men by 26 percent. République Hellénique, Ministère de l'Économie Nationale, Statistique Générale de la Grèce, *Résultats statistiques*, 293; figures for 1939 indicate that many of them were widows. See Papaioannou, "Georgooikonomiki erevna," 152 and 155.

in the habit of emigrating annually to the Morea, during the harvest season; they brought home the pecuniary produce of their labors, but too frequently they also imported with them the germ of fever of the remittent kind, occasioned by their exposure to the sun, sleeping in the open air, and feeding on bad bread and other food devoid of nutrition, while subjected to the malarious vapours arising from marshy ground, especially in the districts of Elis and Arcadia.[89]

In the late nineteenth and early twentieth centuries, peasants from Zakynthos and Lefkada who migrated to the Peloponnese and Akarnania, respectively, continued to return home with malaria.[90] Similarly, Thessaly attracted workers from Cephalonia to work on railroad construction; these men also returned home sick with malaria. Crossing over to the coast of Epirus to fish in the waters of the Vouthroto (Butrint) lagoon increased the amount of malaria in the Mandouki district in the town of Corfu.[91] Migration to the United States late in the nineteenth and early twentieth centuries relieved the demographic pressure and, at the same time, provided much needed remittances to the island, which reduced the pressure to migrate on those who had stayed behind; as a result, their exposure to malaria from continental Greece decreased.[92] On the other hand, some landowners in Thessaly blamed the disease for their failure to hold on to their migrant labor force in the summer.[93]

Labor arrived in Copaïs even from across the frontier. In the 1870s, when owners of tobacco- and cotton-growing estates were unable to find cheap farm hands to dig irrigation canals and harvest the crop, they negotiated with Muslim Albanian band leaders and hired their men, who were satisfied with a fraction of what the Greek peasants were demanding; the impoverished Albanians then, invariably, fell ill with fevers.[94]

Selecting underprivileged social groups for antimalarial labor was not an approach unique to farming. In June 1931, the deputy governor general for Crete tried to address the severe problem of malaria in the town of Georgioupoli, where malariologists had reported a 100 percent malaria

---

89 Hennen, *Sketches*, 324–25.
90 Livieratos, "I elonosia," 168; "1905," 449–502.
91 Savvas, Kardamatis, and Dasios, "1906," 604.
92 Livieratos, "I elonosia," 168–69; Savvas, Kardamatis, and Dasios, "1906," 591–92.
93 Manoussakis, *To elonosiakon provlima*, 3.
94 Belle, *Trois années en Grèce*, 133–36.

prevalence. Having drawn up a drainage project with the help of the state engineer, the department health officer and the local director of the Anti-malarial Service, he agreed with the director of the prison farm at Agia to have him send its inmates, some hundred men, while Georgioupoli offered accommodation. However, the plan ran against the reluctance of the Justice Ministry in Athens to provide guards for these convicts in such a dangerous place.[95]

Villains in a Tragedy of the Commons

In the early twentieth century, that is, when they became convinced of the implication of *Anopheles* in the transmission mechanism of malaria, physicians became concerned about the effect of agricultural and, indeed, all kinds of outdoor labor on public health. What or, perhaps, who was responsible for the failure to control mosquitoes?

In September 1933, a speech by malariologist Konstantinos Dimissas to a malaria congress organized by the Thessaloniki Medical Society is indicative of the blame game that went on at the time. In his conference paper, Dimissas began by laying the responsibility for malaria on the Greek peasant and then proceeded to present a comprehensive rural, urban, sociopolitical, and, finally, cultural landscape. His account started literally at ground level, namely at the disastrous tiny pools produced by small rivers and streams, whose irregular flow passed by the villages en route to the larger river. "There exists practically no village that does not have its *'rema,'*" he emphasized. At a distance of about 500 meters from the village, the *"rema"* spread out wherever it found a disturbed surface, and, in the process, collected the surplus water from the village fountains.

"Indeed, the peasants dig up everything," he went on, "inside the banks of these *'remata'* [streams] to collect sand; they dig by the banks of these *'remata'* to manufacture bricks, each for his own house or in common to build their village (refugee settlements). They also dig to collect water for their flock and domestic animals." They used the water to cool their geese, swine

---

95 Perdikaris, Deputy Director General for Crete, to E. Venizelos, Khania, 20 June 1931, 109/20, Venizelos Archive (unit 173), Benaki Museum Historical Archives. On an earlier recommendation favoring the use of prison labor for malaria control work, see letter to the editor, Kastorkhis, "Eli–Fylakai"; I wish to thank Helen Katsiadakis for bringing it to my attention.

and buffaloes and, when they no longer needed it, the water remained in small collections in pools and ditches

or, as the people call them, *"kolymbes, gournes, batakia, ghioles,* etc." But this is not all. For the Greek farmer, when the water has fulfilled its destiny and moved the mill or irrigated the field, it is then free "to go wherever it wishes," with no limitations, no regulation of its flow and no care on the part of the landowner, inhabitants, merchants, or, eventually, the state itself. The water is free to accumulate at the lowest point by the village, and occasionally around cities, and gives rise to the local swamp. Unfortunately, the ill-effects of digging do not cease here. The same peasant, often by force of circumstance and thanks to rising urbanism, comes to the city, becomes a man of responsibility and influence, a municipal officer, lawmaker, businessman, air defense officer. He remembers that he used to dig, and dig far and wide. He is sympathetic to anyone digging.

In a position of authority, without having shed his peasant mentality, he now negotiated public work projects. "Permits are thus granted, ostensibly exceptionally, but invariably whenever they are persistently demanded: to the contractor, who will build the settlements, to the brick or tile manufacturer and finally, for twelve drachmas per cartload, to the cart driver who will extract sand from the river bank."[96] Public health was delivered its coup de grâce by the large and small public works companies and contractors and their road, drainage, and other projects, Dimissas continued: "Nowhere may one find clearcut, unambiguous, terms relating to the obligations of all these contractors to observe certain rules; even though rules may exist, they seek to find ways to be always formally totally in order even while they are breaking the law."[97]

Dimissas summarized a pervasive culture consistent with the notion of a "tragedy of the commons," as defined in 1968 by Garrett Hardin,[98] for situations in which each individual benefits from a positive outcome, in this case covering requirements in irrigation and materials, while the harm, in this case exposure to the risk of malaria, is distributed to all, none of whom has a personal incentive to shoulder the cost of redressing the damage.

---

96 The leading agronomist Petros Kananginis, indeed, highlighted Greek bureaucrats' gross indifference to the lives of refugees regarding the draining of the Almyros marshlands, in an article in the newspaper *Eleftheron Vima* (27 September 1924); it is reproduced in Panagiotopoulos, *Petros Kananginis,* 207.

97 Dimissas, "Eisigisis epi tis epidimiologias tis elonosias en Makedonia kai Thraki," 26–27.

98 Hardin, "The Tragedy of the Commons."

Colonization

"To colonise a plain often means to die there," wrote Fernand Braudel, referring to the taming of marshes to claim new farmland.[99] The restructuring of Greek agriculture after independence intensified the spread of malaria. Indeed, until the 1860s, apart from the colonization of the national lands[100] by peasant families, a large number of uprooted peasants moved around the countryside, between mountains and plains, in search of available land. The large number of landless peasants, whose labor could not justify its cost in lands of low productivity, with a yield of three or four to one, were forced to move to areas of higher productivity in the plains, with a yield of between eight and twenty-five to one, such as Amyklai south of Sparta, Pamisos in Messinia, Marathon, Lake Copais, and Akheloos in western Greece, and as far away as Thessaly and Asia Minor. "On the roads one encounters whole caravan trains of these migrants. Men, women and children carry their last pan while cocks and pigeons travel with them," noted Friedrich Thiersch. "When their situation improves, they take with them their donkeys and oxen, loaded with plows and mattresses and with their wives and children."[101] These individuals, however, were an epidemiological time bomb, primed to go off each spring. It is, therefore, reasonable to associate the documented epidemics of intermittent fevers which broke out in the Greek countryside, for instance in 1833 and 1834, partly with the phenomenon of itinerant landless peasants.[102]

Furthermore, the economic attraction of currant viticulture, particularly in the second half of the nineteenth century, increased the rate of population growth in the northwestern and southwestern Peloponnese. Not only were these settlers exposed to lowland fevers, but, naive as they were, they were most vulnerable to malaria. Moreover, they posed an additional risk for the entire region to an indeterminable degree in that a number of these peasants continued to return to their original villages, when no longer busy in the lowlands, where they set fresh malarial fires among the *Anopheles* mosquitoes

---

99 Braudel, *The Mediterranean*, vol. 1, 66.

100 "National lands" was the term used for the estates abandoned by the fleeing Muslim landowners, mostly in the Peloponnese, when the Greek national revolution broke out.

101 Thiersch, *De l'état actuel*, vol. 1, 304.

102 Soutsos, *Dokimion*, 48, quoted in Petmezas, *I elliniki agrotiki oikonomia*, 40 and Thiersch, *De l'état actuel*, vol. 1, 297–98.

of the hills and highlands.[103] Conversely, discontinued exposure to malaria would prevent peasants from building up and maintaining their immunity, a likelihood that must have increased the instability of the disease and contributed to more or less severe epidemics, for, as noted by Randall Packard:

> Extended interruptions in exposure to malaria parasites reduced resistance. An interval of 1 to 2 years without reinfection would be enough to make an individual susceptible again to the full impact of a malarial infection. While such interruptions would have been unusual in areas of stable, continuous, transmission, they occur during extended periods of drought.[104]

As an indication of the demographic dynamics in nineteenth-century Greece, it is worth noting that between 1861 and 1888 the population in the lowlands of the northwest and southern coast of the Peloponnese increased at average annual rate of 1.87 percent against 0.9 percent for the rest of Peloponnese. Also, between 1861 and 1896 no single province of the Peloponnese increased at a rate even equal to that of currant producing provinces, which grew at 1.97 percent (Ilia) and 1.51 percent (Messinia).[105] In fact, V. Valaoras estimated that during the nineteenth century the national average natural rate of population growth was more than 1.5 percent.[106]

Evidently, the epidemiological impact of colonization is also related to the settlement of refugees. For the most part, colonization projects were laid out without taking into account local disease history. The case of the settlement of the Eastern Rumelian refugees in Almyros is a case in point. Arguing against the selection of that marshy location before draining it, P. G. Politis attempted to alert the leaders of the refugee communities, with whom he had visited the site, and produced a list of earlier attempts at colonization which had been dashed by fever epidemics.[107] "Even ignorant and uncouth a man as Veli Pasha," commented Politis, "a century ago acknowledged this need, and, before building Yenikoy and Tsingeli, attempted to open a large ditch, whose traces are still preserved, known as 'the ditch of Veli Pasha,' and to construct small canals, also known as 'soudes.'"

---

103 Franghiadis, "Peasant Agriculture and Export Trade," 4, 30–31, and 76.

104 Packard, *The Making of a Tropical Disease*, 29.

105 Franghiadis, "Peasant Agriculture and Export Trade," 31.

106 Valaoras, "A Reconstruction," 128.

107 On one of his visits an elderly peasant advised Politis against taking a postprandial nap in the shade of a tree, warning him that he would "inevitably catch fevers." Politis, "To agrotikon zitima," 5.

A second project to colonize the coastal area of Almyros with Muslims "from Asia" in the second half of the nineteenth century at a location called Orman Kavak, meaning "poplar forest," also failed. In 1907 the names of the old Ottoman beneficiaries were still preserved in the title deeds of neighboring properties. Generally, the Ottoman landlords avoided the coast of Almyros from bitter experience, testified by the "innumerable Turkish tombstones strewn over the Almyros plain," and had learned to construct their tenants' houses away from the coast. One Mehmet Ali Pasha built Karambasi on a hill, Arif Bey built his Akici, present-day Mikrothivae, at 6 kilometers from the coast. Aidini and Kourfali were even further away. Husein and Mehmet Bey, the owners of Tsingeli, which was closer to the coast, preferred to have their tenants settle in the town of Almyros, rather than see them "suffer from fevers" at Tsingeli.

Following the annexation of Thessaly by the Greek kingdom in 1881, a number of transhumant shepherds, or *vlakhopoimenes*, who leased the meadows of Almyros for winter grazing, requested the government to establish a settlement in a meadow called Ustup for their use. However, having spent one summer in the plains, they abandoned their settlement to return to the Pindus range and their healthier seminomadic way of life after the winter rains, in April 1882.

Alexandros Kassavetis, a wealthy local landowner, who had purchased the Aidini estate, drew up a settlement plan for a "coastal settlement" within his estate, with housing for himself and his tenants, warehouses, stables, etc., which he called Dimitrias, in honor of his father. He went on to purchase a small ship that would provide communication between Dimitrias and the city of Volos. However, according to Politis, none of his tenants left their old homes to settle by the coast. Kassavetis was obliged to sell Dimitrias at a loss. A subsequent owner of the estate, Topalis, took care to provide quinine to his tenants and even supervised its distribution personally.

Interestingly, the government created a small settlement at the end of the bay of Almyros to accommodate the customs authority.

It was believed that this settlement would soon thrive. However, while throughout the Pagasitikos area one could observe a general tendency on the part of the population of the various mountain villages to move to the coast, a tendency that threatened the villages with depopulation; the coastal settlements of Volos, Agria, Kala Nera, Afyssos, Khorto, and Milina developed to an amazing degree at the expense of their "mother towns." In that particular corner of the Pagasitikos Gulf, in this sole seaport for the entire province, no private house was constructed and it was left with the heads of the civil services as its sole inhabitants. Even the boatmen, who are indispensable for the port operations, prefer to live in Amaliapolis, at two-hour distance, and to come to the coast of Almyros only on days when steamships approach.[108]

In 1906, the year immediately preceding the settlement of the Eastern Rumelian refugees, the district of Almyros had been relatively dry with a low level of malaria; yet, the communities of Akici, Dimitrias, Kainourgia, and the Farm School were badly hit.[109] But malaria hit the refugees in 1907 at alarming rates. In the town of Almyros, some 72.66 percent of the refugees told Kardamatis they had fallen ill between May and August, but mostly in July; among them he noted a heavy burden of *falciparum* malaria.[110]

In northern Greece, the decision to relocate refugees from the Ottoman Empire in 1914 and 1922 in a program of colonization became a serious sanitary challenge, complicated by the fact that the French and British armies of the First World War had come to western and central Macedonia, respectively, and gone, having destabilized a landscape where malaria was already endemic. Amid treeless mountains, major lakes, and sluggish streams abounded in western Macedonia, where they produced dangerous swamps, such as that formed on the southern side of Lake Kastoria, at an altitude of 687 meters. Lacking an outlet and surrounded by high mountains of up to 1,500 meters on all other sides, the lake had a surface of 30 square kilometers and its water was polluted by the town effluvia. The medical team of the French Armée d'Orient who studied the area noted that spleen rates among the local population varied in direct proportion to the proximity to the lake; some ten villages a few hundred meters from the shoreline had the highest spleen rates of more than 35 percent. In villages between 500 to 1,000 meters away and at an altitude of less than 50 meters above the surface, spleen

---

108 Politis, "To agrotikon zitima," 5.

109 Savvas, Kardamatis, and Dasios, "1906," 622.

110 Kardamatis examined 252 blood samples and found 108 positive cases: twenty cases of *vivax* malaria, seventy-two cases, that is, 67 percent, of *falciparum*, fourteen cases of *malariae*, and two mixed infections. Kardamatis, "Ekthesis peri ton en Volo," 221–22.

rates dropped considerably, while malaria was practically nonexistent in villages located more than a kilometer from the lake.[111]

At the center of the Eksissu (now Xino Nero) region lay a landscape of four interconnected lakes, namely Sari-Giol (north of Kozani, now drained), Ostrovo (present-day Vegoritida), and Rudnick (Kheimaditida), connected by a slow meandering stream, with an inclination of 0.003 per meter, to Lake Petrsko (now Petron); this stream also powered two watermills and overflowed into a large marsh of 40 square kilometers northeast of Rudnick. By August, the marsh, "whose entire surface is invaded by an abundance of aquatic flora, sinter, water lilies, rush, aquatic fern and reeds 4 to 5 meters tall," retreated and peasants would come to collect reeds for mat making and allow their animals to graze. Downwind from the marsh and the lake, there was considerable endemic malaria with spleen rates as high as 64 percent in the villages of Rudnick (present-day Anargyroi) and Rakita (present-day Olympiada). Apart from the distance factor, malaria incidence around Lake Rudnik was additionally influenced by northwestern winds that blew over the lake and its marsh, thus blowing the mosquitoes and spreading malaria more heavily to the south of the lake. The marsh was particularly dangerous for travelers on the road between Monastir (Bitola) and Kozani, Sotir (Sotiri) and Sorovitch (present-day Amyntaio) or on the train between Monastir and Thessaloniki.[112]

When the Asia Minor refugees of 1922 began pouring into northern Greece, an already critical situation reached a point of collapse. A telegram published in the October issue of the *Epidemiological Report* of the League of Nations Health Section sounded an alarm about the sanitary situation in Thessaloniki, whose population was suffering from dysentery, pneumonia, malaria, an imminent danger of typhoid and "other epidemics" but had "no disinfectants, quinine or drugs." In Thrace, further to the east, numerous, urgent pleas for quinine from the Komotini office of the High Commission for Refugees arrived at the head office in Constantinople and at the British Red Cross in Athens in anticipation of an April epidemic.[113]

---

111 Bussière, "Paludisme et drainage," 519–21.

112 Ibid., 523–24.

113 Treloar to Lt. Colonel J. Procter, Gumuldjina [Komotini], 24 January 1923, Reports to the Deputy High Commissioner for Refugees, Gumuldjina Office No. 19, External missions, offices, delegations of the High Commissioner, the Balkan collection (1920–1938), box c 1129 (25) 12 (files 1922–1923), Nansen office for refugees, Refugees Mixed Archival Group—Fonds Nansen—Commission files (1919–1947),

Experience with malaria appears to have informed the selection of settlement points for the Greek refugees that poured into Thrace after the country's defeat in the war with Turkey in September 1922. Colonel G. D. Treloar, the League of Nations officer of the High Commissioner for Refugees in Komotini, warned as early as January 1923 about the urgent need for additional quantities of quinine for the refugees in Thrace in anticipation of the annual malaria outbreak expected in April.[114] Likewise, in mid-February 1923, Czesław Wroczyński, the League of Nations Epidemic Commission director in Thessaloniki, reported that malaria was "the greatest danger" to the refugees in Western Thrace and Macedonia and called for immediate preparations to protect them.[115] Treloar made sure to establish the refugees in his charge in villages and new settlements on hillsides, "high up or on the tops of slopes," rather than in the plains.[116] Although by no means a watertight solution to the malaria problem, it is quite likely that this policy spared the refugees in Thrace the horrific suffering and loss of life due to malaria experienced by those who settled in the Macedonian lowlands.

A health bureau had been set up in Macedonia in 1912.[117] In December 1923, the General Directorate for the Colonization of Macedonia, which had been established to settle incoming refugees between 1913 and 1920, was incorporated into the new Refugee Settlement Commission as part of a nationwide restructuring.[118]

Many of the fresh wave of refugees from Asia Minor in 1922 contracted malaria "immediately" from the indigenous population, albeit at higher rates, for instance at Toumba and Langadas, and in villages in the Strymon val-

---

League of Nations Archives; Treloar to Sir James Stewart, British Red Cross, British Legation Athens, Gumuldgina, 15 March 1923 (telegram copy), telegrams outgoing, Gumuldjina Office, File 3, box C 1128 (24) 11 files 1920–1923, Nansen office for Refugees, 1924–1925.

114 G. D. Treloar to J. Procter, Gumuldjina, 24 Jan 1923, Reports to the Deputy High Commissioner for Refugees, Gumuldjina Office No. 19, External missions, offices, delegations of the High Commissioner, the Balkan collection (1920–1938), box C 1129 (25) 12 (files 1922–1923), Nansen office for refugees, Refugees Mixed Archival Group—Fonds Nansen—Commission files (1919–1947), League of Nations Archives.

115 League of Nations, Health Organisation, Health Committee, *Rapport*, 9.

116 [G. D. Treloar] to the Deputy High Commissioner for Refugees [Gumuldjina, 1923], Geneva Correspondence, Gumuldjina Office, n. 4, Delegation in Greece, Commission Files, Nansen Office for Refugees. High Commissioner for Refugees, Archives de l'office Nansen, divers 24, C1128, 1923, External missions, offices, delegations of the High Commissioner, the Balkan collection (1920–1938), Nansen office for refugees box C 1128 (24) 11 (files 1920–1923), Refugees Mixed Archival Group—Fonds Nansen—Commission files (1919–1947), League of Nations Archives.

117 Kontogiorgi, *Population Exchange*, 265.

118 Ibid., 91–92.

ley, as reported by Norman V. Lothian, a Scottish medical entomologist, who had also served as an antimalaria officer in Macedonia during the Great War. "This occurred several times with new groups of refugees, so that it was necessary to give up concentrating them in the villages." In autumn 1923, a malaria epidemic in Toumba affected 90 percent of the refugees, killing 7 percent of them. Malaria mortality in the village and plain of Langadas was 5–7 percent.[119] In fact, the agronomist Petros Kananginis, Director of the Colonization Bureau, noted the reluctance of ethnic Greeks to colonize the sparsely populated plains and marshlands of East Macedonia. As a consequence, the government colonization schemes and the social engineering that marked them, were doomed until the arrival of the 1922 refugees from Asia Minor breathed new life into them.[120] In the Strymon valley, according to local sanitary officers, the average mortality from malaria was 2.5 percent among the indigenous population and "at least" 3.5 percent among the refugees.[121]

In the late Ottoman years, the Strymon region had been sparsely populated and comprised several Muslim-owned landed estates in the more productive plain, which experienced frequent floods that often destroyed the crops; these estates also raised horses. Most of the plain, however, was winter grazing land which nomads used when descending from the surrounding mountains. In the early twentieth century the Ottoman government attempted to settle Bosnian Muslim refugees but failed. The Greek government had, likewise, failed to generate viable settlements of Christian refugees after the Balkan Wars. Flooding kept destroying both their income and health. "The floods threaten people's lives and render crops insecure, malaria and the unsuitability of most of the land for cultivation and its suitabil-

---

119 Rapport provisoire sur le voyage de la Commission du Paludisme en Yougoslavie, Grèce, Bulgarie, Roumanie et Russie du 29 mai au 10 août 1924, présenté par le (Hamburg, Institut für Schiffs-und Tropenkrankheiten), 17, Commission du Paludisme, Geneva, 16 September 1924, Organisation d'Hygiène, Health Committee (H.C.) 227 (vol. 245), League of Nations Archives. Aimé Gauthier of the Red Cross reported similar levels of malaria mortality for the refugee camps around Thessaloniki, where at any time about 20 to 30 percent of the occupants were in bed with fever. In the other towns and villages, the situation was much worse, complicated by tuberculosis and dysentery. Conférence faite le 3 juillet 1924 à Paris devant Sir Claude Hill, directeur général de la Ligue des Sociétés de la Croix-rouge et les membres du secrétariat général de la Ligue par M. Le médecin principal de 1ère classe Aimé Gauthier, de l'Armée française, délégué de La ligue des Societes de la Croix-rouge auprès de la Commission mixte d'echange des populations grecques et turques, 9, doc 33668, dossier no. 26426, box R 858, 12B (Social-Health), League of Nations Archives, A (1919–27).

120 Panagiotopoulos, *Petros Kananginis*, 67–73.

121 "Rapport du voyage d'étude collectif, été 1924" (C.H./E.P.S./66), p. 31, Commission de la Malaria, Organisation d'Hygiène, Société des Nations. Also, Kontogiorgi, *Population Exchange*, 268.

ity only for grazing have hampered the density of small-scale farms of free or tenant farmers."[122]

In 1924, Lothian observed the interaction of the "tremendous extent of anophelism" with the arrival of new people, "the two factors combining to produce widespread outbreaks in this endemic area." Lothian also noted that there was very little antimosquito work and that mechanical protection was limited to soldiers and railwaymen but that quinine was distributed on a "lavish scale." He added: "It is very doubtful whether anything less than major schemes would be effective."[123] He paralleled the influx of nonimmune refugees both in 1914 and 1922 with the arrival of the foreign armies in Macedonia during the First World War, both producing "explosive outbreaks of severe malaria."[124] Indeed, according to information from Health Minister Dimitrios Pazis, as a result of deadly malaria epidemics in some villages of the Strymon valley, successive groups of refugees occupied and subsequently abandoned them, further exacerbating the situation with their increased mobility.[125]

As the refugees were settled in the plains outside the villages, they were exposed to mosquito-rich marshes, lakes and dangerous irrigation canals. In the Vardar (or Axios) valley, there was the Giannitsa marsh with its fishermen's channels; in the Strymon valley there were small and large swamps. "The villages in this region have all been malarious for a long time," noted the Malaria Commission report.[126]

In the interwar years, the area around Lake Langada (Koroneia) consisted of maize fields, vegetable gardens and, mostly, grazing land full of goats as well as reeds and rushes.[127] In the wider Langadas area, half the pop-

---

122 Anagnostopoulos, "O Kampos ton Serron," 596–98.

123 Lothian to Rajchman, Bucharest, 1 July 1924, doc 35133, dossier no. 28002, box R 870, 12B (Social-Health), League of Nations Archives, A (1919–27).

124 Lothian to Rajchman, Salonika, 18 June 1924, doc 35133, dossier no. 28002, box R 870, 12B (Social-Health), League of Nations Archives, A (1919–27); "Rapport du voyage d'étude collectif, été 1924" (C.H./E.P.S./66), p. 37, Commission de la Malaria, Organisation d'Hygiène, Société des Nations.

125 "Rapport du voyage d'étude collectif, été 1924" (C.H./E.P.S./66), p. 20, Commission de la Malaria, Organisation d'Hygiène, Société des Nations. On the mobility of the Asia Minor refugees and their information networks that extended to the 1913–14 wave, see Kontogiorgi, Population Exchange, 256–57. Dimitrios Pazis (1875–1953) was health minister from March to June 1924.

126 Rapport provisoire sur le voyage de la Commission du Paludisme en Yougoslavie, Grèce, Bulgarie, Roumanie et Russie du 29 mai au 10 août 1924 (Hamburg, Institut fur Schiffs-und Tropenkrankheiten), 18–19, Commission du Paludisme, Geneva, 16 September 1924, Organisation d'Hygiène, H.C. 227 (vol. 245).

127 G. Pittaluga, "Observations sur le paludisme en Macédoine grecque," Geneva, 26 September 1924, p. 8, C.H./Malaria/23, Health Organisation, League of Nations.

ulation were refugees. Gustavo Pittaluga, member of the League of Nations Malaria Commission, offered the following description:

> Near the lake one only finds huts, cabins and cottages, where the cultiva-
> tors spend consecutive days and nights. One of these cottages we visited con-
> tained several *Anopheles*. The road from Langada[s] through the countryside
> and around the lake is sandy and difficult for cars and must at several points
> cross the streams, torrent beds with pools of water and ponds fed by small
> streaks of water or springs. We also observed reservoirs of rainwater in the
> shape of more or less irregular ponds, excavated by the side of the road, and
> meant to irrigate the neighboring fields by rudimentary canals which cross
> the road at many points, or pass under the road through small culverts where
> the water gets blocked and forms sheltered points. Personally, we have not
> observed any *Anopheles* larvae.[128]

In the nearby mountains there were also malarious villages at altitudes of around 600 meters, with *A. superpictus* in many streams and wells. In some villages of Mount Hortiatis, located close to Thessaloniki, Pittaluga said that "the peasants construct small lakes, rainwater tanks, which freeze dur-ing the winter, the ice then being sold in Thessaloniki. With the arrival of spring, the remaining ice forms small collections of stagnant water which provide shelter to *Anopheles*."[129]

In Giannitsa, malaria had been heavily endemic long before the influx of the refugees. After their arrival in October 1922, there was a "large ex-plosion of malaria" in the following year. According to local doctors, most of the sick were from the ranks of the refugees, who had been infected lo-cally. Among 8,500 inhabitants, 200 died of malaria. In June 1924, the team from the Malaria Commission of the League of Nations examined the lo-cal schoolchildren in three groups to investigate the effect of social factors on local malaria epidemiology. They found that the spleen rate of the group of indigenous, well-off children, who lived in the more prosperous, elevated quarter of the town, was zero. However, that of the group of refugee chil-

---

128 G. Pittaluga, "Observations sur le paludisme en Macédoine grecque," Geneva, 26 September 1924, p. 8, C.H./Malaria/23, Health Organisation, League of Nations.

129 G. Pittaluga, "Observations sur le paludisme en Macédoine grecque," Geneva, 26 September 1924, pp. 9–10, C.H./Malaria/23, Health Organisation, League of Nations. This was an old practice in Mount Hor-tiatis documented in travelers' accounts, for instance, in Walpole, *Memoirs*, 274; Cousinéry, *Voyage dans la Macédoine*, vol. 1, 110, who related that Ottoman officials received their ice gratis; everyone else had to pay.

dren residing in town for more than ten years, some of whom even born in Giannitsa, was the highest in town, 76 percent, a reflection of the effect of endemic malaria. Finally, the children of the recent refugee wave had a spleen rate of 46 percent.[130]

In Konitsa, a town of 2,000 inhabitants, from where most of the indigenous men had emigrated, 600 residents were refugees. Among this population malaria prevalence was about 20–30 percent, except for the students of the local agricultural school, which was located on the plain of the River Aoos, who all contracted malaria. Near Ioannina, in the refugee settlement of Nea Kaisareia, malaria prevalence was also 100 percent. There was no winter grazing ground there. Poverty generated emigration and a low birth rate.[131]

In 1924, two League of Nations missions to Greece—one led by Norman White of the Health Committee at the request of the Greek government, and the other by Gustavo Pittaluga on behalf of the Malaria Commission—reported on the malaria situation in Macedonia, offered their recommendations and assistance and emphasized that, before tackling the sanitary questions, it was important to first address the social and economic aspects of the refugee settlement and to improve the living conditions of refugees.[132] For the Malaria Commission team, which also toured other countries in the region, the malaria situation in Greece overall was far more difficult than in Yugoslavia, "owing to unfavorable socioeconomic conditions."[133] Pittaluga, however, distanced himself from the orthodox League of Nations view expressed by the commission. For him, the gravity of the endemic situation they encountered in Macedonia could only be understood in the light of the malaria epidemics suffered by the allied forces and the German and Bulgarian armies during the previous war.[134] In a separate report, he recom-

---

130 G. Pittaluga, "Observations sur le paludisme en Macédoine grecque," Geneva, 26 September 1924, p. 20, C.H./Malaria/23, Health Organisation, League of Nations. The situation among the Giannitsa school children had not changed in 1930. M. Ciucă, "Organisation de la lutte antimalarique en Grèce," Geneva, 14 February 1931, p. 7, Commission du Paludisme, CH/Malaria/154, Organisation d'Hygiène, Société des Nations.

131 League of Nations, Health Organisation, Health Committee, *Visite dans la province d'Épire*, 12.

132 League of Nations Health Organisation, Geneva, 4 October 1924, C. 573. 1924III (C.H. 257.1925) Report on the work of the third session of the Health Committee, pp. 6–7, doc 33668, dossier no. 26426, box R 858, 12B (Social-Health), League of Nations Archives, A (1919–27).

133 "Rapport du voyage d'étude collectif, été 1924" (C.H./E.P.S./66), p. 34, Commission de la Malaria, Organisation d'Hygiène, Société des Nations.

134 G. Pittaluga, "Observations sur le paludisme en Macédoine grecque," Geneva, 26 September 1924 (C.H./Malaria/23), p. 2, Organisation d'Hygiène, Société des Nations.

mended solutions focusing on the disease and its vector that were closer to the Italian model of *bonifica*:

> In Greek Macedonia, the problem of agricultural colonization in the two large malarious plains of Strymon and Vardar, a problem whose solution was imposed as an inevitable social and historical phenomenon, implies and demands a prior or contemporary solution of the malaria problem by measures of grand sanitation. Such processes, whose excellent examples we have in Italy (Venice, Ferrara, Ostia, etc.), are in themselves agricultural and sanitary processes, on condition that they are always under the control and surveillance of the malariologist, who must continuously intervene with all his authority, during the entire length of the project, and apply all subsidiary measures he deems necessary, to protect, first, the workers and, then, the peasants from infection.
>
> We believe that the moment has already come for Greece to envisage the concession or enterprise of such projects of grand sanitation in the low-lying basins of Strymon and Vardar. This makes it even more necessary to coordinate the economic and technical efforts of the state to combat malaria.[135]

Five years later, in April 1929, Pittaluga returned to the Strymon project and witnessed the harmful effect of its execution on the local indigenous and refugee population and the influx of workmen.[136]

When the Asia Minor refugees began arriving after September 1922, the Greek authorities had already prior experience with displaced nationals, their particular health problems, as well as colonization issues, albeit on a much smaller scale.[137] Phokion Kopanaris, the director of public health in Macedonia, for one, knew that quinine was an urgent priority, since the refugees had become malaria carriers. In December 1923, he estimated that Macedonia alone would require 8 tons of quinine to treat cases throughout the winter. Treatment of malaria at any cost, he argued, would pay off in agricultural production in only a few years. Otherwise, Macedonia would inevitably decline "as proven by the futile attempts by different foreign peoples to settle in these locations, which have always been most fertile and

---

135 G. Pittaluga, "Observations sur le paludisme en Macédoine grecque," Geneva, 26 September 1924, p. 39, C.H./Malaria/23, Health Organisation, League of Nations.

136 G. Pittaluga, "Rapport sur le problème du paludisme et l'assistance aux réfugiés en Grèce," 15 April 1929, pp. 24–26, C.H./grèce/26 (C.H./Malaria/139), Organisation d'Hygiène, Société des Nations.

137 Kontogiorgi, *Population Exchange*, 91–92; see also p. 220 in this book.

productive, but on which reigned destruction due to malarious infection," he wrote in a report, implying that the Greeks wished to succeed where their national rivals had failed.[138]

Indeed, before the Greek authorities decided to put into effect their bonification program for Macedonia that would feed the colonized Asia Minor refugees, the regional director for public health commented: "Most parts of Macedonia, more fertile than any other land, remained fallow and uncultivated, not because the people were stupid, but because of their natural instinct to avoid death that prevailed in those locations."[139]

Henry Morgenthau, the first chairman of the Refugee Settlement Commission, which was set up in September 1923, wrote quite openly about the origin of the commission's plan to settle the hundreds of thousands refugees in northern Greece. Before arriving in Greece, Morgenthau paid a visit to Eleftherios Venizelos in Paris in November 1923 to seek his advice. The former Greek prime minister laid out two priorities: first to speed up the population exchange between Orthodox Christians and Muslims, already agreed to between Greece and Turkey in January, so that the Greek refugees could settle on the Muslim-owned estates in Macedonia.[140] Venizelos then invited Morgenthau to encourage plans to drain the marshlands along the course of the Axios and Strymon rivers, as well as the plains of Philippi north of Kavala, in order to deliver the refugees from the threat of death from endemic malaria and to allow them to settle and cultivate the newly sanitized fertile lands. The British experience with Copais had convinced Venizelos that the drainage of agricultural land was a financially viable project, sufficient to feed the refugees.[141] The experience at the Copais project with housing schemes and malaria, "one of the greatest difficulties in the resettlement question," was mentioned in October 1922, just as the refugees were pouring in, to promote British engineering interests in the Vardar and Strymon drainage plans, had been conceived long before the Greek defeat.[142]

---

138 Kopanaris, *I dimosia ygeia en Elladi*, 51–53.

139 Ibid., 51–53.

140 Kontogiorgi, *Population Exchange*, 65–68, explains in detail the reasoning behind the compulsory nature of the population exchange.

141 Morgenthau, *I Was Sent to Athens*, 87–88.

142 Kontogiorgi, *Population Exchange*, 279.

Clearly, the sanitization and colonization plans for northern Greece that Greek engineers had drawn up from 1919[143] were being adapted in Venizelos's mind to the new national, social, and demographic realities after 1922. Indeed, the argument that prioritized economic development, also held true. According to Elisabeth Kontogiorgi: "The British and French companies which negotiated with Venizelos between 1917 and 1920 for the undertaking of the construction of infrastructure works had pointed out such a need and suggested the employment of Slavs from neighbouring states."[144] Morgenthau's response to Venizelos's advice was to cable the members of the commission to meet him in Thessaloniki for a firsthand appraisal of the Axios and Strymon plains.[145]

Morgenthau noted that lack of immunity among the refugees in Macedonia exposed them annually to severe seasonal attacks of malaria that left them unable to work for four weeks at a time, and vulnerable to tuberculosis. Their only hope lay in the drainage contracts; only after their completion, Morgenthau estimated, would malaria control measures become effective.[146]

One suggestion from the Health Committee of the League of Nations to the Refugee Settlement Commission was to consider relocating refugees to more suitable permanent villages. "The removal of a village to a site only a few hundred yards away may have a pronounced effect upon health conditions," wrote Norman White of the committee, to John Campbell, the chairman of the Commission in May 1925.[147] The refugees themselves in 1926 tried to improve their lot by draining small marshes with their own labor and the assistance of army engineers; in Khalkidiki in the following years, eucalyptus trees were planted and Paris green was sprayed on the marshes.[148]

The main large drainage projects in Macedonia involved major sanitary engineering issues. The drainage work in the Strymon valley would temporarily affect the local population by disturbing the terrain and by unsettling the stability of the local endemic situation through the introduction

---

143 Ibid., 278; Karadimou-Gerolympou, "Poleis kai ypaithros," 75.

144 Kontogiorgi, *Population Exchange*, 109–10.

145 Morgenthau, *I Was Sent to Athens*, 97.

146 Ibid., 273–74 and 308.

147 [Norman White] to J. Campbell, Chairman, Refugee Settlement Commission, Geneva, 5 May 1925 (carbon copy), doc 33668, dossier no. 26426, box R 858, 12,B (Social-Health) League of Nations Archives, A (1919–27). On the recommendation of the RSC a network of dispensaries was organized, mostly in Macedonia and Thrace. See Kontogiorgi, *Population Exchange*, 269–70.

148 Ibid., 272–73.

of recruited labor, comprising some 1,000 to 3,000 men across three work-sites. These men were expected to cause local malaria epidemic outbreaks, thus increasing malaria virulence. The workers themselves would constitute a source of new infections, a matter that clearly required expert sanitary services. This was the recommendation of Gustavo Pittaluga, who visited the area in 1929 in a second visit to Greece to advise the John Monks & Sons and Ulen Company, the American companies contracted with the drainage project, on sanitary matters, primarily malaria.[149]

Indeed, Daniel E. Wright, the sanitary engineer with the Rockefeller Foundation, paid his first visit to the Vardar and Strymon project as soon as he arrived in Greece, after a stay in Italy, where he had benefited from Lewis Hackett's approach to, and experience with, the Italian reclamation and irrigation projects. Interested in the health aspects of the Vardar and Strymon projects, he noted that, from the point of view of health improvement, the success of these developments depended on their maintenance by the Greek government, as other drainage schemes had failed owing to neglect.[150] Indeed, the experience with Copais, a failure from a malariologist's perspective, and the spectacular, albeit selective, Italian example of the Fascist regime, suggested the benefits of *bonifica integrale* for the Greek peasantry, a general social improvement that would also target health, in preference to simple programs of *bonifica idraulica* and *bonifica agraria*.[151]

MALARIA AND MANUFACTURE

Whether it took place in towns or the countryside, manufacturing activity generally involved increased malaria risk. For instance, construction opened up fresh breeding sites. In the town of Karditsa, as in other towns

---

149 G. Pittaluga, "Rapport sur le problème du paludisme et l'assistance aux réfugiés en Grèce," 15 April 1929, pp. 24–27, C.H./grèce/26 (C.H./Malaria/139), Organisation d'Hygiène, Société des Nations. "The health officer must always have at his right hand a drainage engineer," prescribed Lewis Hackett, in *Malaria in Europe*, 269. In the course of the diversion of the Strymon in the 1930s, the river flooded the fields in a number of settlements in the region of Serres and destroyed the crops. Kontogiorgi, *Population Exchange*, 284.

150 D. E. Wright, to F. F. Russell, Athens, 30 May 1930, folder 25 (Health Services) 1929–1936, 1939, box 3, 749 K, 1.1, RAC.

151 Snowden, *The Conquest of Malaria*, 149–73; Dimissas, *Engkheiridion*, 124–25. On the example of the Tennessee Valley Authority in the United States and its integrated hydro-electric and social development plan with an innovative malariological component, see Humphreys, *Malaria*, 103–6. Also, Stapleton, "Internationalism and Nationalism."

lacking in stone, clay bricks were used as building material. This necessitated digging pits to obtain clay, which caused a malaria epidemic in 1905.[152] A small rural brick industry some 500 meters from the Ypati springs in Central Greece, on the estate of the Khatziskos family at Keramaria, also became a focus of infection. In that location around a dozen workmen from the island of Skopelos arrived with their families on 1 May 1907 to find employment in the works. By mid-June, they had all fallen victim to the attacks of *A. superpictus*, which were breeding in the pools of water drawn from the River Sperkheios for the mixing of clay.[153] Even Athens had its share of malaria problems caused by stagnant pools around brick and marble plants in the outskirts of the city.[154] All through the country, riverside excavations for sand obstructed and delayed the water flow.[155]

Mining was an industrial activity that literally opened up new and unanticipated opportunities for malaria, both by generating mosquito breeding sites and by attracting a naive workforce from elsewhere. The case of the Kakavos magnesite quarries of the Anglo-Greek Magnesite Company, an industrial mining enterprise on a plateau about 180 meters above sea level,[156] located about 10 kilometers southeast of Limni in Euboea, reveals the particular social context involved in this type of malaria foci. In September 1907, the company's workers were abandoning the mine in a state of "panic," according to the local manager. Approximately 20 or 30 percent of the workforce had contracted "the fever and others were afraid of catching it" and management was anxious not to lose any more men. It appears that the company had been expanding its production and recruiting men from a wider area. This had the double effect of heightening the risk of malaria and of creating a housing shortage, leaving many workers with no choice but to sleep out in the open. In the words of the manager, "there appears to be plenty of water there, although no running brook, because, if we dig down 15/20 feet, water very soon collects at the bottom of the pit."[157]

---

152 "1905," 459.

153 Kardamatis, *Ai Athinai*, 22–23.

154 Ibid., 40–42.

155 Dimissas, *Engkheiridion*, 130.

156 Society for Ecology and Development and la Documentazione e l'Educazione Ambientale Agenzia per la Ricerca, *Programme*.

157 Eugene Steiger, Manager, Anglo-Greek Magnesite Co. Ltd., to Ross, 4 September 1907, Ross papers/89/02/44, LSHTM. Ross explained that the infection in the mine was unrelated to malaria in Copais, which was far beyond the mosquito flight range, recommended the immediate administration of

In the mining villages around Lavrio, southeast of Athens, men, women, and children contracted malaria at the pits, but their residences were in villages further away. The mining companies hired doctors to keep them healthy,[158] and, in addition, the Greek Lavrion Metallurgy Company ran an infirmary.[159] The lignite mine in the village of Khalkoutsi, in northern Attica, employed three doctors; the place had become so notorious for its bad health that it was dubbed the "yellow village" (*khorion ton kitrinon*).[160]

The metal ore company at Larymna also employed a doctor for its staff and workers. Located only half an hour away from the malarious plain of Copais, it was surrounded by its own set of marshes. A malaria epidemic hit the mine, which attracted a workforce of 700 to 800 workers, in 1903, the year that it began operating. A railway track leading to the mine also caused much malaria, and half the local population fell ill with the disease the year the plant opened. The company doctor believed that these cases were imported from Lavrio, Aliveri, Larissa, Lamia, Levadia, and the Copais plain. Many of the infections were consistent with *falciparum* malaria. In 1905 about 70 percent of the population caught malaria.[161]

On the malarious Aegean island of Milos during the German occupation, which, contrary to the rest of the country, lasted until the end of the war in Europe, the local barite mining company had managed to control malaria at its site by "conscripting" local labor.[162]

---

quinine to the workers and suggested the company invite Ioannis Kardamatis to inspect the site for a fee. Ross to Eugene Steiger, Manager, Anglo-Greek Magnesite Co. Ltd., copy, 7 September 1907, Ross papers/89/02/47, LSHTM.

158 Savvas, Kardamatis, and Dasios, "1906," 464–65.

159 Kardamatis, *I apostoli tou Syllogou en ti Lavreotiki kata to ear tou 1909*, 37 and 40.

160 Livadas, "Araiosis," 4.

161 Georgiou, "I elonosia en to metalleio Larymnis eparkhias Lokridos."

162 "Report of the Sanitary Inspector Mr. Lazaropoulos Fotios about breeding malaria areas on the island of 'Milos'" [May 1945], General Sanitation July 1944–November 1945, PAG-4/3.0.12.2.3.:44 [S-0527-0708], UN Archives. Papastefanaki (in *Stis stoes*, 113–14) refers to an Allied report on the future of Greek mines written in 1943 that mentioned the Milos mine. According to the history timeline on the official website of the mine's owners, the Silver and Baryte Ores Mining Company, the company shut down in 1941, owing to the German occupation, and reopened in 1946; see Imerys Metallurgy Division, "World Locations. History." An additional factor that may have contributed to the high incidence of malaria among mining workers is suggested by Shanks and White in a recent article, namely that heightened levels of physical stress may provoke a recrudescence of *falciparum* malaria among workers harboring asymptomatic parasitemias and precipitate an epidemic; the two authors cite what was dubbed as "tropical aggregation of labour" in "any major construction and mining project" in India. See Shanks and White, "The Activation of Vivax Malaria Hypnozoites." Papastefanaki's book appeared as *I fleva tis gis. Ta metalleia tis Elladas, 1900s–2000s aionas* [The vein of the earth. The ores of Greece, 19th–20th centuries], Athens: Vivliorama 2017, too late to be consulted in this study.

Apart from accelerating communications and reducing distances, the laying of railway tracks resulted in innumerable small pools of stagnant water along the lines, which placed neighboring communities at risk. Railroad companies consistently assumed responsibility for their own employees by hiring the services of local doctors along their network on a permanent basis, while engineers and technical staff were obliged to take prophylactic quinine, because of their work outdoors. Railroad workers were particularly exposed.[163] One physician in Livadeia complained that malaria incidence in the town increased since the railway to Larissa generated "extensive swamps" along the line.[164] In the central Peloponnese town of Tripoli, the railway staff suffered in particular,[165] while the railway line contributed a considerable amount of malaria incidence in the town of Kalambaka in Thessaly.[166]

In 1924, the Anti-Malaria League targeted all railway companies for its antimalaria propaganda and sent out 3,500 copies of its guidelines to be distributed to staff members living and working in malarious locations.[167] According to the statistics of the largest railway company, the Hellenic State Railways, between 1933 and 1937 each railway employee on average cost the company two sick days annually due to the disease.[168]

Apart from disturbing the environment and involving a large amount of open-air work, railway lines also resulted in greater mobility, which transported malaria very effectively. In 1906, a local doctor explained that virulent *falciparum* malaria exchanges, primarily in the blood of the railroad workers themselves, occurred between Marathon and Boeotia after they were connected by rail.[169]

Other public works also generated malaria epidemics by disturbing the soil. Thus, the workers at the Corinth canal in the 1880s and early 1890s suf-

---

163 Georgiou, "I elonosia en to metalleio Larymnis eparkhias Lokridos," 317.

164 Savvas, Kardamatis, and Dasios, "1906," 467–70.

165 Ibid., 547.

166 Ibid., 611–12.

167 Kardamatis, "Pepragmena kata to 1924," 403. The Hellenic State Railways received 1,500 copies of this publication, the Piraeus, Athens, and Peloponnese Railways (SPAP) received 1,000, and the Thessaly Railways and Northwestern Greek Railway another 500 each.

168 Livadas and Sfangos, *I elonosia en Elladi*, vol. 1, 59–60. Kardamatis had estimated the national mean annual loss of work days to thirty per malaria patient, not per the entire population. See Kardamatis, *Statistikoi pinakes*, 250.

169 Anastasopoulos, Kapanidis, and Dimitriou, "Ai elodeis nosoi en to dimo Marathonos kata to 1906," 280.

fered "serious epidemics."[170] Eventually, malariologists realized that "to enter the path of the mosquito, you shall follow the engineers."[171]

Industrial plants often unintentionally blocked the runoff of water from higher ground. One example was the New Ship Yard of Ermoupoli, which obstructed the water flowing from Ano Syros and produced a marsh, perceived in the 1860s as a source of noxious gasses and disease, particularly for the residents of Ermoupoli. The swamp of accumulated water behind the Kaloutas tannery also was thought to have increased mortality in the neighborhood.[172] In Athens, tanneries made life unbearable for the western neighborhoods of Agios Daniil and Rouf, primarily because of their stench but also on account of the *Anopheles* breeding sites they generated.[173] In Volos, a marsh that had emerged after heavy flooding in 1893 was sustained by water runoff from a neighboring hostel and the town gasworks.[174]

URBAN MALARIA

Malaria may be primarily associated with swamps, saturated fields, and meadows. Nonetheless, towns presented a special type of natural and social environment for mosquitoes to breed. More importantly, however, towns are sites of heightened social pressures, which first gave rise to the hygienist movement that aimed at treating the sanitary implications of urban growth.[175]

Urban malaria was to a large degree imported from the rural hinterland or through the broader town network to which the town in question belonged. Although the mortality rates of urban malaria were low, it assumed a central importance which related to the centrality of diseases, in general, within the urban social environment. Acknowledging the primacy of urban malaria as a fact of social life, Wright of the RF adopted the following tactic for tackling the formidable malaria problem in Thessaly, where malaria control work only began in 1936. He recommended to Grigorios Livadas, the head of the Malariology Division of the Athens School of Hygiene, and the

---

170 Kardamatis, *Pragmateia*, 52.

171 Manoussakis, *To elonosiakon provlima*, 271.

172 Salakhas, Mayor of Syros, to [G. Drakopoulos], Cyclades prefecture, Syros 24 May 1868, T/Public works/37/9, Ermoupoli State Archive; D. Vafiadakis, Mayor of Ermoupoli, to Cyclades prefecture, Ermoupoli, 24 June 1886 (draft), T/Public works/34/8, Ermoupoli State Archive.

173 Kardamatis, *Ai Athinai*, 45–47.

174 Kardamatis, "Ekthesis peri ton en Volo," 218.

175 Baldwin, *Contagion and the State in Europe*, 540–41.

staff of the state's Malariology Service to begin their attack on urban nuisance mosquitoes. Success in the towns soon drew praise from mayors, doctors, lawyers, and other influential groups, who then pledged support and funds for the larvicide campaign of the following year.[176]

Within a town's spatial context, as Lewis Hackett noted, "the centre of a large town is protected by its own periphery rather than by our control measures."[177] For instance, visiting Thessaloniki in May 1938, malariologist W. C. Sweet was informed that the city was surrounded by swamps with *A. sacharovi* and streams with *A. superpictus* and that the spleen rate was 40 percent in the periphery and 17 percent in the city center.[178] Therefore the rate of urban growth as well as urban activities were particularly relevant to the spread and control of the disease.

As demonstrated in table 3.1 and figure 3.3, between 1834 and 1896, Athens absorbed most of the country's urban growth, with an annual rate of 4.68 percent. Most of the other major cities grew at a checkered pace controlled by economic conjuncture. As Socrates Petmezas has noted, before the First World War, Greece does not seem to have experienced a rural exodus. For most of the nineteenth century, surplus labor, rather than migrate to the towns, mostly turned to the colonization of the plains of western Central Greece and the coastal plains and slopes of the currant-producing northern and western Peloponnese. "By contrast," he writes, "the urban population of the newly established towns often originated from the 'horizontal' movement of people from other urban centers in decline. Only toward the end of the century, in parallel with the currant crisis, did a serious wave of transatlantic and internal migration appear (toward neighboring urban centers)." Overall population growth, nonetheless, responded to the capacity of the Greek economy to import grain in exchange for the export of cash crops, primarily currants.[179]

---

176 D. E. Wright to Andrew J. Warren, Ankara, 8 December 1939, 1936–1941, folder 3 Health 1930–1934, box 1, 749 I, Projects Series 749 Greece, RG 1.1, RF, RAC. A similar experience with malaria control in towns of the American South is found in Humphreys, *Malaria*, 92–93.

177 Lewis W. Hackett to F. F. Russell, Rome, 18 October 1934, folder 14, box 2, Series 749, Sub-series I, RG 1.1, RF, RAC. Hackett was commenting on malaria measurements in the town of Tirana in Albania.

178 W. C. Sweet, "Diary of a European trip" 1938, entry 10 May 1938, 100 I, folder 511 Swe-1, box 51, Series 100, RG 1, RF, RAC.

179 Petmezas, "Agrotiki oikonomia," 113 and 129.

	Year	Population	Annual growth
Athens	1834	7,200	
	1896	123,001	4.68%
Patras	1834	5,115	
	1896	37,985	3.29%
Volos	1858	400	
	1896	16,788	10.33%

Table 3.1. Urban growth in major Greek cities, 1834–96
Source: Greek census data.

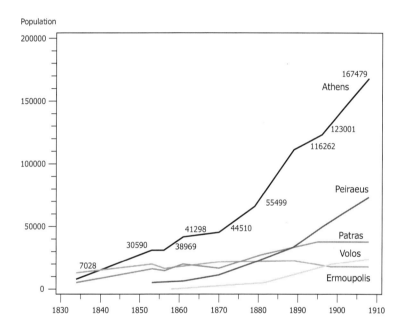

Figure 3.3. Urban growth in major Greek cities, 1834–1907

In terms of morbidity, overall Greek towns experienced a much lighter malaria burden than the countryside. Balfour compared urban and rural localities, that is, settlements above and below a thousand inhabitants, and found a spleen index of 27.8 percent and a parasite index of 13.3 percent in the former and a spleen index of 56.7 percent and a parasite index of 27.7 percent in the latter.[180]

---

180 Balfour, "Malaria Studies in Greece," 322.

Before Athens became the Greek capital in December 1834, the seat of government moved several times for security reasons. The capital transferred from Nafplio to Aigina and back before finally settling on its final location. This fluctuation inflated each temporary capital with government officials, office seekers, government offices, and housing[181] and had serious sanitary implications. When the British traveler Thomas Alcock visited Aigina in 1828, he took note of the fever epidemic caused by overcrowding: "When I was in Egina fever was at such a height, that from ten to fifteen persons on average died each day; and, for fear of increasing the consternation, the church bells were not allowed to be tolled. It was at the end of September before the usual autumnal rains had commenced, and until the atmosphere is refreshed by heavy falls, that period of the year is very liable to an epidemic disease."[182] Although Alcock did not specifically refer to intermittents—most likely, the fevers were a disease mix due to a more general breakdown of sanitation, which must have also included waterborne diseases such as typhoid fever—the seasonal peak in September suggests that at least some of the fever epidemic could have been due to *falciparum* malaria.

In the first years of Greek statehood, the population began to rebuild, redesign, and resettle their towns, which had been damaged during the War of Independence. Corinth, for one, at the time an inland town, had the potential to become a thriving commercial center if it could gain safe access to Lekhaio, its ancient port, which over the centuries had become a large, unhealthy marsh. Sea traffic was the only choice for trade, since overland communication was extremely difficult. The construction of a harbor at Lekhaio, however, would require draining the extensive marsh. As Konstantinos Mavrogiannis argued in 1840,

> Drawing closer to the sea, will be a double benefit for Corinth and will perhaps encourage its inhabitants to settle there, because, it must be said, to imagine Corinth as a commercial town without Lekhaion is just as absurd as to figure Athens without Peiraeus. Corinth needs the port in order to form a crucial link in the chain of maritime commerce in a country, where overland communication is, as yet, difficult, slow and expensive. If Lekhaion were to

181 About, *Greece and the Greeks of the Present Day*, 157–58.
182 Alcock, *Travels in Russia, Persia, Turkey and Greece*, 184.

be restored, it could become the hub of a commercial town, in which living will perhaps become far less unhealthy.[183]

The same author, nonetheless, was skeptical about the rush displayed by his "ignorant" contemporaries to settle close to the sea. The residents of Megara, Sicyon (Kiato), Corinth, and Patras before the revolution, and those of Argos and Athens, during the revolution, had been forced from their towns by violence and war, but they all returned to rebuild their homes at the original locations, where ancient topography had proven its wisdom that the climate was healthy. Thus, with Corinth in mind, he recommended rebuilding new towns on ancient sites. In his words: "Now, as long as greater interests do not attract townspeople to move toward the shores, whenever they wish to live in the locations occupied by old towns, the plans of the new towns should be drawn on the basis of the ancient places."[184]

In Athens itself, fevers, although not exclusively malarial ones, had a considerable impact on the original city plan of the new town and caused its reorientation: the relocation of the site for the royal palace on higher ground than originally planned, and shifts in land values.[185] It suffered a fever epidemic in 1835, the first summer after the transfer of the capital. It was so severe that it drove the members of the Athens Medical Society out of town, forcing it to temporarily suspend its operations.[186] The intensive construction activity and road works generated by the transfer of the capital and the new town plan must have spawned an unprecedented number of mosquito breeding sites across the city. The next fever epidemic on record, which began in June 1842 and ended the following January, attacked one-third of the inhabitants.[187] As long as Athens was relatively small and compact in size, it remained a unified malarious zone.[188] By 1861 it had become a city of 41,000 inhabitants, growing but not yet large enough to afford malaria-free neighborhoods.

Thanks to the Athens Medical Society and the records of the Astykliniki, the University of Athens outpatient clinic, Athens was the first Greek city

---

183 Mavrogiannis, "Paratiriseis epi ton klimaton tis Ellados," 349–50.

184 Ibid., 351–52.

185 Biris, Ai Athinai apo tou 19ou eis ton 20on aiona, 65–66.

186 [Introduction], Asklipios (1836): iv.

187 Mavrogiannis, "Protai grammai mias topografias," 542–43.

188 Kardamatis, Ai Athinai, 9.

where numerical data on malaria was recorded. Although mostly treated at home, malaria was nonetheless responsible for most hospital admittances. On the basis of statistics from hospital and university clinics between 1860 and 1910, Ioannis Kardamatis compared the relative malaria morbidity to general morbidity in Athens. Thus, in the two decades from 1860 to 1880 one in every three patients was hospitalized for malaria. In the 1880s malaria morbidity shot up steeply; half of all patients had malaria; then in the 1890s, this rate fell to one in every five, whereas in the first decade of the new century it dropped even further to one in every ten patients hospitalized.[189] Taking into account the fact that most malaria sufferers remained at home, what is important is not the proportions themselves but their declining trend since the 1890s. Indeed, in a comment on the general state of public health in 1882, as malaria morbidity was peaking, Athenian physician Ioannis Valassopoulos warned: "if the population of Athens increases even slightly, and public health continues to be deemed worthless (*en moira karos*), Theseus's erstwhile city will have become completely unhealthy."[190]

Furthermore, as the town expanded, the boundaries of its malaria-free zone gradually moved away from the town center. The 1865 malaria epidemic in Athens hit the city outskirts worst; the center experienced only sporadic cases.[191] After 1875, when the River Ilissos and its tributaries began "gushing water which ran intermittently every summer," its neighboring district suffered in particular. Vatrakhonisi, on the far side of the Ilissos, became so malarious that in the 1870s the outpatient clinic reserved a thousand drachmas' worth of quinine each year specifically for that neighborhood. Until the first antimalarial works in 1906, that is, seventy-two years after it became the capital, Athens had suffered twenty-nine malaria epidemics, most of them confined to specific neighborhoods. The most severe outbreaks occurred in 1875 in the neighborhood of Agios Konstantinos and in 1886 in the neighborhood of Gazokhori. Later on, large-scale excavations caused epidemics along Alexandras Avenue and the adjoining neighborhood of Tsakagiannis.[192]

189 Kardamatis, "I elonosia en Athinais," 128.

190 Valassopoulos, "Nosologiki geografia," 73.

191 Writing in the early 1880s, Professor Georgios Karamitsas attributed this difference to the exposure of the surrounding zone to unhealthy, miasma-bearing winds. See Karamitsas, "Peri elodon i eleiogenon nosimaton," vol. 2, 734.

192 Kardamatis, "I elonosia en Athinais," 123–25; Kardamatis, *Ai Athinai*, 8–10; Kardamatis, "I kata to theros tou 1907," 6. In October 1907, Kardamatis examined blood slides of 157 "individuals of various ages" who lived in the neighborhood of the Averof prison and found 118 positive cases, i.e., 83 with *falciparum*

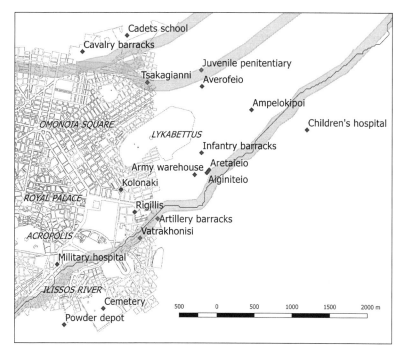

Map 3.1. Malaria in Athens, 1908
Source: "I okhri panoukla."

Subsequently, as the city spread eastward, more malaria foci emerged along the Ilissos, effectively no larger than a stream, and its tributaries, particularly among large concentrations of confined people, for instance in hospitals, barracks, and prisons. In this recent area of the city malaria struck particularly heavily at the turn of the century with severe epidemics in 1901 and 1907. A newspaper account delineated an arc that effectively encompassed one-third of the city and began from the artillery depot, "through the nurses quarters, Rigillis street, the artillery barracks, Lykabettus, the cadets barracks, and reaching from the Children's hospital to Vatrakhonisi," a zone it dubbed "the domain of shivers" or "the domain of fever."[193] It was in this developing eastern region of Athens that the Anti-Malaria League performed its first beneficial, small-scale annual interventions in 1906.[194]

---

malaria (70 percent), 21 with *vivax* malaria, 5 with *malariae*, 6 with *vivax* and *falciparum*, 2 with *falciparum* and *malariae*, and 1 with *vivax* and *malariae*. Kardamatis, "I kata to theros tou 1907," 14.

193 "I okhri panoukla." See map 3.1.

194 An itemized account of *Anopheles* breeding sites in Athens in 1915 may be found in Kardamatis, *Ai Athinai*.

In 1901, the entire town of Aigio in northern Peloponnese, which had previously benefited from the effects on cultivation by the sanitization of the countryside, now suffered renewed malaria epidemics owing to railroad ditches and frequent flooding. The 8,500 inhabitants of the town had a malaria prevalence that reached 90 percent, and were particularly affected in the outskirts of the town among those who worked in the fields and those who "descended from the mountains for the first time."[195] By 1930, however, malaria must have retreated from the town center to the outskirts. This can be deduced from the spleen rates among schoolchildren examined in May and June 1930, which were as follows:

School No. 1	26%
School No. 2	36%
School No. 3	34%
School No. 4	49%

Assuming that schools were numbered in the order in which they were founded, School No. 1 was the oldest school and closest to the town center, while School No. 4 was the most recent one, and was probably closer to the edge of the town and, thus more exposed to *Anopheles* breeding sites.[196]

A deadly malaria epidemic hit Nafplio in 1886 when the old fortifications were pulled down. After that, however, with the help of drainage works, the situation improved considerably.[197] The town of Argostoli on the island of Cephalonia was exposed to the Koutavos lagoon, which fed from a freshwater spring that presumably reduced its salinity. Drainage and filling works executed by the British for the sake of their troops improved the situation, but only temporarily. By the early twentieth century, the whole town was again in the grip of severe malaria epidemics.[198] In small towns surrounded by marshes like Agrinio, malaria was endemic in all neighborhoods.[199] In 1901, Kalamata, where some drainage work had started but remained incomplete, was also surrounded by rivers and

---

195 "Apantiseis ton k. Iatron," 214–16.
196 M. Ciucă, "Organisation de la lutte antimalarique en Grèce," Geneva, 14 February 1931, p. 5, CH/Malaria/154, Commission du Paludisme, Organisation d'Hygiène, Société des Nations.
197 "Apantiseis ton k. Iatron," 207.
198 Ibid., 249.
199 Ibid., 205.

swamps with "no neighborhood remaining unaffected" and malarial cachexia on the increase.[200]

Even lay contemporaries were aware that the urban environment was exposed to infecting agents from the countryside. Arta, a town in western Greece which had an estimated morbidity rate of 30 percent, was surrounded by rural communities with a rate of 80 percent. In an effort to protect the urban population the town authorities purchased quinine to distribute free to the rural communes.[201] However, in the light of later knowledge about the properties of quinine, namely that it does not kill the gametocytes of *P. falciparum* in circulation and fails to reach the hypnozoites of *P. vivax* in the liver, this attempted public health measure was of limited effect. Treatment with quinine merely relieved individual cases and controlled mortality rates but did not prevent carriers from infecting mosquitoes.[202]

Urban malaria was one of the two initial causes for data collection on disease, the other being malaria in the army. Urban malaria is, therefore, a convenient field for cross-country comparison. Since malaria, unlike many other acute infectious diseases, was not a notifiable disease until 1950,[203] it is not possible to determine malaria morbidity nor to improve on the imprecise estimates of the medical surveys. However, a broad assessment puts the number of nationwide malaria cases to between 1,500,000 and 2,000,000, depending on the year.[204] It is indicative of the size of the problem that in the eight years between 1924 and 1931, out of the 767,225 patients admitted to all hospitals (public and municipal, including mental), 152,642 (20 percent) were malaria cases, an average of 19,080 per year, with a case mortality of 1.25 percent, or 5 percent of all hospital deaths. In 1925 malaria admittances peaked with 22,175 cases. 1929, with 20,488 malaria cases, was also a particularly bad year.[205]

---

200 Ibid., 229.

201 Savvas, Kardamatis, and Dasios, "1906," 610–11.

202 On the limitations of quinine consumption as a public health measure, see chapter 4.

203 Information on the malaria control program in Greece, 8 May 1956, p. 2, Inter-Regional Conference on Malaria for the Eastern Mediterranean and European Regions WHO/Mal/163-8, WHO.

204 Cholera became a notifiable disease in 1911 (royal decree of 18 May 1911), smallpox in the same year (royal decree of 2 December 1911), plague and typhus in 1915 (royal decrees of 30 March 1915 and 20 July 1915, respectively). Typhoid fever, paratyphoid, dysentery, scarlet fever, diphtheria, spinal meningitis, recurrent fever, rabies, glanders, anthrax, influenza, leprosy, puerperal fever, lethargic encephalitis (trypanosomiasis) by royal decree of 3 May 1921 and poliomyelitis by royal decree of 18 August 1930. A ministerial decree also made pertussis, dengue, erysipelas, brucellosis, leishmaniasis, measles, tetanus, and chickenpox notifiable. Kopanaris, *I dimosia ygeia en Elladi*, 158.

205 Kopanaris, *I dimosia ygeia en Elladi*, 200, 296–97, 298–313, tables 77–84.

By contrast, city authorities counted malaria deaths. The table below presents a comparison of mortality figures in the twelve largest Greek cities at the turn of the century and the 1920s for general mortality, malaria, and tuberculosis.

	1899–1908 (Old Greece)	1921–30	Difference
Malaria	7.50	2.54	-66.12%
Tuberculosis	78.14	31.64	-59.51%
General	257.73	190.21	-26.20%

Table 3.2. Annual deaths per 10,000 inhabitants in the twelve largest cities, 1899–1908 and 1921–30

Source: Kopanaris, *I dimosia ygeia en Elladi*, 3. The annual mortality for malaria for the years 1921–30, "in the last decade," was 9.14 per 10,000 inhabitants, i.e. considerably higher than the urban figures. For the years 1930–38 malaria mortality had fallen to 6.92 per 10,000. Ibid., 4–5, 200. Between 1933 and 1937 the contribution of tuberculosis to general mortality in Greece was 8.95%; for malaria, the figure was 3.67%. Valaoras, *Stoikheia viometrias kai statistikis*, 145 and 157.

The following chart represents malaria and tuberculosis mortality per 10,000 inhabitants in the 1930s with malaria deaths increasing slightly after 1934.

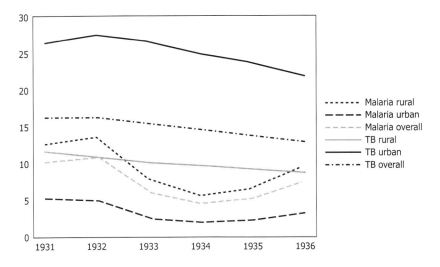

Figure 3.4. Mortality per 10,000, 1931–36
Source: Alivizatos, "Georgiki Ellas," 314.

Despite the fact that the respective sources of these figures stem from different sources,[206] the reduction in urban malaria deaths in the 1920s to one-third of the rate at the beginning of the twentieth century remains impressive. It could be attributed to the extensive use of better quality quinine that became available after the 1908 quinine law. Furthermore, considering the fact that there was a similar reduction in deaths from tuberculosis and a significant drop in general mortality in the same cities, one may also assume a general improvement in medical services, even in the face of the country's postwar hardships.

Among the twelve largest towns of Greece before the Balkan Wars and the ensuing accession of Macedonia to Greece, Volos was the town with the highest malaria mortality per 10,000 inhabitants and as a percentage of general mortality. Malaria deaths peaked in July, with the city in 1907 recording almost twice as many deaths as Athens (figure 3.7). Larissa and Trikala, also in malaria-ridden Thessaly, with Pyrgos and Kalamata in the southwestern Peloponnese were not far behind, as shown in figures 3.5 and 3.6.[207]

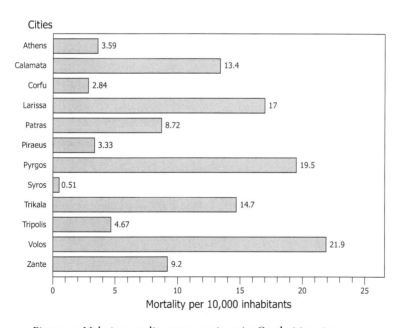

Figure 3.5. Malaria mortality per 10,000 in major Greek cities, 1899–1907

206 The provenance of the 1899–1908 figures is the Medical Council; that of the 1920s is the General Statistical Service of Greece. Kopanaris, *I dimosia ygeia en Elladi*, 11.
207 Hadjimichalis and Cardamatis, "Report on the Work of the Greek Antimalaria League."

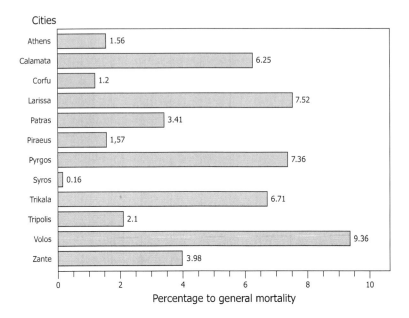

Figure 3.6. Malaria to general mortality (%) in major Greek cities, 1899–1907

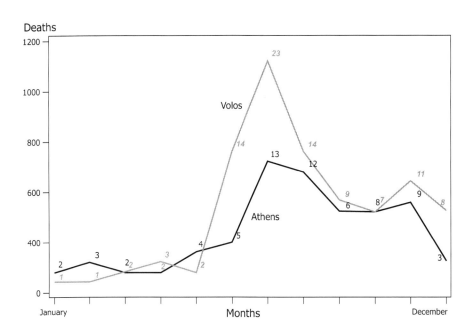

Figure 3.7. Malaria deaths in Athens and Volos, 1907

As for the national figures for malaria deaths in the 1920s (1921–31), the mean for recorded urban malaria deaths was 7.75 per 10,000; recorded urban malaria deaths shot up steeply in 1923 and 1924 to a rate of 19.94 (or 2.23 times the 1922 rate) and 11.63 per 10,000, respectively, clearly as a result of the presence of thousands of refugees and recorded urban malaria death rates returned to pre-1922 levels by 1925. The respective national mean for rural areas in the 1920s was considerably higher than the corresponding figure for cities, that is, 10.07 recorded malaria deaths per 10,000 inhabitants. Recorded rural malaria deaths, on the other hand, shot up to 11.09 (or 1.71 times the 1922 rate) and 11.53 deaths per 10,000 in 1923 and 1924, respectively, and remained above the pre-1922 level until at least 1931.[208]

PEACE AND MALARIA ERADICATION

As noted by Mary Dobson in her seminal work *Contours of Death and Disease in Early Modern England*, the growth imperative drives populations to incur risks that reduce the quality and even the length of their lives, whether in pursuit of opportunities in the city or in productive and even marginal areas of the countryside.[209] The intensity of malaria in Greece after independence, as in much of the developing world today, should be seen in this light. It is, moreover, a common theme in the literature on the social and economic parameters affecting the spread of malaria in postcolonial Africa and a critique of the view labeled as "malaria blocks development." This critique suggests that the relationship between malaria and economic development is far from linear or necessarily discrepant.

It is, indeed, interesting to note that in nineteenth-century Greece, the choice to resettle in marshy plains and restructure Greek agriculture in favor of currant viticulture was a free choice on the part of peasant families to improve their own living standards and to abandon "their traditional occupations, namely grain cultivation and flock-herding."[210] It is, moreover, rea-

208 Kopanaris, *I dimosia ygeia en Elladi*, 225, table 59. On the gradual reduction of malaria deaths per 100,000 inhabitants between 1930 and 1938, see Valaoras, *Stoikheia viometrias*, 157. According to the same author, the refugees compensated for the heavy toll mainly of malaria, tuberculosis, dysentery, and malnutrition by a large number of marriages and an increased birth rate. Valaoras, *To dimografikon provlima*, 24–33. On the recommendations of the League of Nations Health Committee team for Thessaloniki in 1929, see Kontogiorgi, "I katastasi tis dimosias ygeias sti Thessaloniki."
209 Dobson, *Contours of Death*, 147 and 182.
210 Franghiadis, "Peasant Agriculture and Export Trade," 71.

sonable to hypothesize that, even as this new environment often provided increased opportunities for malaria, improved income would, in turn, make access to quinine and medical advice more affordable to the peasants. Leaving individual choices and income aside, however, in 1924, Kardamatis was the first observer to actually discuss the economics of the malaria burden incurred by Greece and to put an annual price tag on the cost of the disease. He thus estimated the annual cost of malaria to the Greek economy in 1923 at 860,193,350 drachmas.[211] In February 1945 Daniel E. Wright put the annual tag at 4,636,000,000 drachmas or US$46,360,000,[212] while, in the 1960s, Livadas and Athanassatos put the benefit from eliminating the annual cost of malaria at US$26 million.[213]

Beyond the direct implications for Greece's national economy, demographer Vasileios Valaoras calculated the cost of malaria in terms of life expectancy. By drawing up life tables with and without malaria deaths and adding up the differences in life expectancy at birth through the age of five, the most vulnerable age group, he estimated that "malaria . . . deducts approximately one year from all Greeks up to the age of four, in other words overall it shortens the life of our country's population by five full years."[214] This estimate, however, does not take into account loss of life from the indirect effect of malaria on other serious diseases, most notably on deaths from tuberculosis, that occurred in adult life. In the 1930s, this was estimated annually at around 2,000 deaths.[215]

In 1951, Greece introduced a surveillance experiment that was adopted as a control policy the following year. The United States ended its financial support for the malaria control program through the Marshall Plan's Economic Cooperation Administration (ECA), and then Mutual Security Agency (MSA), in 1953. Surveillance became even more important when, in 1957, Greece adopted the WHO malaria-eradication campaign.[216] However,

211 Kardamatis, *Statistikoi pinakes*, 249–50.

212 D. E. Wright to Finances and Administration, Athens, 3 February 1945, Medical Care and Sanitation Malaria October 1943–July 1946, 651 Health, PAG-4/3.0.12.3.1.0.:8 [S-0527-0729], UN Archives.

213 Livadas and Athanassatos, "The Economic Benefits," 181.

214 Valaoras, *Stoikheia viometrias*, 194–96. Valaoras calculated life expectancy at birth in 1928 at 49.09 years for men and 50.89 for women; life tables in ibid., 182–83. For the island of Mykonos, where malaria was not a problem, Violetta Hionidou has calculated life expectancy at birth at "at least" forty-five years in the mid-nineteenth century and at fifty-seven in the 1950s. See Hionidou, "The Demographic System," 13–14.

215 Livadas and Athanassatos, "The Economic Benefits," 178–79.

216 Vassiliou, "Politics, Public Health, and Development," 266–87. For a critical view of surveillance services and bureaucratic impediments to action, see Nájera, "Malaria Control," 69.

the country failed to reorganize its malaria service, to enforce measures, and to stem a general complacency toward the campaign.[217] Despite these serious failings, however, as Maria Vassiliou has convincingly demonstrated, the elimination of malaria in Greece by the mid-1970s was the combined effect of improved socioeconomic conditions and the rise in living standards in the 1960s—in turn, partly resulting from the decline of malaria—a consistent vertical campaign that reduced morbidity dramatically, as well as foreign aid in the form of the Marshall Plan.[218]

The eradication of malaria from Greece was a peacetime achievement of applying DDT technology to a country that had received substantial foreign aid and advice. The last indigenous malaria cases were recorded in 1973 among a Roma community in Imatheia and, in the northern Evros region in 1976 and, possibly, in 1978.[219] Unlike Bulgaria in 1965 and Yugoslavia in 1973, the WHO never formally declared Greece malaria-free.[220] Nonetheless, by the mid-1970s malaria in Greece had effectively disappeared. However, while the Greeks are no longer a reservoir of malaria parasites and have lost their immunity to malaria, after 2009 KEELPNO, the national disease control agency, has detected indications of local transmission of imported *vivax* malaria cases, attributable to migrants, at several older heavily malarious locations.[221]

MALARIA AND WAR

In his *Man's Mastery of Malaria*, the RF malariologist Paul F. Russell devoted just over one page on war and malaria, concluding: "war heightens endemicity."[222] In any malarious country, military life under wartime conditions exposed large numbers of susceptible individuals to the disease. Indeed, the exposure of the British troops to malaria in Macedonia in the First World War provided C. M. Wenyon, the British malariologist, the opportunity to give his Macedonian experience a global scope by comparing it to

217 Vassiliou, "Politics, Public Health, and Development," 300–306, 311–13.
218 Ibid., 315–16.
219 Ibid., 311, 314; Bruce-Chwatt et al., "Sero-Epidemiological Surveillance"; Bruce-Chwatt and De Zulueta, *The Rise and Fall of Malaria in Europe*, 41.
220 Vassiliou, "Politics, Public Health, and Development," 312–13.
221 Piperaki et al., "Assessment of Antibody Responses," 156 and KEELPNO, "Ekthesi epidimiologikis epitirisis."
222 Russell, *Man's Mastery of Malaria*, 185.

China, India, and Africa.[223] On the basis of centuries of British experience with colonial warfare, another medical officer, William Hunter, warned with regard to the measures required in Macedonia: "They extend to all aspects of the problem of combating malaria under war conditions—admittedly as the experience of military history shows—one of the most—if not the most—difficult problem with which military operations can be faced."[224]

Armies may be wartime machines. Nonetheless, most of the time they are on a peacetime footing. From the perspective of this study, therefore, soldiers share much of the environment that affects civilians, whose experience with malaria, in turn, they influence. Consequently, I will avoid drawing a sharp distinction between army life in peacetime and times of war by also looking into the relationship between army and civilian life.

Fevers in the military camps and barracks of the British-ruled Ionian Islands and, later, of the Greek mainland initiated the systematic collection of evidence on local malaria. After independence, in the mid-1880s, it was the Greek Army physicians who first mobilized to face the collapse of the public health system of the 1830s, by targeting malaria in the Greek Army. This response coincided with the military reforms of the Trikoupis governments, which included universal conscription and made the army the center of public attention and national expectations.[225] This development is not, of course, unique to Greece and reflects a general trend in Europe to set the army into the public sphere. For instance, under the scrutiny of the press and the reports of William Russell in the *Times* from the Crimean War, the British public began to take a closer interest in the fate of the common soldier.[226]

From the perspective of scientific research, military forces exposed to malaria in the Greek lands provided medical officers with enough evidence to formulate hypotheses on the nature and causes of intermittent, remittent, and continuous fevers. A substantial amount of medical writing on the subject was prompted by the British and French military presence and the exposure of troops to the local disease regime. In fact, as demonstrated by medi-

---

223 Wenyon, "Malaria in Macedonia," 51. Wenyon, however, believed that Macedonian malaria was extensive but not particularly virulent.

224 William Hunter, AMS (Army Medical Service), Medical Advisory Committee for Prevention of Epidemic Diseases (Mediterranean and Mesopotamia), Salonika, to H. R. Whitehead, Director of Medical Services (DMS), Salonika, 26 February 1917, Salonika Army, March and April 1917, British Forces Salonika, WO 95.

225 Kostis, *Ta kakomathimena paidia tis istorias*, 459.

226 Harrison, *The Medical War*, 2.

cal historian Bernardino Fantini, the significant corpus of wartime medical research during the First World War threw into question many of the certainties that had emerged from advances in malariology since 1898 and the discovery of the role of the mosquito in transmitting malaria.[227]

In terms of public discourse, the relationship between human societies and malaria was generally perceived in battlefield terms and affected the discourse about the disease. This was particularly true until the end of the First World War, when "most of the doctors in the field saw themselves at war; the language of battle came easily to their minds and pens," wrote malaria historian Gordon Harrison. Alphonse Laveran and Ronald Ross, the two pioneers in malaria research, were army physicians serving their respective country's tropical empires. Beyond the symbolic use of wartime terminology, however, waging a war against the *Anopheles* was a crucial component of the military competition among imperialist countries.[228] Greece, however, unlike Italy, which was a latecomer in the imperialist race, possessed neither an interest in the tropics nor a tradition in scientific research. Nonetheless, its own as well as invading foreign armies experienced malaria very intensely, often to a greater degree than local civilians, who were protected by various degrees of immunity. After the First World War, the battlefield metaphor was replaced by one of a full-scale international confrontation, as "the fight against malaria, yellow fever, and dengue increasingly resembled a pitched battle against mosquitoes."[229]

The effects of war on malaria in Greece must include army mobilization, wartime exposure to disturbed environments, population displacement, contacts between people of different disease experiences and disease pools imposed by war, the importance of lines of communication, and the impact on malaria research.

Foreign Troops in the Local Environment

By disturbing the soil, military preparations, operations, fortification works, and, even on occasion, measures designed to control malaria, all increased the extent of mosquito breeding sites and, thus, the risk of malaria for fight-

227 Fantini, "Malaria and the First World War," 242.
228 Harrison, *Mosquitoes, Malaria, and Man*, 2–3.
229 Anderson, *Colonial Pathologies*, 225; Fantini, "Malaria and the First World War," 269.

ing men in the field as well as for civilians returning home in the aftermath
of wartime devastation. Additionally, even after the role of the mosquito in
malaria transmission had become established, defeating the enemy invariably took precedence over controlling the mosquito population. This may
be illustrated by the following instances from the Greek lands.

Malaria in the Ionian Islands

South of the Venetian-held town of Corfu there was a large marshy lagoon,
the remnants of an ancient harbor. Having lost its original depth, it had
turned into a fishery and salt pans, and become the property of the Venetian government. The French, who occupied the island in 1797, exchanged
the lagoon with the island of Vido, which had been in the possession of the
Corfiot noble family of Khalkiopoulo. The lagoon, which assumed the name
of its new proprietor, kept diminishing in size and the salt pans lost much of
their yield as agriculture encroached on the lake.

The French envisaged a military role for the spot. To fortify their communications and "strengthen their position in the town of Corfu," they decided
to create a fortified communications canal that would connect the lake of
Khalkiopoulo to the bay of Kastrades, present-day Garitsa, on the other side
of the town. The Kastrades end of the project started 343 meters from the
sea and reached Fort St. Salvador (Lofos Sotiros) along a line of 2,745 meters surrounded by swamps and low-lying vegetable gardens that supplied
the town. In the meantime, the canal had been accumulating all kinds of
animal and vegetable refuse and stagnant water. With the ground drasti-
cally disturbed by the works, the ditch had added to the area's fever load.
The men working on the canal lived nearby in wooden barracks; one-fifth
of the total force of 10,000 men lost their lives as a result of fevers—an early,
small-scale Panama Canal disaster. Still, when the French evacuated Corfu
in July 1814 they left the project incomplete. Interestingly, when handing
over the island, General François-Xavier Donzelot, the French commander,
informed Sir James Campbell, his British counterpart, "of the unhealthiness
of the spot," in a gesture noted "for the honour of human nature." Yet, the
first British troops occupied the very same spot, only to find out for themselves the risk they were in and soon to abandon the place. Eventually, the
British authorities decided to fill up the ditches, and on 16 July 1819 they is-

sued a proclamation ordering all residents within ten miles of Kastrades to provide one day's labor per week to undo the work of the French. Within forty days of corvée labor, some 1,250 meters, less than half the distance, had been covered by the forced labor of 9,368 Corfiot peasants, or a daily average of 234 laborers.[230] Unlike the French, the British refrained from exposing the lives of their own troops, when they could unload the work and the risk of malaria on the locals, a practice that was repeated with consistency.[231]

In the British-controlled Ionian Islands, British soldiers died of fevers in significant numbers. John Davy, the inspector-general of army hospitals, who published an account of his service in the Mediterranean, saw the islands as a relatively salubrious place, were it not for the extensive prevalence of fevers. In his words: "these islands would be superior even to our own country, and to most parts of Europe, in general healthiness, and I believe on a par, or nearly so, in regard to lowness of mortality."[232] Yet, he and his medical colleagues attributed half of the deaths of British troops in the territory between 1822 and 1835 to fevers.[233] Although hospital admissions of fever cases rose with the increase in the size of the British military presence, particularly between 1827 and 1831, mortality fell slightly, as shown in figure 3.8.

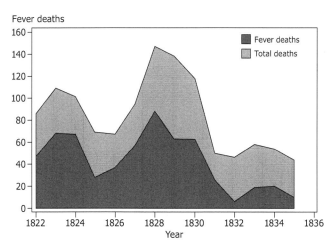

Figure 3.8. Fever mortality in the Ionian Islands, 1822–35
Source: Davy, *Notes and Observations.*

230 Hennen, *Sketches*, 149–51.
231 As will be seen, the French subsequently also learned their lesson.
232 Davy, *Notes and Observations*, vol. 2, 218.
233 Ibid., 220; Laskaratos, "I katastasi tis ygeias," 145.

The irregular and unpredictable behavior of the disease over the years of observation, both as regards to its geographical distribution among the islands and to the varying intensity with which it affected the British troops, baffled these early scientific observers. According to Davy:

> Our troops in the garrison of Santa Maura [Lefkada] suffer more from fever than in any other of the islands; the ratio of deaths annually there, per 1000 mean strength, appears to have been 37.6 from fever alone, during a period of twenty years; yet in 1832 the reverse happened; in all the other islands they suffered more; that year, in Santa Maura, the ratio of mortality, from all diseases, was reduced to sixteen, and this without any obvious cause; in 1828 it was as high as 170, chiefly from fever.[234]

Variables	Mean	Standard deviation	Coefficient of variation
Army strength	3601.21	495.44	13.76
Fever deaths	42.36	25.14	59.34
Total deaths	84.36	34.36	40.73
Fever admissions	1621.64	641.82	39.58
Fever mortality to admissions (%)	2.46	1.03	42.00
Fever deaths to strength (%)	1.14	0.64	55.70

Table 3.3. Hospital admissions and deaths of fever in the Ionian Islands, 1822–35
Source: Davy, *Notes and Observations.*

Table 3.3 reflects the variability of the disease over a fourteen-year period. Thus, over a period of fourteen years, a relatively stable number of troops demonstrated a remarkably variable exposure to fevers despite a background of declining trends in mortality.[235]

The chances, moreover, of dying from fevers were unequally distributed. Over a period of twenty years the average annual mortality per thousand British soldiers in the Ionian Islands exceeded that of British officers by 22:1.

---

234 Davy, *Notes and Observations*, vol. 2, 244–45. See also chapter 2; Hennen, *Sketches*, 366.

235 The degree of variability is suggested by the coefficient of variation of fever hospital admissions (39.58 percent of the fourteen-year mean) and an even greater variability in fever deaths (59.34 percent of the mean). On average, 2.46 percent of hospital patients admitted for fever (or 1.14 of the total military strength) lost their lives, but over the years this percentage varied significantly, i.e., by 42 percent of the mean (or by 55.70 percent of the mean in the case of deaths per mean strength).

Increased exposure to fevers was indeed a fate soldiers shared with the local peasantry; both were at a disadvantage to their social betters, British officers, and local landlords, respectively. "The common soldiers, like the peasantry, are much exposed to the night air—the officers little; the former on duty on guard—and independent of this, which is unavoidable, many of them, from the crowded state of the barracks, and from the rooms being infested with fleas and bugs, are tempted to come out and sleep in the open air."[236]

Each year, one-fifth of the locals in British-ruled Cephalonia suffered from intermittent and remittent fevers. In 1816, a bad year, that number rose to one in four. In the same year, the British garrison had 307 troops sick with fever, of whom more than 80 died, a huge proportion when compared to the mortality of the locals of whom about 12,000 had fallen ill with remittent and intermittent fevers, but no more than 50 died. The difference in mortality between the locals and the British garrison was "most striking."[237]

Although the properties of the place were generally thought to cause fevers, contact with the natives was also seen as a probable source of risk. In his account of sanitary conditions in the British garrison of Lefkada, John Hennen suggested that confining the men inside the fort protected them from the emanations of the lagoon and from the "pestilential" heat and effluvia in the streets of the neighboring town but also from "intoxication from the poisonous ardent spirits retailed by the natives." The town barrack, however, which was located near the lagoon, "has ever been found more inimical to health than the barracks within the fort." Lefkada also had several outposts manned by a handful of men on an irregular basis. These were considered highly dangerous, with one such post, Catechori, a rocky location some 15 miles to the south of the fort, abandoned "in consequence of the whole detachment, consisting of sixteen persons, being taken ill of remittent fever of the most malignant type, in 1817, of whom three died, and the remainder very narrowly escaped." For want of a convincing explanation, another military observer, cited by Hennen, vaguely hypothesized that there was "something in the nature of the soil itself, sufficient to produce the disease, added to a particular constitution of the air, which rendered the summer of 1817 so sickly throughout the whole of the Mediterranean."[238]

236 Davy, *Notes and Observations*, vol. 2, 251.
237 Hennen, *Sketches*, 274 and 283.
238 Ibid., 379–81.

The endemic nature of malaria notwithstanding, the fact remains that it is impossible to estimate retrospectively precisely how much of these Mediterranean fevers corresponded to the post-1880 concept of malaria. Davy indeed admitted his inability to identify the nature of malaria, in which he sought, not a disease in itself, but the probable cause behind an array of diseases framed in the medical paradigm of his time, namely intermittent, remittent, and continued fevers. He pondered:

> I shall now proceed to offer a few remarks on malaria, the presumed cause of intermittent and remittent-fever, and, according to some medical men, of the continued and ephemeral fevers also of warm climates. What is malaria? I apprehend were it not for the fevers above mentioned [remittent and intermittent], the word would not be in use; and that the only idea we can at present with propriety connect with it, is that of a certain something, an agent in the atmosphere, the cause of these fevers.[239]

The Devastation of the Peloponnese

Although the evidence from the Greek War of Independence is scant and eclipsed by more violent events, the fact that Greek fighting men suffered from fever is evident from the fact that government officials in Tripolitsa (Tripoli) ordered cinchona powder from contacts in Zakynthos in October and November 1822, whereas others, like Georgios Koundouriotis, the statesman from Ydra in 1827, ordered their quinine from the port city of Ermoupolis.[240]

After more than seven years of warfare, the Peloponnese lay in ruins. When the third brigade of General Nicolas Joseph Maison's French army entered the city of Patras in late October 1828, leaving behind the heavily malarious swamps of their camp at Gialova,[241] north of Navarino (Pylos), they witnessed the appalling effects of protracted warfare on the most prosperous city of the Peloponnese. Until early October, when the first French military units took over the city, Patras had been in the hands of Ibrahim

---

239 Davy, *Notes and Observations*, vol. 2, 241.

240 *Tomos ogdoos*, 58, 63–64 and 204–5; Leivadaras, "To proto nosokomeio," 30.

241 Bory de Saint-Vincent wrote of that camp: "this camp of misfortune, where, a few months ago, so many French soldiers died victim of a bad choice of location, for which no one since then wishes to admit having had the disastrous idea." Bory de Saint-Vincent, *Relation*, vol. 1, 221.

Pasha's Egyptian Army, which then capitulated to the French, except for a small contingent of local ağas, who held out against the French at Rio castle, or Château de la Morée; thus, the newly arrived units from the Gialova camp were ordered to besiege the fortress. However, beyond its military purpose, thanks to the scientific interest of the French physicians who took part in the Expedition, the French military presence in the Morea became an opportunity for French medicine to study the local medical geography. Upon their return home, a number of these physicians went on to produce doctoral theses, books and scientific articles on fevers, cholera and the plague.[242]

Guillaume Gaspard Roux, the chief medical officer of the campaign, attributed the state of health in the city of Patras both to the state of a place itself that was rife with putrid matter and to fevers imported from other locations. According to his account, all that was left of the city were a few dilapidated houses and abandoned huts, extreme filth, and stench: everywhere lay rotting organic matter, decomposing animal carcasses, and moldy rags that "harbored harmful miasmas or exhumed evil smells, soon to become the source of miasmatic poisoning." The French soldiers began by clearing up the desolation. For Roux, the worst sources of miasmatic emanations were, on the one hand, the numerous cemeteries within the urban confines, which, presumably, contained some recent hasty and shallow burials, and on the other, in the extensive treeless land surrounding the city.[243] As the number of sick French soldiers peaked, and mortality increased, between the end of October and the first fortnight of November, the city's mosques served as makeshift hospitals. By the end of November 1828, 312 soldiers had been admitted with mostly intermittent, quite often pernicious, fevers,[244] while seventy-seven patients died in hospital in the first fortnight of November, some while in a coma on the day they were admitted or on the following day.[245] In Patras, patients with fevers outnumbered the wounded, in terms of hospital sick days, by twenty-five to one, in October and by twenty-seven to one in November.[246] While some of these men had transmitted their infection from the marshes of the Gialova camp, others, presumably those who fell ill ten days or so after their arrival in the city, had been exposed to the

---

242 Stavropoulos, "I nosologia tis Messinias," 6–7.
243 Roux, *Histoire*, 57n1.
244 Ibid., 40.
245 Ibid., 44 and 66.
246 Ibid., 166–68.

hardships of the siege of the fort of Rio, which eventually fell to the French on 30 October.[247] Regrettably, noted one of the French physicians, although on the basis of his experience in Spain and Corsica he was convinced of the efficacy of quinine in treating endemic intermittent and remittent fevers, the French Army had only enough for the officers.[248]

In Modon (Methoni), Bory de Saint-Vincent also encountered similar sites of wartime destruction that contributed to malaria prevalence in the area, where he also found signs of abandoned settlements. At the center of a marsh, around the few surviving masonry supports of an ancient aqueduct, were mounds of soil containing the remnants of an old brick kiln that would have served the local communities in better times. The unhealthy site had in the past been populated by hamlets that had all but disappeared, plundered for ready building material for the Ottoman-Egyptian camp, thus leaving behind little else than rubble. The old olive groves had also disappeared; even the tree roots had been unearthed "to help heat the Barbarians."[249] Oval traces of their barracks where grass failed to grow, were still visible in the marshlands of southwestern Peloponnese for two or three years after their departure.[250]

Livestock had also suffered the effects of war. In fact, certain areas like the extensive swamps of the River Pamisos,[251] where mud dried up completely in the summer to become "as hard as iron," was suitable only for grazing. In the past, Bory de Saint-Vincent noted, the locals had used buffaloes to work the land, but "these animals completely disappeared during the last war."[252] It is therefore quite likely that, by losing their livestock, the locals also lost whatever protection these animals could offer against mosquito bites and malarial infection.

---

247 The capitulation of the fort of Rio to the French army signaled the evacuation of the last Turks and Egyptians from the Morea by 5 November 1828.

248 Roux, *Histoire*, 65–66.

249 Bory de Saint-Vincent, *Relation*, vol. 1, 192–93. The author mentions the hamlets of Osphino, Metaxidi, "Dia-ta-Bathani," "Theiflik," "Keupritchu-kévi," and Agatchau (Agajíki/Agantzíki, now Foiniki).

250 Ibid., vol. 1, 224. The need for local medical facilities must have been such that, as the evidence suggests, the French established a military as well as a marine hospital in the area overlooking the camp site of Gialova and a convalescence unit half way between Navarino and Methoni. I wish to thank Professor Jack L. Davis for pointing out his article "Prosper Baccuet and the French Expédition Scientifique de Morée," which elucidates the topography of these units.

251 The swamp extended over a distance of more than a league (about 5 km), and during the rainy season completely blocked the road connecting the towns Nisi (Messini) and Kalamata.

252 Bory de Saint-Vincent, *Relation*, vol. 2, 63.

Roux blamed the miasmas of Patras on the urban filth and the surrounding swamps.[253] However, he was unable to reconcile inhaling miasmatic particles in the atmosphere by the respiratory tract on the one hand, with his observations that these miasmas were in fact affecting the digestive tract or the nervous system.[254] Clearly, the French soldiers, nonimmune to the local strains because they had previously served mostly in the south of France and Spain, had visited some of the potentially most harmful locations at the peak of the *falciparum* season: they had landed on 31 August 1828 by the mouth "of a small river named Caracasilli," north of Petalidi,[255] camped at Gialova in September, and carried out the siege of Rio for the greater part of October.

With the Peloponnese free of Ottoman and Egyptian forces by November 1828, the French reduced their military activity. Raymond Faure, another French Army physician, remained in Greece for a total of two years, treated a few local patients besides French soldiers, toured a large part of the countryside and witnessed the country's sanitary situation after the effective end of hostilities.[256] In a two-volume medical textbook on intermittent fevers published upon his return to France, he contended that marshes were not the only source of intermittent fevers.

Drawing from his experience in the interior of the Peloponnese, he argued that extreme heat was at least as responsible as marshes.[257] Besides the locations of the French camps in Navarino, Koroni, and Methoni, to which the Patras contingent had returned by July 1829, arid places, such as Mani and the Megalopoli plain,[258] locations that British topographer William Martin Leake had visited on his tour of the Morea in 1805, had also become heavily malarious in the meantime. Likewise, in postrevolutionary Mani, in the villages facing east "intermittent fevers are extremely common" with annual outbreaks "since time immemorial," despite the arid nature of the land-

---

253 Roux, *Histoire*, 57–60. On his visit to the fort in 1806, Leake had observed "marshes intermixed with a few plantations of currants" and unhealthy-looking inhabitants. Leake, Travels in the Morea, vol. 2, 149.

254 Roux, *Histoire*, 58n1.

255 Ibid., 2–3.

256 Faure, *Des fièvres intermittentes et continues*, vol. 1, 129. Some ninety years later, his colleague on the Macedonian Front of the First World War remembered the French losses to malaria in the 1828 campaign. Armand-Delille et al., *Le paludisme macédonien*, v.

257 He also blamed other excesses such as drinking and overindulgence at the cabarets of Navarino. Faure, *Des fièvres intermittentes et continues*, vol. 1, 63.

258 Ibid., vol. 1, 64.

scape, whereas at a few miles distance the villages facing west were healthy in that respect.[259] Reflecting the prewar situation, by contrast, Leake seemed indifferent to the state of health of the Maniots; he even traveled through Elos in early April without ever mentioning fevers.[260] In his account, serious malaria trouble lay further to the west; there, marshes like those at Anaziri (present-day Eva), in the district of Androusa, were pasturelands, unsuitable for cultivation.[261]

Indeed, the French Army topographers who ventured into the interior of the Peloponnese in the summer of 1829 put their lives at serious risk. In Faure's words: "The heat was the most powerful cause of these diseases to such a degree, that the staff officers in charge of making the topography of the Morea, who wished to continue their work during this season in the arid and mountainous interior of this country, were almost struck by severe and stubborn intermittent fevers: two died of gastro-encephalitis."[262]

As for the local population, in September 1829 the residents of Siderocastro, a village on the road to Phigaleia, about 300 meters "in the mountain," told a French topographer, who found them exhausted by annual attacks of periodic fever, that they had made up their minds to abandon the place.[263] Although there is no word of disease in Leake's account of February 1805— in fact in May he painted an idyllic picture of the area of Megalopoli[264]—the medico-statistical tables of 1838 reported that the 304 inhabitants of Siderocastro were "mostly weak and pale" and that "in almost all villages of the municipality of Avlon (Avlonas) periodic fevers are endemic."[265] A century and a half later, in August 1945, the end of the war found the village still heavily malarious with a 50 percent malaria rate. Thanks to its energetic doctor, even during that war, it had become a distribution center from

259 Ibid., vol. 1, 87.

260 Leake, *Travels in the Morea*, vol. 1, 222–33.

261 Ibid., vol. 1, 359.

262 Faure, *Des fièvres intermittentes et continues*, vol. 1, 62. By "gastro-céphalites," Faure was referring to acute, often terminal symptoms of *falciparum* malaria.

263 Ibid., vol. 1, 54–55. The French phrase is *"placé à une hauteur de cent cinquantes toises dans les montagnes."* In contrast, their neighbors in the village of Cara-Mustapha (Avlonas) were free of fever. It is unclear whether the inhabitants of Siderocastro acted on their resolution. Even if they did indeed resettle their village, it became the principal town of the municipality of Avlonas in the administrative reform of Greece in 1833. Diligiannis and Zinopoulos, *Elliniki nomothesia*, vol. 2, 454.

264 Leake, *Travels in the Morea*, vol. 2, 31–32.

265 Manousos, "Idiaiteros pinax ton dimon Trifylias."

which a whole region of around 5,000 to 6,000 people in remote malarious villages received drugs from the Swiss Red Cross.[266]

From a sanitary perspective, Leake's record of Ottoman Peloponnese in the 1800s as a well-cultivated, productive land is irreconcilable with that of Faure and Roux, the two French physicians, and of Bory de Saint Vincent, although they all covered much of the same ground, unless one takes into consideration the effects of warfare and devastation and, to some extent, season, given that Leake does not record traveling in the Peloponnese beyond the month of May. Interestingly, without directly attributing the health situation specifically to the effects of the recent war, Faure implied that the high prevalence of intermittent fevers among the Greeks was related to adverse social and political factors and that, once peace returned to the country, the Peloponnese could hope to recover and restore the health of its inhabitants. "To the extent that this country will be rebuilt," he wrote, "that the villages and the density of the houses will increase; to the extent that wealth will spread among the inhabitants, it is probable that these diseases shall become a great deal less frequent, and that the Peloponnese will become once more what it once was, that is, a country favorable to health, inhabited by a numerous population, as certified by the ruins of its famous towns and the most indisputable pages of history."[267]

The Macedonian Front

For the next eighty years, the Greek lands recovered from the devastation of the War of Independence and were transformed by progress in agriculture. Thus, environmental disruption was related to peacetime activities discussed earlier in this chapter. Irregular fighting in Macedonia, however, in the early twentieth century, the Balkan Wars and, ultimately, the opening of the Southern Front of the First World War in 1915, initiated a major episode in the history of malaria in Greece that had severe implications on the malaria burden of northern Greece and the lives of the refugee colonists, particularly after 1922.

---

266 These villages were Avlonas, Silaveika, Agios Ilias, Tourkaki, Kaponista, Kaimeni Yinaika, Agaliani, Vanadha, Agios Serafim, Bouzi, and Fonissa; the doctor visited his practice by horse or mule. C. Gurney, "Report Methoni District," [?] July, 6 August 1945, Rural Reports Messinia, PAG-4/3.0.12.2.3.:11 [S-0527-0675], UN Archives.

267 Faure, *Des fièvres intermittentes et continues*, vol. 1, 65.

The early twentieth century saw an intensified presence of Greek bandits and undercover army officers as armed band leaders in western Macedonia, a region that was violently contested between Greeks and Bulgarians. The feats of these men against their Bulgarian counterparts became the subject of Penelope Delta's (1874–1941) patriotic novel *Mystika tou Valtou* (Secrets of the swamp), first published in 1937. The plot develops in the marshland surrounding Lake Giannitsa. Both sides of the conflict, particularly the nonnative men among them, suffered from marsh fevers. However, Telos Agras, Delta's fictitious undercover Greek Army officer, heroically, if unrealistically, managed to overcome the clocklike physical suffering of malaria through sheer willpower. When the Greek fighters were overcome by fever-induced exhaustion, they returned to Athens and were replaced by fresh recruits.[268] Indeed, as noted by Patrick Zylberman, cross-border banditry by destitute peasants was closely associated with the spread of malaria in the broader Macedonia region and Albania.[269]

Then the Balkan Wars (1912–13) initiated a ten-year period of wartime, during which the antimalarial work in Old Greece was abandoned.[270] Indeed, the Hygiene Service of the Greek Army ordered Kardamatis to conduct a study of malaria in the lands under its control in Macedonia but the Second Balkan War which broke out in May 1913 put an end to this project.[271] The upheaval, moreover, in northern Greece marked a watershed in the population structure of the region. As noted by Elisabeth Kontogiorgi:

> The Balkan wars, though short, set new standards for cruelty and destruction in Macedonia, a region known for its political turbulence. Specifically, the phenomenon of the uprooting of local populations had in fact occurred previously but never on such a scale as during the wars of 1912–13. Massacres were widespread and these bitter conflicts were accompanied by the movement of many thousands of refugees travelling in opposite directions, seeking safety in their respective national states.[272]

---

268 Delta, *Ta mystika tou Valtou*.

269 Zylberman, "Mosquitoes," 310.

270 Konstantinos Moutoussis's statement at Conférence de l'échange entre personnels sanitaires spécialisés dans la lutte contre le paludisme, Procès verbal provisoire de la 1ère séance tenue à Genève le jeudi 14 juin 1923, CH/EPS/PV1, p. 21, document 28980, dossier 25944, box R 849,12B (Social-Health), A (1919–27), League of Nations Archives.

271 Kardamatis, *Statistikoi pinakes*, 9.

272 Kontogiorgi, *Population Exchange*, 37. Estimates of populations fleeing from hostile territory to new

The years following the Balkan Wars exacerbated the preexisting malaria situation in the region owing to the extensive military presence of Greek and foreign armies, conflict, and population displacement, particularly in Macedonia. These activities "intensified the epidemic and occasionally pandemic outbreaks of the disease," according to Phokion Kopanaris, as large numbers of naive humans entered the habitats of susceptible *Anopheles* mosquitoes and became exposed to the risk of malaria.[273] After years of armed conflict and war, peacetime colonization, treated in earlier in this chapter, completed the burden of suffering and death.[274]

British and French military presence in Macedonia in the First World War resulted from the region's strategic importance for the allied Southern Front after the British failure in Gallipoli. Therefore, in October 1915 both the British and the French landed troops in Thessaloniki, from where they contributed toward winning the war only in the final offensive in September 1918. From the perspective, however, of malariology, the three years spent in malaria-ridden Macedonia both altered the local disease environment and shaped that field of medicine.

Military presence and actual fighting also affected the civilians in the region; some were displaced, while others simply fled. In the Prespa basin, for instance, the survey team of the French Army recorded relatively high spleen rates in villages where displaced villagers had found refuge, such as (Agios) Germanos, inhabited by Macedonian Slavs, Albanians and Gypsies, that also hosted refugees from Krani, Harvati (Arvati), and Nakolec; the village of Strkovo (Platy), that also gave shelter to evacuees from Opaja (Opagia); and the village of Dupeni, inhabited by Macedonian Slavs and Albanians, that also hosted evacuees from Krani and Nakolec. More affected by malaria, with a recorded spleen rate of 22 percent in the summer of 1917, was the Albanian village of Vineni (Pyli) at the foot of Mount Soua Gora, the site of a "concentration camp for the inhabitants of the peninsula of Soubagora [Soúa Góra]."[275]

The French team conducting the survey in the Prespa valley noted that the marsh indicated on the Austrian map had given way to fields of maize

---

homelands as a consequence of the Balkan Wars range in the tens of thousands. Kontogiorgi, *Population Exchange*, 39.

273 Kopanaris, *I dimosia ygeia en Elladi*, 202.

274 This point is made in Zylberman, "Mosquitoes," 326–27.

275 Delamare and Robin, "Carte du paludisme des confins albano-macédoniens," 490.

and watermills, whose runoff created pools of stagnant water. There were no more than some thirty poor villages "about a third of which had been evacuated or destroyed by water or fire."[276] More importantly, though, the relative centrality of the region had shifted; an otherwise inaccessible mountainous location, the Prespa basin had become a communication hub on the supply routes of the occupying French troops and therefore an important site of interest for malaria control.[277] The Jelova and Brenitsa valleys were likewise equally important for the French Army for comprising heavily used, poorly drained roads leading to Florina, Biklista (Bilisht), and Kastoria along the river.

Evacuation and displacement also affected mountain villages, previously untouched by malaria. In the Koritza (Korçë) region, the children of Selenitza (Selenicë) were found to have enlarged spleens. The locals explained to the French Army team that during the first years of the war the villagers had emigrated to Valona (Vlorë) on the Adriatic coast, where they had, presumably, been exposed to malaria, and returned two years later.[278]

Malaria in Macedonia during the First World War is far better documented than any previous war in the area. Despite the fact that British and French military presence intensified the malaria burden in the region, the medical teams of the French Armée d'Orient and the British Salonika Army of the First World War were the first to study the malaria situation in Macedonia systematically, albeit in a different paradigm than their predecessors in the Peloponnese in the late 1820s. Besides conducting geographical surveys, each army set up research teams and laboratories to study local entomological and epidemiological facts. When it came to medical research output, the physicians of the Royal Army Medical Corps (RAMC) in Thessaloniki published their conflicting medical opinions in the *British Medical Journal*.[279] The Macedonian Front became a site where the medical battle between the advocates of quinine prophylaxis, on the one hand, and the proponents of the ideas of Ronald Ross and *Anopheles* control, on the other, was played out, with the latter eventually gaining the upper hand.[280]

---

276 Ibid., 489.
277 Ibid. The same also applied to the valley of Kolomnati. Invaded by French troops in September 1916, it had since become an army supply center. Ibid., 500.
278 Blanc and Heckenroth, "Répartition du paludisme," 477–78.
279 Fantini, "Malaria and the First World War," 246–49; Harrison, *The Medical War*, 237.
280 Ibid., 231.

As part of their landing operations in Thessaloniki in October 1915, and in anticipation of the malaria season of the following year, the French and British called on the expertise of Alphonse Laveran and Ronald Ross respectively, both legendary figures in tropical medicine.[281] Both the British and the French, moreover, established laboratories and mechanisms for medical observation and surveillance as part of their local military apparatus, collaborated with the Greek medical authorities in Thessaloniki, set up the International Hygiene Committee (IHC) with the regular participation of the Greeks and the occasional presence of Italian, Serbian, and Russian representatives, and, in 1917, a special Antimalarial Commission.[282] Throughout the war years, the IHC met in Thessaloniki every Monday to exchange medical intelligence and agree on common procedures. According to the French physician Raphaël Blanchard, the British troops suffered less than the French because, from the start, they had "rightly considered the Macedonian campaign as a colonial war, as a *medical war*, according to their own picturesque as well as exact expression."[283]

The French had a laboratory in place from the beginning of their operations in Macedonia with Major Paul-Félix Armand-Delille at its head.[284] In December 1916, the Pasteur Institute in Paris sent out brothers Edmond and Etienne Sergent of the Pasteur Institute in Algeria on a mission to conduct an "in-depth study" of malaria on the Macedonian Front for the protection of the French Army. The two brothers recommended creating a specific service to carry out the antimalarial measures they were proposing. Accordingly, a French special antimalarial mission was sent over to Thessaloniki in March 1917 and operated under the French Army's health services directorate. The antimalarial mission was headed by chief army physician Fernand Visbecq, who had a long experience in Indochina. They also set up a laboratory at the camp of Zeitenlik, directed by biologist Pierre Abrami.[285] In ef-

281 Ronald Ross, British Consultant in Malaria, was kept informed on the malaria situation in Thessaloniki in 1916 and 1917 and contributed his expertise. Ronald Ross, London, to Assistant Director General (ADG), Army Medical Department (AMD2), 20 October 1917, WO 32/5112; "Travaux et résultats," 456.

282 Niclot, "Le paludisme," 766. The French antimalarial mission in Thessaloniki created a permanent inter-Allied Antimalarial Commission which also held weekly meetings presided over by Fernand Visbecq.

283 Blanchard, "Le danger," 661, quoted in Fantini, "Malaria and the First World War," 250.

284 Salonika, 21 December 1915, War Diary of the Director of Medical Services (DMS), Salonika Army, Salonika, 1–31 December 1915 (vol. 2), WO 95/4770. Armand-Delille, *Malaria in Macedonia*, 6, fig. 3; Niclot, "Le paludisme," 756.

285 "Travaux et résultats," 456–60; Fantini, "Malaria and the First World War," 244.

fect, the allied effort to protect the troops on the Macedonian front from malaria brought about an "international network of information-exchange" among scientists with colonial and laboratory experience.[286] Furthermore, the doctors of the Armée d'Orient shared their research data and results at the weekly meetings of the Salonika Medical Society, the international, collaborative scientific space they had created for themselves.[287]

In his account of the mission's preparation, René Legroux of the Pasteur Institute, who had been responsible for organizing the mission, noted that

> the measures that the mission put in place aim at anopheline prophylaxis and quinine prophylaxis. With these two concepts in mind, the campaign plans of the Pasteur Institute of Algeria, those of Ronald Ross and those established by the Americans in Panama were profitably consulted: no measure that had given a good result, however minimal, was neglected by the mission of the Armée d'Orient. The mission held foremost the use of mosquito nets and the daily preventive administration of quinine."[288]

The preference for quininization reflected a French and Italian national bias that differed from that of the British, who were divided among the proponents of quinine prophylaxis following J. W. W. Stephens and S. R. Christophers, and those who favored antilarval measures, following the opinion of Ronald Ross. However, both the French and the Italians soon modified their positions in favor of a more selective approach that also included antilarval work, mosquito nets, and winter treatment of cases.[289]

British malaria research in Macedonia began with ad hoc missions sent out by the War Office to investigate the effect of local malaria on the troops. Apart from two visits by Ronald Ross, one in November 1915 and one in 1917, such missions included the Anti-malaria Mission, the Malaria Commission, and the Malaria Enquiry Unit. On 5 August 1918 the War Office created a fully-fledged Malaria Enquiry Laboratory in Thessaloniki with C. M. Wenyon, a lieutenant colonel in the Royal Army Medical Corps connected with the Wellcome Bureau of Scientific Research, as its officer-in-command. The laboratory, which consisted of a chemical, an entomological, a hematological,

---

286 Mikanowski, "Dr Hirszfeld's War," 111–12.
287 Ibid., 111.
288 Legroux, "Présentation," 422.
289 Fantini, "Malaria and the First World War," 265; Harrison, *The Medical War*, 229 and 238.

and a pathological unit, was additionally given 400 beds in the 52nd General Hospital at Kalamaria for research purposes.[290] In their evaluation of the antimalarial work carried out in Macedonia, Wenyon, and his colleagues conceded that, despite all the "expenditure of energy," this work may not have contributed any "appreciable reduction in infections"; they had, however, improved "our knowledge of aetiology of disease, its prevention and treatment."[291]

The new scientific approach brought the British and the French medical researchers and services into contact with the indigenous population and the newly established Greek Public Health Service of Macedonia, both in combating malaria and in collecting data from 1915 to 1920.[292] Phokion Kopanaris, the head of the Greek service, believed, for his part, that contact with the foreign medical missions changed the way the Greek medical authorities dealt with malaria as a public health issue among the refugees. Thanks to foreign military influence, a humanitarian problem acquired, for Kopanaris, an additional, broader social meaning. According to him: "without the presence of the allied armies in Macedonia, which, particularly, by employing many thousand refugees as laborers in various public works and by encouraging overall development, largely rescued the refugees from famine and misery, the refugee problem would have simply come to a pitiful end already by 1915 and 1916."[293]

Already in November 1915, Surgeon General W. G. Macpherson, the director of medical services of the British Army in Thessaloniki, a Canadian who had gained experience with vector control in Cuba, the Panama Canal, India and Palestine,[294] noted: "This place will be unhealthy in summer, and more so with tents. Mosquitoes will abound. Sir Ronald Ross, who was here, reported that we need have no fear of malaria for the next 5 months (April) and should take precautions in February."[295] Anticipating the threat of malaria, Ronald Ross, then a consulting physician in malaria, visited Thessaloniki on his return to Britain from Alexandria, and reported that he believed

---

290 C. M. Wenyon, [Thessaloniki], 21 September 1918, to March 1919, Medical Malaria Enquiry Laboratory, 5 August to 31 August 1918, Malaria Enquiry Laboratory, August 1918–March 1919, British Forces. Salonika Army Troops, Vol. 1 BSF War Diary, WO 95/4807 (War Office diaries). For more on the research carried out at the lab, see Wenyon et al., *Malaria in Macedonia*.

291 Ibid., 1.

292 Kopanaris, *I dimosia ygeia en Elladi*, 202n.

293 Ibid., 45.

294 Mikanowski, "Dr Hirszfeld's War," 110.

295 DMS, Salonika, 30 November 1915, Vol. 1, Salonika Field Force War Diary 27 November 1915 to 30 November 1915, folder "Salonika. Director Medical Services," November–December 1915, WO 95/4770.

malaria "would become prevalent in June and July, 1916, and still more prevalent in 1917." Macpherson had formulated an antimalarial plan in January 1916, which also drew on information provided by the local Greek health authorities.[296] Indeed the IHC heard from a Greek military physician that the Greek Army began distributing quinine daily to its men starting in June, a decision adopted by the British in keeping with Ross's recommendations; they were satisfied that treating the Greek refugees in the adjacent Lembet (present-day suburb of Stavroupoli in Thessaloniki) barracks would provide British troops with adequate protection.[297] The French troops, for their part, may have begun receiving prophylactic doses of quinine already in January, quininization of the entire French force began on 1 March, but "prophylactic measures, as should be applied against malaria, failed to be executed." The Mission antipaludique sent to Macedonia a year later attributed this failure to the disruption that followed the collapse of the Serbian Front in November 1915 and the need of the Serbs to also set up camp in Thessaloniki.[298]

In the same spirit, after Ross's first visit to Thessaloniki at the start of the campaign, in November 1915,[299] the Medical Advisory Committee that arrived in Thessaloniki in May 1916—consisting of Lt. Colonel Andrew Balfour of the Royal Army Medical Corps, the renowned physician who had founded the Wellcome Bureau of Scientific Research in 1913, Colonel William Hunter and Lt. Colonel George Buchanan—made similar recommendations. The committee spent four weeks in Macedonia and conducted a malaria and entomological survey of the areas occupied by the British troops.[300]

---

296 H. R. Whitehead, Report on the incidence of malaria in the Salonika Army in 1916; on the measures taken for its prevention; on the measures proposed for its prevention during 1917, Salonika, 20 November 1916, pp. 7–8, WO32/5112; Ross, *Memoirs*, 518–19.

297 IHC proceedings, 27 March 1916, Appendix 355, DMS Salonika M.E.F. (Surgeon General W. G. Macpherson CB KCMG) January–August 1916, Phase "B," Vol. War Diary of DMS, Salonika Army. 1–31 March 1916, WO 95/4770.

298 IHC proceedings, 20 March 1916, Appendix 351A, DMS Salonika M.E.F. (Surgeon General W. G. Macpherson CB KCMG) January–August 1916, Phase "B," Vol. War Diary of DMS, Salonika Army 1–31 March 1916, WO 95/4770; Summary page Phase "B" [page] 31 prior to operations of autumn of 1916, 7 February 1916, DMS Salonika M.E.F. (Surgeon General W. G. Macpherson CB KCMG) January–August 1916, Phase "B," Vol. War Diary of DMS, Salonika Army 1 to 29 February 1916, WO 95/4770; IHC proceedings, 22 May 1916, Appendix 403, Vol. War Diary of DMS Salonika Army 1–31 May 1916, WO 95/4771; "Travaux et résultats," 456–57.

299 See p. 225 in this book.

300 11 May 1916, Vol. War Diary of DMS, Salonika Army, 1–31 May 1916, WO 95/4771; 15 May 1916, Vol. War Diary of DMS, Salonika Army, 1–31 May 1916, WO 95/4771; 20 May 1916, Vol. War Diary of DMS, Salonika Army, 1–31 May 1916, WO 95/4771 and Appendix 400, cable to War Office from DMS, [Whitehead], Salonika, 26 May 1916, Vol. War Diary of DMS, Salonika Army, 1–31 May 1916, WO 95/4771.

The British records of military movements are informative concerning the spread of the disease. Until the summer of 1916, the British troops had been deployed on the hills south of Lake Langaza (Langadas) and Lake Besik (Volvi), on the hills toward Kilkis and to the west of Thessaloniki along the road leading north toward Monastir (Bitola). At the end of June, when, for strategic reasons the army advanced to low-lying grounds, malaria shot up to reach an "appalling magnitude." The disease then spread with the advance of previously infected men.[301]

Surveys and sanitization works continued throughout the war. Even before the outbreak of the June 1916 epidemic, there had been surveys, spleen indices of the local population in the Langadas valley, and drainage works, particularly along the road leading from Thessaloniki to Monastir. As the war effort progressed, however, it became clear that some of the locations presented incredible difficulties and the work to be done was so extensive that, in Wenyon's words, "an arbitrary limit had to be fixed to any work here, so that the good results which might have been expected were spoilt by the vast extent of breeding ground immediately beyond."[302]

The work involved the marshy, waterlogged shores of Lake Besik, which had an expanse of 40 square kilometers; it lay in the front line and therefore could not be treated. Lake Langadas was smaller; along it ran the main road that crossed through the army camps. The shore was full of tall rushes and other vegetation. "Nothing short of a large and costly scheme could render this marsh free from the mosquitoes which abound there," wrote W. G. Willoughby, adding his fear "that the magnitude of the work, the expense and the difficulty of getting labor are prohibitive as regards this swamp." To reduce the larva population to some extent, Willoughby recommended oiling the lake surface and cutting down some of the vegetation and channeling, filling and draining pools. Oiling alone, however, required repeating the work three times a week and would pollute water otherwise used for animals, bathing and washing. Pools at a lower level than adjacent streams should be filled with sand and earth and raised to a higher level that would prevent the sinking of animal hooves, where larvae could live in very wet sand or mud, he warned.[303] For Wenyon, though, a slight reduction in the

---

301 See p. 228 in this book.
302 Wenyon, "Malaria in Macedonia," 12.
303 Willoughby and Cassidy, *Anti-Malaria Work*, 41–45.

number of mosquitoes meant nothing. "It would thus appear that the clearing measures undertaken in the long line of swamp regions in the valleys can have done very little to reduce the number of mosquitoes and practically nothing to lessen the incidence of infection."[304]

The French, who occupied the territory west of Thessaloniki, also suffered as their operations were rolled out. In order to protect their own troops, they sent out research teams to explore even the remotest areas of Epirus and Macedonia. As one French medical team reported, expanding their data collection area was dictated by constantly shifting military expediency.

> From a practical point of view, this habit is somehow imposed by the conditions of military life on the campaign: one village that in May does not have a garrison, may have an important one in July; territories that seem too remote from the occupation zone to be at risk of being dangerous are, in fact, visited frequently by supply parties, surveillance patrols, etc. Finally, it would be foolish to believe that the soldiers don't stop in houses other than at official stopping points; small detachments camp mostly to suit their fancy, large units wherever they can. During major troop movements, there is not a point, even among the most unhealthy places along a line of stopping points, that does not have passing guests for one or two nights.[305]

As noted above, a true epidemic broke out for the British following the movement of their troops from the healthier hills into the low-lying valley of the Strymon River at the end of June 1916. The situation worsened in July.[306] Cases more than doubled in the second week of July 1916, from 332 cases on 8 July to 686 on 15 July with a similar leap to 1,127 cases at the end of the following week (22 July) and 2,264 hospital admissions by the end of the last week (29 July).[307] This epidemic of "appalling magnitude," according to We-

---

304 Wenyon, "Malaria in Macedonia," 12–14.

305 Delamare and Robin, "Carte du paludisme des confins albano-macédoniens," 485–86.

306 Wenyon, "Malaria in Macedonia," 27. The French, who mostly occupied hilly grounds to the west of the British, complained of a notable increase of malaria among their ranks. According to M. Niclot, who considered the year 1916 one of normal malaria incidence, primary cases developed from 8, 4, 7 cases each ten days in May to 7, 10, 150 cases in June, 357, 837, and 1,191 cases in July and 1,021 cases in August. See Niclot, "Le paludisme," 759–60.

307 International Hygiene Committee (IHC) proceedings, 10 July 1916, Appendix 442, Vol. War Diary of DMS, Salonika Army, 1–31 July 1916, WO 95/4771; IHC proceedings, 17 July 1916, Appendix 444, Vol. War Diary of DMS, Salonika Army, 1–31 July 1916, WO 95/4771; IHC proceedings, 24 July 1916, Appendix 450, Vol. War Diary of DMS, Salonika Army, 1–31 July 1916, WO 95/4771 and IHC 31 July 1916, Appendix 456, Vol. War Diary of DMS, Salonika Army, 1–31 August 1916, WO 95/4771.

nyon, even spread to the hospital area of the high Khortiatis plateau east of Thessaloniki.[308] H. R. Whitehead, the principal medical officer of the British forces at Thessaloniki, requested help from the Medical Advisory Committee. Andrew Balfour and William Hunter, who had already been in Thessaloniki in May, were once more sent by the Committee from Egypt.[309]

The malaria outbreak of late June 1916 and the extensive requirements for prophylactic use for refugees and locals depleted the British stock of quinine. By the end of July, the British were ordering a monthly consignment of 3,000 lbs, triple the original estimate.[310] By mid-August, they had run out of quinine bichloride for injections and were purchasing it on the local market at a higher cost, presumably exacerbating local shortages and fueling price increases.[311] The French also used quinine heavily; by 12 August they had received and mostly distributed 13 tons of pills, almost a ton of other forms, and were expecting more at a cost of approximately 130 francs per kilogram.[312] Indeed, in the first year in Macedonia, M. Niclot, the French chief medical officer, believed that by following the work of Celli in Italy, M. Léger in Corsica, and the Sergent brothers in Algeria, they could "eradicate" malaria with quinine.[313]

Quinine arrived with difficulty. The shortage was felt again in 1917, heightened by the unrestricted submarine warfare at sea. Until he had sufficient amounts, Whitehead had to delay the distribution of quinine to the troops until after the end of May, with the exception of "the personnel and prisoners of war at Arakli [Irakleio] potato farm." Meanwhile, quinine was being shipped from wherever it could be found: from India, some of it was gleaned from the Italians, some from Malta, and elsewhere.[314] The shortage of quinine also affected the Germans; the British blockade cut them off from shipments from Java.[315]

---

308 Wenyon, "Malaria in Macedonia," 5–6.

309 Entry 22 July 1916, Vol. War Diary of DMS, Salonika Army, 1–31 July 1916, WO 95/4771 and entry 23 July 1916, Vol. War Diary of DMS, Salonika Army, 1–31 July 1916, WO 95/4771. For the last days in June (25 June to 1 July) the British reported 171 cases and the French (21 to 30 June) 160 primary and 117 secondary cases. IHC proceedings, 3 July 1916, Appendix 435, Vol. War Diary of DMS, Salonika Army, 1–31 July 1916, WO 95/4771.

310 Entry 30 July 1916, Vol. War Diary of DMS, Salonika Army, 1–31 July 1916, WO 95/4771.

311 Entry 14 August 1916, Vol. War Diary of DMS, Salonika Army, 1–31 August 1916, WO 95/4771.

312 Niclot, "Le paludisme," 771.

313 Ibid., 766.

314 H. R. Whitehead, DMS, [secret report], Salonika, 30 May 1917, WO 95 and entry 20 May 1917, Vol. War Diary of DMS, Salonika Army, 1–31 May 1917, WO 95/4774.

315 Migliani et al., "Histoire," 358.

The malaria season of 1917 was longer than expected, and by October the British authorities were alarmed, particularly about what this might mean for the following year.[316] They decided to carry out an extensive program of winter quininization to sanitize the chronic and relapsing malaria cases among their troops and increased the monthly consignment of quinine from 3,000 to 4,000 lbs of powder.[317] Once again the War Office called on the expertise of Ronald Ross, who visited Thessaloniki, via Itea in Central Greece, on a confidential mission. He landed in the city on 14 December 1917, with Captain F. W. O'Connor of the Royal Army Medical Corps.[318]

Ross's mission was to set up the so-called Y scheme to select and repatriate men who were too debilitated by malaria to serve the following summer. The plan was to remain secret in order to conceal the severe health conditions of the British troops in Macedonia from the British public.[319] Repatriation was a measure the French had been applying since 1916, although they also had more hospital admissions for malaria in 1917 than in 1916.[320] Keeping sick men in the force had indeed proved to place the rest of the force at risk. Thus, although in 1916 the British sent their worst cases to Britain or Malta,[321] unrestricted submarine warfare in 1917 prevented them from doing so, a fact that both inflated admissions figures but also the real risk of infections.[322] The army was becoming "saturated with malaria."[323] Ross, with O'Connor, completed their mission and left Thessaloniki for Itea on 6 January 1918, and discussed malaria prevention with Wenyon en route.[324] More than 25,000 men were repatriated from Thessaloniki via the newly opened overland route to Itea and from there to the Italian port of Taranto. Wenyon estimated that these evacu-

---

316 Summary Phase C and D, October 1917, p. 62, 14 October 1917, Vol. War Diary of DMS, Salonika Army, 1–31 October 1917, WO 95/4775.

317 Entry 7 December 1917, Vol. War Diary of DMS, Salonika Army, 1–31 December 1917, WO 95/4775.

318 Entry 20 December 1917, Vol. War Diary of DMS, Salonika Army, 1–31 December 1917, WO 95/4775 and entry 21 December 1917, Vol. War Diary of DMS, Salonika Army, 1–31 December 1917, WO 95/4775.

319 Appendix 750, 26 December 1917, Vol. War Diary of DMS, Salonika Army, 1–31 December 1917, WO 95/4775. Harrison, The Medical War, 233–34.

320 Wenyon, "Malaria in Macedonia," 27–28. The French replenished their ranks with troops from Senegal and labor battalions from Annam, a French protectorate encompassing the central region of Vietnam, thus enriching the local Plasmodia pool with foreign strains. Fantini, "Malaria and the First World War," 258. A similar practice used by the British—who employed Indian, Chinese, Egyptian, and South African labor units on the Western Front—introduced the threat of typhoid and smallpox among the allied troops. See Harrison, The Medical War, 139–40.

321 Wenyon, "Malaria in Macedonia," 7.

322 Ibid., 9–10.

323 Ibid., 10–11.

324 Appendix 766, 6 January 1918, Vol. War Diary of DMS, Salonika Army, 1–31 January 1918, WO 95/4776.

ees would otherwise have contributed an additional 50,000 to 60,000 hospital cases of malaria in the summer months of 1918.[325]

In the first year of the British military presence in Macedonia, from January to 11 November 1916, 29,594 men, or 23.6 percent of the force, were admitted to hospital mostly with malaria, but also with dysentery, typhoid, and paratyphoid. The troops suffered an estimated mortality from malaria of only 0.89 percent, thanks to extensive therapeutic use of quinine.[326] For most of the season, they suffered preponderantly from *vivax* malaria, with *falciparum* malaria prevailing in October and November.[327] The approximate figures for 1917 and 1918, published by Wenyon in 1921 on the basis of some 40,000 positive blood film examinations in the army labs, revealed the relative significance of the monthly infections with *vivax* and *falciparum* malaria.[328] By 1918, the average annual hospital admission rate for malaria corresponded to 300 percent of the British force or an average of three annual admissions per man.[329]

Local Labor, Refugees, and Foreigners

The foreign army physicians mostly feared the local population, whom they suspected of carrying endemic malaria. Regarding the malaria sit-

---

325 Wenyon, "Malaria in Macedonia," 10–11.

326 Estimates of malaria incidence vary, particularly for 1916. Indeed, not only diagnoses would fail to differentiate between malaria and typhoid fever, but, as Shanks and White have suggested in a recent article based on the medical literature on the British Salonika Force, typhoid and paratyphoid C most likely triggered *vivax* relapses, and may therefore have often been causally linked with *vivax* malaria cases. See Shanks and White, "The Activation of Vivax Malaria Hypnozoites." Furthermore, figures for case mortality in 1916 vary accordingly. Improved diagnostics in subsequent years resulted in more accurate figures. Thus, Wenyon, who attributed the higher rates for 1916 to greater hardship and unpreparedness, provides the following case mortality figures:

1916	1.01%
1917	0.37%
1918	0.31%

See Wenyon, "Malaria in Macedonia," 51.

327 H. R. Whitehead, Report on the incidence of malaria in the Salonika Army in 1916; on the measures taken for its prevention; on the measures proposed for its prevention during 1917, Salonika, 20 November 1916, pp. 1–3, 8, appendix III, WO32/5112. In September 1917, the newly created 28 Mobile Laboratory reported the August results for its area of responsibility, No. 3 Area Base Line of Communications: 216 negative, 189 malaria (benign tertian 56, malignant tertian 75, unclassified 58), that is, a slight preponderance of *falciparum* malaria. No. 28 Mobile Bact. Lab, 17 September 1917, 28 Mobile Laboratory, May–December 1917, Vol. 1, Salonika Army Troops, WO 95/4807 (War Office diaries).

328 Wenyon, "Malaria in Macedonia," 47.

329 Harrison, *The Medical War*, 233.

uation in rural Macedonia, the British relied largely on information provided by Phokion Kopanaris.[330] Presumably, however, owing to differences in susceptibility between the local population and nonimmune foreigners, such information could be misleading. For instance, when asked at the IHC meeting of 19 June 1916 about the frequency of malaria in the Strymon valley, where the British had encountered an abundance of mosquitoes, Kopanaris replied that malaria "is observed there but without any particular frequency."[331] Yet, on 9 July 1916, the British soldiers in that valley had still not received orders for compulsory use of quinine and were already being exhausted by *vivax* malaria.[332]

Kopanaris represented the Greek authorities at the regular meetings of the IHC in Thessaloniki. He provided sanitary intelligence to his foreign colleagues[333] and made sure locals and refugees drew on allied supplies of quinine, Greek supplies being, as he said, "extremely limited" and totally inadequate for a refugee population that was dying from the disease.[334]

Upon arrival in Salonika in October 1915, the British and French Army physicians found that their camps were located next to a Greek refugee camp at Zeitenlik, "a small town of some 3,000 souls, highly malarious, a dangerous reservoir," from where the troops were soon infected. When the Zeitenlik camp opened up for the settlement of refugees, the first to settle there were the Greeks who fled the Bulgarian-controlled zone in 1912, followed by Greeks from Western Thrace after the Treaty of Bucharest, which allocated that region to Bulgaria. They were joined by Greeks expelled in 1914 from Asia Minor and Eastern Thrace in a wartime measure of the Ottoman Empire. Greek refugees from the Caucasus were also added to the camp population. The Zeitenlik refugees made up a fraction of the 150,000-strong ref-

---

330 In December 1916, a Major Portokalis, a representative of the Greek Venizelist pro-Entente militia, the National Defense, also joined the International Hygiene Committee and reported on the state of health of its men. IHC proceedings, 24 December 1916, appendix 529, 18 December 1916, Vol. War Diary of DMS, Salonika Army, 1–31 December 1916, WO 95/4772 and IHC proceedings, 25 December 1916, Appendix 530, Vol. War Diary of DMS, Salonika Army, 1–31 December 1916, WO 95/4772.

331 IHC proceedings, 19 June 1916, Appendix 427, Vol. War Diary of DMS, Salonika Army, 1–30 June 1916, WO 95/4771.

332 Entry 9 July 1916, Vol. War Diary of DMS, Salonika Army, 1–31 July 1916, WO 95/4771.

333 Among the pieces of information was a map of Macedonia depicting villages badly, slightly, and not infected with malaria. Kopanaris told his colleagues, however, that practically all villages were infected to some degree. IHC proceedings, 7 February 1916, DMS Salonika M.E.F. (Surgeon General W. G. Macpherson CB KCMG) January–August 1916, Phase "B," Vol. War Diary of DMS, Salonika Army, 1–29 February 1916, WO 95/4770.

334 IHC proceedings, 17 January 1916, Vol. 1–31 January 1916, WO 95/4770.

ugee population that the Greek Refugee Commission was looking after in the city.[335] The large number of malaria deaths in the camp was due to the Greek shortage of quinine.[336] According to the Greek doctors treating the refugees, malaria had in previous years appeared there as early as April or "even in March."[337]

Early January 1916, the IHC asked Kopanaris to jointly inspect the Lembet refugee camp, a place of indescribable filth on either side of the road to Serres.[338] The French health authorities saw in the Greek refugees from Asia Minor a "dangerous reservoir" of severe malaria, assigned one of their doctors to survey these refugees together with the Greek medical authorities. They intended to do the same in the survey of the neighboring villages. The French also undertook to conduct a medical survey of the Serb refugee population.[339]

In March 1916, in the Lembet camp Major Mauban, the French physician, interviewed several and registered some 3,000 Greek refugees living in a hundred huts, 91.5 percent of whom had contracted malaria, mostly during the previous summer in the camp itself. Since most of the adult males were working for the allies and the women were reluctant to present themselves for physical examination, Mauban examined some 300 children and youths and found a large number of enlarged spleens and *P. falciparum* in their blood samples. The Greek physician on the allied medical team examined some 190 refugees, almost all had enlarged spleens. 110 were found with *P. falciparum* in their blood, while the others were negative. The prevalence of untreated *falciparum* malaria already in March formed a reservoir of the disease for the new malaria season. For Mauban, "this clear observation makes one fear the next infection of *Anopheles*, which have already begun to appear in the allied camps." He was referring to the adjacent Greek barracks and the entrance to the British camp. Quinization of all 3,000 refugees was considered urgent as "a work of charity and a measure of prudence for our

---

335 Kontogiorgi, *Population Exchange*, 39; Niclot, "Le paludisme," 767–68. For a topography of the refugee and military camps in Thessaloniki, see Savvaidis, "Thessalonki"; Kourti, "Oi prosfygikoi synoikismoi tis 'dytikis pleyras.'"

336 IHC proceedings, 7 January 1916, Vol. 1–31 January 1916, WO 95/4770.

337 Niclot, "Le paludisme," 760 and 767–68.

338 IHC proceedings, 6 March 1916, p. 3, Vol. 1–31 January 1916, 10 January 1916, WO 95/4770. Also Vol. 1–31 March 1916, WO 95/4771.

339 Commission d'Hygiène de l'Armée d'Orient. Lutte contre le paludisme, War Diary of DMS, Salonika Army, 1–31 January 1916, WO 95/4770.

troops at the same time." To ensure compliance the quinine pills would be administered in the presence of a French or British Army nurse, who would record the intake in the refugee's bulletin. Failure to maintain one's bulletin in order would cost the refugee his meal and the right to employment with the allied army.[340] Distribution of quinine to the refugees began on 18 March 1916 and had an immediate effect on the number of malaria deaths, which fell dramatically.[341]

Besides the refugee camps, villages where malaria prevalence was found to range between 11 and 75 percent[342] were also deemed a threat to the allied forces. As early as February 1916, Macpherson carried out a survey in "the villages," presumably a small-scale operation, and reported splenic indices of 60 to 80 percent, a sign of serious endemicity.[343] For fear of being infected in the next *Anopheles* season, the British troops began leaving some of the villages in which they had been billeted in March[344]; soon they began distributing quinine to residents in the villages they occupied,[345] reducing the distributed dosage at first to accommodate the approximately 27,000

340 IHC proceedings, 6 March 1916, War Diary of DMS, Salonika Army, 1–31 March 1916, WO 95/4771, and 31 March 1916, DMS, Salonika M.E.F. (Surgeon General W. G. Macpherson CB KCMG) January–August 1916, Phase "B," Vol. War Diary of DMS, Salonika Army, 1–31 March 1916, WO 95/4770. The allies also feared that the destitute refugees might try to sell their quinine. IHC, 28 February 1916, DMS, Salonika M.E.F. (Surgeon General W. G. Macpherson CB KCMG) January–August 1916, Phase "B," Vol. War Diary of DMS, Salonika Army, 1–29 February 1916, WO 95/4770. Kopanaris suggested that 50 percent of the Lembet refugees were gametocyte carriers. IHC proceedings, 28 February 1916, Appendix 329A, DMS, Salonika M.E.F. (Surgeon General W. G. Macpherson CB KCMG) January–August 1916, Phase "B," Vol. War Diary of DMS, Salonika Army, 1–29 February 1916, WO 95/4770.
    The idea that *falciparum* malaria was an Indian import rather than a local infection does not seem to be correct, since the Greek refugees were already heavily infected with it before the arrival of the allied troops. Harrison, *The Medical War*, 231.

341 In April, May, and June 1915, there had been ten, twenty-two, and thirty-two deaths; in the corresponding months of 1916 deaths dropped to six, five, and fourteen, respectively. The morbidity rates dropped from 0.8, 1.5, and 2.2 percent to 0.2, 0.83, and 1 percent. 18 March 1916, DMS, Salonika M.E.F. (Surgeon General W. G. Macpherson CB KCMG), January–August 1916, Phase "B," Vol. War Diary of DMS, Salonika Army, 1–31 March 1916, WO 95/4770; Niclot, "Le paludisme," 769.

342 McLay, "Part III," 104.

343 IHC proceedings, 21 February 1916, Appendix 322, DMS, Salonika M.E.F. (Surgeon General W. G. Macpherson CB KCMG) January–August 1916, Phase "B," Vol. War Diary of DMS, Salonika Army, 1–29 February 1916, WO 95/4770.

344 20 March 1916, DMS Salonika M.E.F. (Surgeon General W. G. Macpherson CB KCMG) January–August 1916, Phase "B," Vol. War Diary of DMS, Salonika Army, 1–31 March 1916, WO 95/4770.

345 7 April 1916, Jan.–Aug. 1916, Phase B, Vol. War Diary of DMS, Salonika Army, 1–30 April 1916, WO 95/4771. The French adopted a similar regulation in June, to protect their men from outbreaks of dengue such as the one in Orevitsa (now Pefkodasos). They also calculated that this regulation would also protect them from typhus in the winter. IHC proceedings, 26 June 1916, Appendix 434, Vol. War Diary of DMS, Salonika Army, 1–31 July 1916, WO 95/4771.

refugees in the Greek refugee settlements of Lembet and Zeitenlik as well as in churches and large houses of the city,[346] following an agreement with A. A. Pallis, the secretary of the Greek Refugee Commission for Macedonia. Despite the fact, though, that they ran out of quinine before the end of the first month, there was a notable reduction in the parasite index among the refugees,[347] just as the French and the British were reporting their first fresh malaria cases in April and proving Ronald Ross wrong.[348] Replying to a request "for quinine for prophylactic issue to villagers near Kukush" (present-day Kilkis), the DMS in Salonika stated "that quinine should only be given to inhabitants if places are occupied, or likely to be occupied by our troops, and should be administered in the presence of an army medical officer, not handed over to the people themselves."[349]

The allies considered the local populations as the main source of their initial malaria infections.[350] Evacuations of villages on the front line followed, as a result. "When the troops first occupied the front line," Wenyon later wrote, "the villages dotted along the fertile valleys were still occupied by their native inhabitants, who themselves were ridden with malaria. They undoubtedly constituted the foci from which our troops were infected in the first place. The villages were then evacuated but there were so many infected individuals and carriers amongst our own men by this time that there was ample material for mosquito infection without the necessary intervention of the native."[351]

The British and French issued instructions to their troops not to approach villages between sunset and sunrise during the mosquito season or even to bivouac within a half mile radius from a village. In order to protect their own men earlier in the campaign, they also planned "the treatment by quinine of refugees and inhabitants of villages in the neighborhood of our camps, who

346 19 April 1916, Jan.–Aug. 1916, Vol. War Diary of DMS, Salonika Army, 1–30 April 1916, WO 95/4771.
347 IHC proceedings, 3 April 1916, Appendix 362, Jan.–Aug. 1916, Vol. War Diary of DMS, Salonika Army, 1–30 April 1916, WO 95/4771 and IHC proceedings, 10 April 1916, Appendix 370a, Jan.–Aug. 1916, Vol. War Diary of DMS, Salonika Army, 1–30 April 1916, WO 95/4771.
348 IHC proceedings, 17 April 1916, Appendix 374a, Jan.–Aug. 1916, Vol. War Diary of DMS, Salonika Army, 1–30 April 1916, WO 95/4771.
349 7 April 1916, Jan.–Aug. 1916, Vol. War Diary of DMS, Salonika Army, 1–30 April 1916, WO 95/4771.
350 Migliani et al., "Histoire," 354.
351 Wenyon, "Malaria in Macedonia," 7. Wenyon also noted that A. maculipennis and A. superpictus, the two most efficient malaria vectors in Macedonia, preferred to hibernate in inhabited villages in houses and barns, close to humans or animals, on whom they could feed in brief spells of warm weather; they were almost completely absent from uninhabited villages. See Wenyon, "Malaria in Macedonia," 36–37.

are infected with malaria. The form of infection is pernicious and, in association with the French medical authorities, advised by M. Grall, the medical Inspector General of the French colonial troops," wrote Macpherson in February 1916. He added that he considered this "one of the first and most urgent steps to be taken, but as the Greek authorities are unable to provide the full amount of quinine necessary to carry this out themselves, they have applied to the General Officers Commanding the French and British Forces for assistance in the form of 800 lbs of quinine." The French and British would contribute equally this amount. Macpherson also requested from the medical headquarters in Cairo a monthly consignment of 1,000 lbs of quinine for the protection of the British troops, half of what the French were planning to use for their own men. The French had, in fact, had a bitter experience with malaria from the French Madagascar campaign of the 1890s. The British Army medical authorities in Cairo had difficulties in providing such large amounts. With only 150 lbs of quinine in stock, however, and with the first mosquitoes breeding "along miles of lake country" near troop positions by mid-February, Macpherson was getting impatient: "Salonika and the neighbouring districts in Macedonia are notoriously among the most malarial districts in Europe. Their reputation in this respect is as evil as the Roman Campagna, and the form of malaria here is of a pernicious character."[352]

Already by mid-February 1916, with news of breeding mosquitoes from units stationed by lakes "especially as Indians are stationed in the neighborhood of the mosquito breeding places," pleas for quinine for prophylactic use increased.[353]

The Bulgarians had also suffered from malaria and quinine shortages. "I was informed by a Bulgarian doctor after the armistice," wrote Wenyon,

---

352 W. G. Macpherson, DMS, Salonika, 13 February 1916, to PDMS Headquarters, Cairo; Copies of Cablegrams re: Quinine. DMS, Salonika to PDMS, Cairo, 14 January, 2 February, 4 February, 10 February; PDMS Cairo to DMS Salonika, 8 February, 11 February 1916, WO 95/4770 and Windsor Clive, 12 July, 1916, WO 95/4771. In May, the Medical Advisory Committee instructed the British medical officer to warn troops not to halt in the village of Ajvasil (now Agios Vasilios) "in the evening nor to shelter in barns" and to give quinine to the local children, whom they had found suffering from malaria. 11 May 1916, Vol. War Diary of DMS, Salonika Army, 1–31 May 1916, WO 95/4771; 15 May 1916, Vol. War Diary of DMS, Salonika Army, 1–31 May 1916, WO 95/4771; 20 May 1916; Vol. War Diary of DMS, Salonika Army, 1–31 May 1916, WO 95/4771 and Appendix 400, cable to War Office from DMS [Whitehead], Salonika, 26 May 1916, Vol. War Diary of DMS, Salonika Army, 1–31 May 1916, WO 95/4771. Balfour subsequently published an article on his entomological findings: "The Medical Entomology of Salonika."
353 11 February 1916, DMS, Salonika M.E.F. (Surgeon General W. G. Macpherson CB KCMG) January–August 1916, Phase "B," Vol. War Diary of DMS, Salonika Army, 1–29 February 1916, WO 95/4770.

"that at one time there were 23,000 in hospital with malaria."[354] In fact, on account of lack of quinine in 1918, the Bulgarian Army was compelled to turn to antilarval and antimosquito control on the Aegean, Strymon, and Albanian Fronts or over more than 100 kilometers, using both military and civilian labor, which was paid for with bread rations. Some years later, in a report to the Malaria Commission of the League of Nations, the German malariologist Peter Mühlens (1874–1943) claimed that the Bulgarian approach had been more successful than quininization.[355]

The French and the British jointly planned to repeat the distribution of quinine to refugees in 1917, but only if the British had no shortages in supply. The French also wished to issue quinine to a Gypsy village near the French hospital at Kapoudjilar (present-day Pylaia).[356] The War Office promised generous amounts of quinine for the British troops and for the pro-Entente Greek provisional government in Thessaloniki on credit or "on repayment, financial adjustment to be made locally," but, unlike the previous year, quinine only became available for the refugees on 7 June 1917.[357] With much of the British quinine supply lost in the great fire that burned down most of the city center in mid-August 1917, Whitehead requested further supplies of 3,000 lbs per month.[358] At the end of a difficult malaria year, in November 1917, Konstantinos Angelakis, the mayor of Thessaloniki, also requested and received 28,350 grams of quinine in exchange for a certificate of pay-

354 Wenyon, "Malaria in Macedonia," 28. On the other side of the line Bulgarian villages in the Strumica valley, namely Strumica, Bosiljovo (Bosilovo), Dobilja (Dabilje), Turnova (Turnovo), Sekrinik (Sekirnik), and Yenikoj, were also found to be heavily malarious in October 1918. McLay, "Part III," 104.

355 Peter Mühlens, "Leçons de la querre et de la période d'après-guerre en ce qui concerne la lutte contre le paludisme," p. 40, Renseignements sur l'épidemiologie et la prophylaxie de la malaria en divers pays d'Europe, R873/12B/28002/33686, League of Nations Archives. The German troops also suffered from lack of quinine; yet, although malaria incidence was double that of other diseases, they still suffered less than the Entente allies. The experience of quinine shortages in the First World War led the German scientists to search for synthetic alternatives in the interwar period. See Martini, *Berechnungen*, 7–11.

356 IHC proceedings, 5 March 1917, Appendix 566, Vol. War Diary of DMS, Salonika Army, 1–31 March 1917, WO 95/4773; 29 March 1917, Vol. War Diary of DMS, Salonika Army, 1–31 March 1917, WO 95/4773 and 1 April 1917, Vol. War Diary of DMS, Salonika Army, 1–30 April 1917, WO 95/4773.

357 Summaries Phase C and D 18, 20 April 1917, Vol. War Diary of DMS, Salonika Army, 1–30 April 1917, WO 95/4773; entry 1 April 191, Vol. War Diary of DMS, Salonika Army, 1–30 April 1917, WO 95/4773; Summary Phase C and D, p.23, 16 May 1917, Vol. War Diary of DMS, Salonika Army, 1–31 May 1917, WO 95/4774; entry 1 June 1917, Vol. War Diary of DMS, Salonika Army, 1–30 June 1917, WO 95/4774; entry 7 June 1917, Vol. War Diary of DMS, Salonika Army, 1–30 June 1917, WO 95/4774 and entry 8 June 1917, Vol. War Diary of DMS, Salonika Army, 1–30 June 1917, WO 95/4774.

358 Entry 19 August 1917, Vol. War Diary of DMS, Salonika Army, 1–31 August 1917, WO 95/4774 and entry 26 August 1917, Vol. War Diary of DMS, Salonika Army, 1–31 August 1917, WO 95/4774.

ment.[359] Likewise, in December 1917, Archbishop Gennadios of Thessaloniki received 250,000 5-gram tablets of quinine on similar terms for distribution among the city indigent.[360]

The allied armies required the cooperation of the locals to carry out some of the endless and ephemeral drainage, canalizing, digging, and other antimalarial projects. In one case, a British officer threatened to shut off the water supply to a mill near Salamanli (present-day Gallikos) station, unless the mill owner repaired the leaking millrace within ten days, which he did. On that occasion, Egyptian laborers from British units completed the rest of the work on the stream.[361] Furthermore, the British made sure they distributed quinine to villagers and laborers who came into contact with their troops.[362]

Most of the drainage, canalizing, filling, and other work had to be accomplished in the winter months, before the onset of malaria, and was extremely demanding in man days. Such work, if left for the spring and especially the summer months, was dangerous and primarily assigned to locals. Employment with the allied forces may have fed local families. Still, there was a serious negative aspect to the employment of locals and refugees in some of the works. The area occupied by the British forces comprised a circle of lakes connected by rivers, "surrounded on all sides by high land, except at its south-west corner, where the Vardar loses itself in the extensive Vardar marshes."[363] Malaria prevalence was found "in inverse proportion to elevation."[364] The extensive networks of streams required the deployment of a large workforce, in order to clear the streams of bushes and grass in an effort to reduce the larvae breeding grounds near the British and French camps, and to repeat the same job whenever bad weather destroyed the works.

---

359 Entry 23 November 1917, Vol. War Diary of DMS, Salonika Army, 1–30 November 1917, WO 95/4775 and entry 29 November 1917, Vol. War Diary of DMS, Salonika Army, 1–30 November 1917, WO 95/4775.

360 Entry 17 December 1917, Vol. War Diary of DMS, Salonika Army, 1–31 December 1917, WO 95/4775.

361 Report on the anti-malarial work in No. 2 area, Line of Communications, A . . . son, Sanitary Section RAMC TF to DDMS Base and Line of Communications area, Salonika, 29 June 1917, DMS, Salonika Army, March and April 1917 WO 95/4773.

362 H. R. Whitehead, Report on the incidence of malaria in the Salonika Army in 1916, WO 95/4773; on the measures taken for its prevention; on the measures proposed for its prevention during 1917, Salonika, 20 November 1916, 10–20.

363 Wenyon, "Malaria in Macedonia," 3.

364 Ibid., 4–5.

[A] clear cut channel had to be formed by digging, blasting removal of rocks and boulders, and by opening up pools; water had to siphoned off, areas of depression filled in, the edges of the stream lined with stones—and all this had to be done for every stream and its tributaries right up to the source of each. When the work was completed it had to be constantly watched and repeated, the channel damaged by horses, cattle, sheep and men, but most of all by the sudden downpours of rain which occur in the summer months. A tiny stream would be converted in a few minutes into a roaring torrent, undoing in an hour the work of many weeks. The summer downpours had one advantage. All the streams were suddenly flushed out and millions of larvae were washed away and destroyed. It was always very difficult to find mosquito larvae in the streams for a week or two after a thunderstorm.[365]

Such work was carried out over the whole area of high land occupied by troops in the Doiran–Vardar line, across the country directly south of the Strymon valley and on either side of the Serres Road, on the hills to the west of Lakes Ardzan and Amatova and on the large Khortiatis plateau, the great summer hospital area south of Lakes Langada and Besik.[366]

The French also employed local workers under the command of a French Army engineer for "*travaux du sol.*"[367] One of their projects in 1917 was to drain the marsh around Lake Rudnik (Kheimaditida) and its run off stream into Lake Petrsko (Petron); both put at serious risk their troops on the move along the busiest army routes: the Monastir to Thessaloniki railroad, the roads from Monastir to Kozani, from Sotir (Sotiri) to Sorovitch (present-day Amyntaio), from Sorovitch to Petrsko and from Sorovitch to Eskissu (present-day Xino Nero), a resting place for the troops.[368] At the request of the French in late May, the Greek authorities imposed on all the villages "public services" (*prestations*) or "sanitary corvées" of six to twenty locals working for "free" under French direction. The men received a daily ration of bread, which was sufficient to recruit adequate numbers. Thanks to these "sanitary corvées" the locals provided 2,768 man-days out of a total of 3,801 man-days in forty days to dig, clear, and drain. However, this was a waste

365 Ibid., 16–17.
366 Ibid., 16–17. On exposure to malaria wearing shorts and kilts: William Hunter, AMS, Medical Advisory Committee for Prevention of Epidemic Diseases (Mediterranean and Mesopotamia), Salonika, to H. R. Whitehead, DMS, Salonika, 26 February 1917, WO 95/4773.
367 Niclot, "Le paludisme," 766.
368 Bussière, "Paludisme et drainage," 524.

of effort according to the French medical officer-in-charge because the process would have to be repeated every month in order to be effective. By contrast, digging absorbent sumps and channeling the meandering 2,200-meter-long stream into a deeper bed and a straight 1,500-meter canal, so that it ran downstream from the watermill of Sorovitch, had increased its flow and drained that part of the marsh.[369]

However, draining the entire Rusnik marsh was a larger project, of particular interest to local agriculture, one that also attracted the interest of Ioannis Iliakis, governor of Western Macedonia, who promised to supply additional workforce.[370] The French Directorate of Health Service would provide 300 daily bread rations for the local workforce. The work, which began in mid-July 1917 and stopped at the end of October, saw the daily employment of more than 300 local laborers, corresponding to some 20,000 man-days. As a result, 10 square kilometers of cultivable land were reclaimed, with another four hectares reclaimed from a small marsh were made available as gardens for the French forces, a local watermill and its water rights were preserved and a 5,000-meter-long stream was replaced by a small, straight-edged canal, with a significant decrease in malaria incidence. The same French officer planned to completely drain the marshland in the following year and create a significant area of fertile arable land, with "a layer of humus of several meters," for the benefit of the 100,000 inhabitants of the region.[371]

In early March 1917, the British employed "about 19,000 Macedonians." Besides these locals, the Greek pro-Entente Venizelist provisional government in Thessaloniki, subsequently enlisted a number of "Musselmans" whom they transferred to the British to work under the "same lines as the Macedonian Mule Corps."[372] With regard to the employment of locals the British policy, as spelled out in March 1917, was "to use local labour under British gangers (with native gangers as well) rather than employ soldiers on labour during summer—with view reducing risk sickness. . . . Medical treatment, in case of unenlisted labour to be as at present, i.e., only for wounds,

---

369 Ibid., 524–28.

370 A workforce shortage of soldiers, prisoners, or mobilized Muslims had led the French to even consider employing nurses on the project. Ibid., 529.

371 Ibid., 529–30.

372 This British Army unit was created in 1916 to cover the transport needs or the British Army in Salonika. It consisted, initially, of some 2,000 Greeks; when the Greeks joined the National Defense units in late 1916, they were replaced by muleteers from Cyprus. The National Archives, "Macedonian Mule Corps." I wish to thank Dr. Damian Mac Con Uladh for bringing this information to my attention.

etc." Local workers would not receive treatment from the British for malaria.[373] The French were using their 150 Bulgarian prisoners to canalize the *Anopheles* breeding places by the brickworks of Thessaloniki.[374] When, also in 1917, Greece joined the Entente, Greek laborers were "placed on semimilitary footing" under uniform and as such were entitled to hospital treatment.[375]

The cost of the labor required to deal with such an endless system of streams would be prohibitive and would not justify the expense in peacetime, according to Wenyon. "In times of peace the country is only used as a grazing ground for sheep and goats. The rocky nature of the soil, except in patches here and there, renders it useless of other purposes so that any expenditure of labor from an antimalaria point of view is hardly worth considering. It was only when occupied by an army liable to infection that the question presented itself."[376]

A peace dividend from his wartime service was, however, in the mind of Norman V. Lothian (1889–1925), a Scottish medical entomologist serving on the Macedonian Front, on the eve of the final British offensive against the enemy, in October 1918. He wrote:

I have no further remarks to add except to affirm once again what one perhaps misses the perspective of under "peace" conditions, namely the extraordinary good and valuable results of our campaign this year, as thrown into contrast by experience of the Bulgar side where no work had been done; where as a result mosquitoes swarmed, and where necessarily the efficiency loss must have been very considerable. The success of the 1918 British antimalaria campaign is as promising an omen for the future of Macedonia as the success of the military campaign is for our common cause.[377]

---

373 8 March 1917, Vol. War Diary of DMS, Salonika Army, 1–31 March 1917, WO 95/4773 and 11 March 1917, Vol. War Diary of DMS, Salonika Army, 1–31 March 1917, WO 95/4773; also, Harrison, *The Medical War*, 238–39.

374 The French carried out a survey of urban *Anopheles* breeding sites in April 1917 and found several around the French and other hospitals, farms, and ravines, and near the Catholic and the Orthodox cemeteries. IHC proceedings, 16 April 1917, Appendix 593, Vol. War Diary of DMS, Salonika Army, 1–30 April 1917, WO 95/4773.

375 5 November 1917, Appendix 722, Vol. War Diary of DMS, Salonika Army, 1–30 November 1917, WO 95/4775.

376 Wenyon, "Malaria in Macedonia," 16.

377 N. V. Lothian, Major, DADMS 16th Corps, H.Q. 16th Corps, "16th Corps troops anti-malaria report for September 1918," 22 October 1918, Hygiene 12 51, WO 95/4807. Norman V. Lothian subsequently returned to Macedonia in 1924; he died soon after in Beirut, in 1925, in the same car accident that also killed the American medical entomologist S. T. Darling.

Clearly, however, the Greek colonization plans for northern Greece, set a higher price on the value of antimalarial and reclamation work.[378]

After the removal of King Constantine from the throne and the return of Eleftherios Venizelos to Athens as prime minister in June 1917, the country was unified and the allies were able to begin some antimalarial work in southern Greece as well in places of interest to the allied troops, for instance at Bralos and Itea in Central Greece.[379]

When the Greeks joined the Macedonian Front, the allies realized how heavily the Greek Army also suffered from malaria, apparently with more cases than the allies. There was a Greek battery near Lozista (present-day Mesolofos), a Second Athens Division, and a Greek Regiment, in which, "practically every man in the company had had fever" according to an English speaking Greek soldier, but the reporting British officer thought that "the men did not look sickly; on the contrary they seemed fit and cheerful." Most likely, their immunity was protecting them from serious malaria symptoms.[380] Still, in July 1918, the Greek deputy war minister, Ioannis Athanasakis, requested 4,000 lbs of quinine for the Hellenic Medical Service. H. R. Whitehead, the DMS, was willing to accommodate the Greeks provided the needs of the British medical units were met first.[381]

The final military attack in September 1918 exposed the British troops to additional risks and was carried out in the face of a serious shortage of quinine. Possessing a stock of 20,000 lbs, that had to last until the end of the year or even early spring, and with no additional orders for quinine placed, the British force was to continue prophylactic usage but offers of quinine to third parties "on payment" would cease.[382]

Wenyon's Malaria Enquiry Laboratory followed the allied army in its final attack. For Wenyon, quinine prophylaxis and antilarval measures had proved disappointing and wasteful; nets and other mosquito proofing measures were the only realistic protection.[383] The attack on Bulgaria in late Sep-

---

378 On the colonization of Macedonia see p. 176 in this book.
379 Extracts from a report by DADMS (Sanitary) Base & L. of C. Area, on a visit to Bralos and Itea, 13–16 January 1918, J. T. Johnson, DADMS (Sanitary) Base & L. of C. Area, 19 January 1918, WO 95/4807.
380 Malaria in 1st Infantry Regiment, 2nd Athens division, [July?] 1918, WO 95/4807.
381 Entry 27 July 1918, War Diary DMS, BSF, 1–31 July 1918, WO 95/4778.
382 Entry 20 September 1918, DMS, BSF War Diary, 1–30 September 1918, WO 95/4778.
383 Wenyon, "Malaria in Macedonia," 23–27. By 1917 the failure of quinine to protect the troops from malaria had become evident and caused much disappointment among several of the medical officers and a preference for antilarval measures and mosquito nets. Harrison, *The Medical War*, 232.

tember coincided with the outbreak of influenza among the combatants, which further aggravated the severity of malaria cases. From 1,000 weekly cases at the end of September, malaria figures rose to almost 1,600 cases in the beginning of October and then declined toward the end of the year.[384] In the camp of the Central Powers, the Germans also suffered from malaria, more heavily in 1918 than earlier. On the Balkan Front, their morbidity was particularly high with 92.6 cases per thousand strength in 1917 but 232.4 per thousand in the final year of the conflict.[385]

In 1919, relapses and fresh *vivax* malaria cases continued to infest Thessaloniki as well as *falciparum* later in the year. The war had made of the area along the road to Monastir with its army camps and ordnance depot a particularly dangerous place. Furthermore, a Maltese labor force, newly arrived in the city after the end of hostilities, in 1919, was soon infected locally.[386]

The Greek Army

The pitiful state of health in the Greek forts was revealed as soon as the Bavarian regency assumed authority in the new kingdom. Expectations of, more than experience with, fevers among the military allowed the War Ministry, manned entirely by Bavarian officers and soldiers, to assume a pivotal role in combating malaria epidemics among civilians in the early days of Greek statehood. During the epidemic of 1834, the War Ministry provided medicines, most likely quinine, from army supplies, to the Interior Ministry in September. The Interior Ministry, in turn, sent these medicines to the provinces of Thebes and Livadeia, where a "pernicious disease" struck the area soon after King Othon had toured the region.[387] In fact, the prefecture physician, the chief civilian medical authority, was delayed in Athens, not yet the country's capital, "owing to the number of sick soldiers, whom

384 Wenyon, "Malaria in Macedonia," 11.
385 On the Turkish front the figures were 651.2 per thousand for 1917 and 183.7 per thousand for 1918. *Malaria and Quinine*, 27.
386 Wenyon, "Malaria in Macedonia," 28.
387 Ioannis Kolettis, Interior Minister to King Othon, Nafplio, 28 September/9 October 1834, doc. 003, f 193, Interior Ministry, Othon's administration, GAK; Ioannis Kolettis, Interior Minister to King Othon, Nafplio, 29 September/10 October 1834, doc. 004, f 193, Interior Ministry, Othon's administration, GAK. More on the 1834 epidemic in chapter 2.

he was charged to treat in the absence of a military physician."[388] Before the end of the crisis, the War Ministry had provided 1,318 drachmas' worth of medicine to the visiting doctors sent out by the Interior Ministry to treat the peasants.[389]

Although the military helped out in the crises of the first years, as soldiers also shared the peasants' exposure to malaria, the reverse was also true: barracks developed into sources of degradation for the urban environment by providing a mixed supply of infected and nonimmune recruits. In western Greece, in the town of Vonitsa, close to the Ottoman frontier, fevers were a serious problem. In August 1845, King Othon requested a report from the Interior Ministry on the necessity of draining the swamp surrounding the town, principally because it was harmful for the health of the garrison troops. It speaks a great deal about the mental map of social hierarchy that the king suggested the use of convicts for the job.[390] Six years later, the Greek authorities were still searching in and around the town, by the fort, even across the Greek border, for the source of the intermittent fevers that were befalling Vonitsa. In a report to the Interior Ministry physician A. Mavrogenis interestingly offered no medical recommendations. Rather, the scope of his advice involved extensive, hugely costly engineering projects. Mavrogenis also advised consultation with the Ottoman neighbors over similar issues regarding swamps and fisheries on Ottoman territory.[391]

On some occasions, civilian communities benefited from their proximity to military barracks. Such was the case of Kalpaki, a village in Epirus in the interwar years, whose inhabitants appeared to have a lower malaria incidence, thanks to the illicit trade in quinine tablets by the soldiers.[392] The practice was not uncommon among soldiers; in the First World War quinine was being used for barter by Bulgarian solders. Also in Dalmatia, it was used in exchange for food, tobacco, sugar, but mostly for wine.[393]

388 Ioannis Kolettis, Interior Minister to King Othon, Nafplio, 13/25 October 1834, doc. 005, f. 193, Interior Ministry, Othon's administration, GAK.

389 Ioannis Kolettis, Interior Minister to King Othon, Athens, 21 January/2 February 1835, doc. 013, f. 193, Interior Ministry, Othon's administration, GAK.

390 King Othon to Interior Ministry, Athens, 3 August 1845 (draft), doc. 046, f. 232, Interior Ministry, Othon's administration, GAK.

391 A. Mavrogenis to Interior Ministry, "Medical report on the causes of the endemic and occasionally epidemic diseases and on the measures to be taken for their elimination," Athens, 8 November 1851, doc. 012, f. 192, Interior Ministry, Othon's administration, GAK.

392 Dimissas, "Ekthesis peri tis eis tas perifereias tis Ipeirou," 40.

393 Peter Mühlens, "Leçons de la guerre et de la période d'après-guerre en ce qui concerne la lutte contre le

In Athens, military camps in and around the city interacted with older foci of endemic malaria. In August 1861, a serious epidemic hit the area around Mount Lycabettus (Anchesmos), where the 10th Army battalion had camped, specifically by the Petrakis (or Asomatoi) monastery. As reported to the Athens Medical Society, the monks were aware that their site had been "insalubrious" (*nosodes*) and "fever-prone" (*pyretovrithes*) during the *Tourkokratia*, or "since time immemorial." Eventually, the government relocated the camp to .the city outskirts, in Kypseli.[394]

The occupation of Athens and Piraeus by British and French troops in 1854, during the Crimean War, introduced the Greeks to the prophylactic use of quinine. Having witnessed how the drug had protected the British officers in Piraeus from fever, Greek doctors began administering quinine for its effectiveness and safety. The experience then spread from the army to civilian doctors.[395] The French also noted that the frequency of grave forms of fever among their own troops was rare: only three in a thousand cases were recorded.[396] The beneficial effects of its usage was indeed spectacular. In order to set up a central state depot for delivery of quinine to local doctors, pharmacists or directly to patients in times of shortage, the Greek government lost no time in ordering municipalities nationwide to assess their requirements.[397] Thus, the joint British–French occupation of 1854 left a legacy of preventive use of quinine and introduced some state initiative.

The military reforms of the Trikoupis governments in the 1880s coincided with the steady spread of the germ-theory paradigm and the understanding of the cause of malaria among the medical profession. The first malaria data from Athens military hospitals date to 1882. By 1890 a considerable amount of numerical information was made available in Greek medical journals and other publications.[398] It is conceivable that a sense of na-

---

394 "Praktika tis en Athinais ypo tin prostasian tis A.M. Iatrikis Etairias, Synedriasis tis 22 Noemvriou 1861." If Kypseli had been malaria-free, it now acquired a focus of malaria in the army camp.

395 Afentoulis, *Farmakologia*, vol. 1, 240. See also *Asklipios*, Period II, 1, no. 12 (June 1857): 590.

396 Stéphanos, *La Grèce*, 499n1.

397 Ypourgeion Esoterikon, *Peri promitheias kininou*; Elliniko Logotekhniko kai Istoriko Arkheio (ELIA) 290/D190. Nothing, however, is known to have come from this government order.

398 The army published its own monthly medical review between 1890 and 1897, the *Iatriki Efimeris tou Stratou*. For a list of its content, see Skampardonis, Antonakopoulos, and Skhizas, *Iatriki Efimeris tou Stratou*.

tional emergency[399] generated the disclosure of epidemiological evidence by leading army physicians, for instance, Konstantinos Savvas,[400] who thus paved the way for civilian medical surveys.

The collection of statistical evidence was affected by changes in attitudes toward the disease itself. For instance, physicians correlated the resurgence of cases in 1886 and, again, in 1898 with the two failed Greek war efforts. The Greek Army that was mobilized in response to the Bulgarian Crisis of 1885 was stationed in Thessaly for several months in 1886. Malaria cases hospitalized in the military hospital of Athens doubled in comparison to previous years,[401] then decreased considerably and tripled again in 1898, compared to the 1896 level, following the Greco-Turkish War of 1897, a year for which data are not available, as can be seen in figure 3.9.

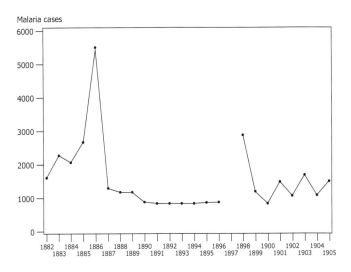

Figure 3.9. Hospitalized malaria cases in the Greek Army, 1882–1905
Source: Typaldos, "Statistikai pliroforiai."

The noticeable drop in malaria cases in proportion to total hospital admittances of troops after 1898 was attributed to a change in attitude rather to a de-

399 Livieratos, "I elonosia," 163. The army often released recruits with severe cachexia. Typaldos, "Statistikai pliroforiai," 387.

400 Savvas soon became physician to King George and later professor of microbiology at the University of Athens. He initiated the series of publications of army data in an article in *Galinos* in 1888 titled "Pentaetis statistiki tou Stratiotikou Nosokomeiou Athinon apo 1882–1887." See Typaldos, "Statistikai pliroforiai," 383.

401 Ibid., 384–85.

cline of infections. In the 1880s, on the basis of the overall quinine consumption of the army, Ioannis Typaldos, an army physician, had estimated that one in two soldiers with malaria was admitted to hospital; by 1898 though sick solders took their quinine in the barrack infirmary without being transferred to a military hospital. Even in the nationwide epidemic of 1905, 35 percent of the armed forces was hospitalized for malaria, relatively fewer both in absolute numbers and in proportion in comparison to the postwar year of 1898, when 45 percent of the Greek armed forces had been admitted for malaria.

Annual patterns of monthly malaria prevalence varied between bimodal and unimodal curves, presumably depending on the annual fluctuation of *falciparum* malaria cases.

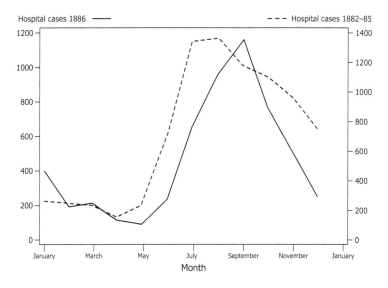

Figure 3.10. Monthly distribution of malaria prevalence in the Army, 1882–86
Source: Typaldos, "Statistikai pliroforiai."

In 1886, one of the most serious nationwide epidemics affecting both soldiers and civilians broke out.[402] As seen in figure 3.10, the 1886 hospital cases almost equaled those of the previous four years together. Subsequently, between 1887 and 1905 the two Athens military hospitals[403] treated 21,310 malaria cases, comprising 21 percent of all admissions (one in every five), an av-

---

402 Ibid.
403 Ibid., 387.

erage representing a range of 14 to 30 percent of all admissions annually. In all, only 24 malaria cases were fatal.[404] The harsh reality in the army between 1896 and 1905, particularly in the western part of the country, is reflected in data from various garrisons, as indicated in figure 3.11.

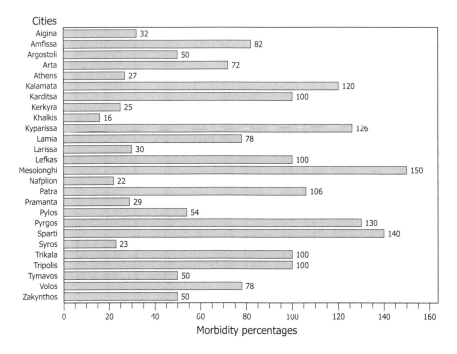

Figure 3.11. Malaria in garrisons, 1896–1905
Source: Typaldos, "Statistikai pliroforiai."

As suggested by the percentages exceeding 100 percent, the figures reflect multiple infections, recrudescences, and relapses. Figures for the heavily malarious garrison of Messolonghi indicate that in 1906 the vast majority of cases received treatment in the camp. Likewise, in Khalkis, an important military installation, practically all malaria incidents were treated without hospitalization, while the surge of cases in July virtually crippled the entire unit, reason enough to keep the total Greek force to a minimum in the summer months.[405] However, throughout the Greek Army, which was clearly in

404 Ibid., 389.
405 Ibid., 407.

the grip of malaria, large volumes of quinine reduced malaria deaths to insignificant numbers.

In the interwar years, the Greek Army continued to be a source of rampant disease, from which conscripted young men returned home in ill health. In his 1932 general election campaign, Eleftherios Venizelos, without alluding specifically to malaria in the army, claimed that his government had halved the general morbidity in the army from an alarming 68.2 percent and had reduced general mortality from around 8 percent to 2.49 percent.[406]

According to one army medical officer, malaria reduced the fighting capacity of the military to 80 percent in some particularly malarious parts of Greece. In those areas the army could only enlist 60 percent of the men of military age. Indeed, the army filled the ranks in the artillery and cavalry first so that sometimes there were not enough healthy recruits to man the infantry units. In the summer, in particular, in endemic zones, the officers gave their men leave and reduced the number of drills to spare their health. The army also spent large sums of money on quinine for the troops. For instance, in 1936, the Larissa garrison alone used 473 kilograms of quinine to treat its malaria cases and lost 41,000 man-days from its training program owing to severe cases of the disease.[407]

In the late 1930s, fear of war took hold of the Athens civilian population. Despite the fact that the water works at the Marathon dam had been completed and Athenians had running water in their homes, they insisted on "keeping storage tanks in their houses. The principal reason for this is the fear of a war which might involve the bombing of the dam." This widespread practice, which, at the time had become unnecessary, nonetheless placed the city at risk by providing breeding sites not only for *Anopheles* mosquitoes but also for the *Aedes aegypti* (*Stegomyia*), the vector that had caused the dengue epidemic in 1927.[408]

Combating malaria in the army became a central goal of the government's health policy toward troops after the end of the Nazi occupation in Greece, and during and following the Civil War. At the same time, the reor-

---

406 *To ergon tis kyverniseos Venizelou*, 245.

407 Manoussakis, *To elonosiakon provlima*, 4.

408 Excerpts from W. A. Sawyer diary notes, entry 22 May 1936, 1934–1938, folder 14, box no. 2, 749 I (Malaria) Projects Series 749 Greece, RG 1.1, RAC.

ganized Greek Army became an integral part of the country's malaria-erad-ication strategy and performed much of the country's antimalarial work. Just as with the national program that had been promoted by UNRRA and then by the Marshall Plan, the army also made heavy use of DDT and made structural adaptations accordingly.

The army set up special antimalarial teams (*anthelonosiakai omades*) headed by reserve officers from the engineers corps.[409] These teams belonged to campaign hygiene sections, which, in turn, were headed by medical officers and were mostly stationed with divisions and brigades in northern Greece.[410] Interestingly, in the case of Eastern Macedonia and Thrace in 1946, the regional antimalarial campaign was drawn up in consultation with the "hygiene advisor" (*ygeionomikos symvoulos*) of the Army High Command of East Macedonia and Thrace (ASDAMT).[411]

The antimalarial teams sent out parties for antimalarial residual spraying, antilarval work, and mosquito collection, in military installations, army training centers, villages, and the countryside.[412] Occasionally, they were required to collaborate with local civilian authorities in undertaking antimalarial measures.[413] Assignment to antimalarial spraying duties was considered particularly harsh treatment and was sometimes used as a disciplinary measure.[414] The teams also became training sites for visiting officers and men who would transfer to other units where they were expected to perform further antimalarial work.[415] In this respect, therefore, they were central to malaria control. Their own men and officers received a short period of

---

409 Order-of-the-day 30 January 1946, film 1, 263/Antimalarial Team (AT) [Anthelonosiaki Omas] 283; 18 January 1948, AT 282 and 22 October 1953, film 3, p. 188, 264/AT 284, Section of Campaign Hygiene (SCH) [Tmima Ygieinis Ekstrateias], Service of Military Archives (SMA). The material is available on 35 mm microfilm.

410 Order-of-the-day 14 March 1946, book 1, p. 48, film 1; 22 March 1946, book 1, p. 52, film 1; 16 March 1946, book 1, p. 54, film 1; 15 April 1946, book 1, p. 75, film 1; 13 April 1948, book 3, film 1, SCH 261, SMA.

411 Orders-of-the-day 23 March 1946, p. 21, film 2; 13 August 1946, p. 72, film 2, SCH 264/AT 284, SMA. There is no indication as to the nationality of this expert in these documents.

412 Order-of-the-day 10 July 1949, book 3, film 1; 25 June 1952, p. 341, book 4, film 1; 17 June 1949, 10 April 1950, 11 April 1950, 23 April 1950, AT 282, SCH 261 and 26 April 1946, 6 May 1946, film 1, SCH 263/AT 283, SMA. The same team received orders to send a party to the road from Thessaloniki to Veroia and another party for the bridge on the Strymon River. Order-of-the-day 19 July 1946, 1 August 1946, film 1; 9 July 1947, book [2], p. 6, film 1; 25 April 1948, film 2; 10 May 1949, p. 16, film 2, SCH 264/AT 284, SMA.

413 Order-of-the-day 27 May 1946, film 1, SCH 263/AT 283, SMA.

414 Order-of-the-day 26 June 1948, p. 94, film 3, SCH 264/AT 284, SMA.

415 Order-of-the-day 1 April 1947, p. 140, film 1, SCH 263/AT 283; 17 April 1947, p. 127, film 2, SCH 264/AT 284, SMA.

antimalarial training, initially at the School of Malariology in Larissa[416] and later on at the newly founded Military School of Hygiene and Malariology in Athens.[417] The Greek Army still used Paris green throughout 1946 and 1947, consumed enormous amounts of DDT in its antimalarial campaign since 1946, and treated its men with quinine and Atabrine.[418]

Second World War

The disruption of social life that resulted from the German occupation after April 1941 unleashed unprecedented levels of suffering on the Greeks. With the technical and material intervention of the allies, however, the end of the war finally saw the turning of the tables on malaria.

Among other occupation hardships, Greece experienced a serious malaria epidemic.[419] Much of the progress in malaria control of the 1930s was due to the scientific approach of the RF mission, which had also been adopted by the Greek Army. This, however, was wiped out by wartime developments. When Greece entered the war in October 1940, peacetime control work ceased and civilian malariologists were seconded to the heavily malarious zones in Albania for the protection of Greek troops. To offset this setback, Greek expatriates came to the assistance of Greece; the GWRA came into being in November in New York, and in February 1941 it ordered 5 tons of Paris green to make up for supply shortages that were threatening that year's control campaign. In a similar spirit of concern, the foreign director of the Near East Foundation (NEF), Laird Archer, appealed to the RF to send its sanitary engineer, Daniel E. Wright, back to Greece.[420]

---

416 Order-of-the-day 25 February 1946, 13 March 1946, film 1, SCH 263/AT 283, SMA.

417 Order-of-the-day 26 March 1949, book 3, film 1; 28 February 1954, 14 March 1954, p. 372, book 4, AT 281, SCH 261; 26 March 1949, p. 78, film 3; 19 March 1953, p. 162, SCH 264/AT 284, SMA. I wish to thank Professor Dennis Cokkinos for pointing out the existence of the Military School of Hygiene and Malariology in Athens.

418 Daily administration order 3 June 1946, 5 July 1946, 9 August 1946, 31 August 1946, 2 October 1946, 31 October 1946, p. 98, film 2; 31 December 1946, 1 February 1947, 1 March 1947, 31 March 1947, 30 April 1947, 31 May 1947, 30 June 1947, 31 July 1947, 31 August 1947, 30 September 1947, 31 May 1948, 30 June 1948, 31 July 1948, 31 August 1948, 30 September 1948, 3 November 1948, film 3, SCH 264/AT 284; 30 April 1949, 30 September 1949, 31 October 1949, 30 November 1949, 31 March 1950, 30 April 1950, p. 3, AT 282; 15 October 1947, pp. 73–74, film 1, SCH 263/AT 283, SMA.

419 This section is largely based on my article "Relief Work and Malaria in Greece, 1943–1947."

420 Laird Archer to E. C. Miller, 15 February 1941, quoted in E. C. Miller to A. J. Warren, 7 April 1941, folder 15, box 2, series 749 I, RG 1.1, RFA, RAC; G. Livadas to A. J. Warren, 21 December 1940, folder 15, box 2, series 749 I, RG 1.1, RFA, RAC.

The war, however, prevented the RF medical directors from taking any immediate action.[421] By the time the annual antimalarial campaign was scheduled to begin, Greece had been occupied by the German forces. As a result, civilian services and international communications broke down.

The division of the country into three occupation zones by the Germans, Italians, and Bulgarians, in June 1941, and the Allied blockade disrupted the internal market; possibly hundreds of thousands of civilians perished in the famine of the following winter.[422]

The disruption of antimalarial control work combined with the winter famine unleashed a nationwide malaria epidemic in the summer of 1942, which touched the remotest mountain villages and islands.[423] Its intensity and extent have been associated with the famine and the reduction of people's resistance, shortages in antimalarial medication, the collapse of mosquito-control measures, extensive population mobility, and cyclical climatological conditions.[424] Epidemics, however, are often fueled by famines which compel their victims to consume their domestic animals, which otherwise would have largely protected the human hosts from the bites of anthropophilic *Anopheles*. This additional factor, in all likelihood, was at play in the case of the 1942 malaria epidemic.[425] Most of these adverse factors still produced high levels of malaria mortality and morbidity even after 1942. The following table represents indices of malaria mortality, presumably mostly from *P. falciparum*, in Thessaloniki, its suburbs, and rural Macedonia between 1939 and 1943, taking 1940 as a base year.[426]

---

421 A letter from A. J. Warren, Assistant Director of the RF IHD, to Grigorios Livadas, Director of the Malaria Department of the Athens School of Hygiene, left New York on 4 March 1941 and returned undelivered almost nine months later, intercepted by the Wehrmacht, which had occupied Greece in April. In the letter, Warren regretted that he could do little but wait until "the situation in Greece has returned to normal" and pledge the services of the RF for "when this period arrives." A. J. Warren to G. Livadas, 4 March 1941, folder 15, box 2, series 749 I, RG 1.1, RFA, RAC.

422 Mazower, *Inside Hitler's Greece*, 24–41; Hionidou, *Famine and Death*, 158; Thomadakis, "Black Markets."

423 Comité International de la Croix-Rouge, *Ravitaillement*, 475.

424 Hionidou, *Famine and Death*, 163; United Nations Relief and Rehabilitation Administration, Health Division, Region EG, Christos Damkas, Chapter X: "Malaria," 559, folder Greece 38, Region EG, Health Division Final Report, box 36, PAG-4/4.2.:36 [S-0524-0060]; J.M. Vine, "Malaria control on a national scale—Greece, 1946," p. 26–27, Malaria and Sanitation, folder Greece #22, box 35, PAG-4/4.2.:35 [S-0524-0059], UN Archives.

425 Barber, *A Malariologist in Many Lands*, 82; Snow and Gilles, "The Epidemiology of Malaria," 93; Vassiliou, "Politics, Public Health, and Development," 173, also points to this factor.

426 Mandekos, "I ex asiteias kai elonosias thnisimotis eis Thessalonikin."

Year	Thessaloniki	Suburbs	Rural Macedonia
1939	56.41	36.36	—
1940	100.00	100.00	100.00
1941	207.69	181.82	110.23
1942	1,825.64	2,522.73	511.36
1943	323.08	450.00	137.12

Table 3.4. Index of malaria mortality in Thessaloniki, its suburbs, and rural Macedonia, 1939–43 (1940 = 100)

Source: Mandekos, "I ex asiteias kai elonosias thnisimotis eis Thessalonikin."

The short-term immunity of the survivors, improved weather coupled with a small amount of malaria control, and, more importantly, the distribution of antimalarial medication, may explain the decline of mortality in 1943.[427] As for 1944, the final year of the occupation in Greece, the Red Cross estimated at least 2.5 million cases in a population of 7 million. This represents a morbidity level comparable to, if not higher than, the early-twentieth-century peacetime epidemics.[428]

The relief effort mounted by the Greek government-in-exile in London and the GWRA in the United States, under the auspices of the International Committee of the Red Cross (ICRC) in Geneva, entailed a relaxation of the British blockade. Following an agreement with the occupying forces at the end of March 1942 and the establishment of a Joint Red Cross Relief Commission, food and medical supplies began to trickle into the country that November. The Swedish Red Cross became responsible for food shipments, while the ICRC was in charge of medical supplies.[429] The distribution of these life-saving supplies—quinine and Atabrine being the most pressing need—became a highly contested subject among the Greeks.[430]

---

427 Snow and Gilles, "The Epidemiology of Malaria," 99–100. Weather conditions in subsequent years were also reported to have contributed to a decline in the anopheline population. J.M. Vine, "Malaria control on a national scale—Greece, 1946," p. 26–27, Malaria and Sanitation, folder Greece #22, box 35, PAG-4/4.2.:35 [S-0524-0059], UN Archives.

428 Excerpts from UNRRA Medical and Sanitation Program 1944 in W. J. Carroll, "Greece. Medical and sanitation program," 1, folder Bureau of Supply, Medical 10, box 14, PAG-4/4.2, UN Archives.

429 Comité International de la Croix-Rouge, Actions de Secours, 500–509; Kazamias, "Turks, Swedes and Famished Greeks," 306.

430 Comité International de la Croix-Rouge, Actions de Secours, 508; Comité International de la Croix-Rouge, Ravitaillement, 464–65; Commission de Gestion de Secours à la Grèce, Comité de Haute Direction, Procès-Verbaux, 31 March 1943, 3, Secours/Grèce, 1940/1946, SG11, ICRC Archives, Geneva.

The Joint Relief Commission in Athens created a nationwide network of more than 3,000 local Red Cross distribution subcommittees, which survived beyond the end of the occupation and were incorporated into the UNRRA distribution structure. They became the target of violent attacks and persecution by the Security Battalions, the militia of the collaborationist government. Before the end of the occupation, the most powerful resistance groups had their own distribution committees.[431] As the battle lines of the Greek Civil War were being drawn, these relief structures and the selection of relief recipients emerged as a contested political issue after liberation.[432] Finally, a Joint Medical Supply Committee was agreed on in January 1945, which was technically an agency of the Greek Health Ministry and was staffed by representatives from UNRRA, the Greek Red Cross, regional committees, and local subcommittees.[433]

Antimalarial drugs were in short supply, sold on the black market, and used as currency. In September 1943, after the capitulation of Italy and the looting of Italian warehouses, medical supplies entered the black market, which became the source of antimalarial drugs for both the Germans and the Greek resistance groups. Supplies became even scarcer after the illegal importations of antimalarials by the Italian and German military practically ceased at the end of 1943.[434]

The Joint Red Cross Relief Commission set the country's annual requirements for antimalarials at almost equal to prewar levels. With the Wehrmacht itself, though, suffering from antimalarial shortages, this was clearly far below demand.[435] As in the case of food relief, the geographic dis-

431 Kazamias, "Turks, Swedes and Famished Greeks," 304; Hionidou, *Famine and Death*, 137; Laiou-Thomadakis, "The Politics of Hunger," 29; Comité International de la Croix-Rouge, *Ravitaillement*, 62–64; "The Hygienic and Social Welfare Problems of Greece," Report Greece, Medical Summary, 30 July 1944, 1, folder Greece 42, box 36, PAG-4/4.2.: 36 [S-0524-0060], UN Archives.

432 Kazamias, "Turks, Swedes and Famished Greeks," 306. As regards the political interference with the UNRRA distribution subcommittees see, for instance, the historical report prepared by the Office of the Regional Director, 22, folder Greece 45, Region EG, Office of the Regional Director, box 36, PAG-4/4.2.:36 [S-0524-0060], UN Archives; also, Close, "The Changing Structure of the Right," 132.

433 Comité International de la Croix-Rouge, *Ravitaillement*, 465; Health Division, UNRRA Greece Headquarters, Historical notes, General, 1, 6–7, folder Greece 20, Report of the Director, Health Division, box 35, PAG-4/4.2.:35 [S-0524-0059], UN Archives.

434 Report Greece, Medical, General summary [date of information: March 1944], 10 May 1944, 2, 3, folder Greece 43, Health Division, Intelligence Reports, box 36, PAG-4/4.2.:36 [S-0524-0060]; Report Greece, Medical Summary, 30 July 1944, 1–2, folder Greece 42, The Hygienic and Social Welfare Problems of Greece, box 36, PAG-4/4.2.:36 [S-0524-0060], UN Archives.

435 Until its withdrawal in early 1945, the Red Cross Joint Committee had distributed approximately 50 million tablets of Atabrine, 4.4 million tablets of Plasmoquine, and 1.3 million tablets of quinine. Comité

tribution of antimalarials depended on local security conditions. In western and central Macedonia, for instance, where the Greek authorities cooperated closely with the Germans, distribution improved, but even there only one-fifth of the "normal requirement" of quinine was available. The areas where the activity of the resistance groups remained intense, like in the northwestern Peloponnese and the mountains of Epirus and Thessaly, however, were cut off from relief distribution centers, particularly during the final year of the occupation. Even before British liberation forces arrived in the country, British military intelligence reported on the urgent need for antimalarials.[436]

In the winter of 1943/44, the Greek Red Cross organized three missions in trucks, supplied by the International Red Cross, to distribute relief, food, clothing, and medicines to villages that had been destroyed by the Germans in Thessaly, Central Greece and Epirus. The mission to Epirus, headed by Helli Adossides of the Greek Red Cross, received permission from the Germans for only two such villages, Sanovo (Aetopetra) and Mazi (Polydroso). Adossides left the following chilling account of the hardship people endured.

The following day, doctors Tsapras and Zervos, accompanied by Ms. Adossides, visited the sick of the burned villages of Sanovo and Mazi, whose inhabitants took refuge in the marshes of the River Aoos, at a distance of one and a half hours from their village. We left the truck on the main road and crossed the marsh on horseback. The animals often sunk knee-deep in the mud and crossed with difficulty the numerous streams which interrupted the track. On a mound hidden behind brambles and trees miserable huts of braided branches coated with mud on the interior give the impression of a village of some primitive tribe. We entered several cabins, sometimes on all

---

International de la Croix-Rouge, *Ravitaillement*, 465 and 475; Mazower, *Inside Hitler's Greece*, 65; Eckart and Vondra, "Malaria and World War II." Atabrine, also produced under the name Mepacrine, was an antimalarial produced both by German and Allied industries. It contributed critically to the positive outcome of the Allies' war effort after they lost Java to the Japanese thereby losing access to more than 95 percent of the world's quinine. Harrison, "Medicine and the Culture of Command," 445; Greenwood, "Conflicts of Interest," 859 and 864–65.

436 Health Division, UNRRA Health Division Monthly Bulletin, 1, 2 (October 1944), 11, box 16, PAG-4/4.2, UN Archives; Abstract from report on Health conditions submitted by the Military Intelligence Service, September 1943, United Nations Relief and Rehabilitation Administration, Health Division, Region EG, History, Chapter VIII: "Diseases," 477–478, folder Greece 38, Region EG, Health Division Final Report, box 36, PAG-4/4.2.:36 [S-0524-0060], UN Archives.

fours. There was no floor; bare soil with patches of mud here and there show-ing that the "roof" left much to be desired. Within 3 square meters were hud-dled families of five to eight persons. A tree trunk across the "floor" sepa-rated the family "bed," which consisted of a few rags laid out on the beaten earth. Behind the "bed," a sort of rack made of branches contained the small quantity of maize that the family managed to salvage. In a corner, the hearth which burned day and night, as there are no matches and this fire serves for heating, cooking the meager pittance of a meal, and for lighting the room. In terms of furniture and utensils, it was the most absolute bareness. These people, who used to live in stone houses, often two storied, and were pro-vided with the necessities of life, particularly with heavy woolen blankets and warm clothes, now have nothing, absolutely nothing. The look of the women in particular was lamentable. One felt they were overwrought, inca-pable of any more suffering and of struggling against a fate that seemed to torment them with no respite. Even these pitiful huts they were often obliged to abandon at night, persecuted, carrying the children across the marshes to take refuge in the mountain. Eighty percent are crippled with rheuma-tism. The children, of whom there are many, all carry the signs of malaria and undernourishment. . . . The distribution of semolina rations of 20 drams [c. 64.06 g] per child per day (3 okas [3.846 kg] for two months), sugar (about 100 drams [c. 320.3 g] per baby), and soap began. Rice was given out parsi-moniously to sick people and very debilitated children. Then clothes were handed out, preferably to large families. In this marshy country, the clogs of the Hellenic Red Cross are an unanticipated success. We were almost taken by assault. At nightfall, we returned to Konitsa.[437]

In Thrace and eastern Macedonia, the Bulgarians annexed the area and estab-lished their own occupation administration. They persecuted the Greek Ma-lariological Service personnel, abandoned all prewar work and equipment and conducted no malaria control of their own. As a result of neglect, the area be-came inundated with large expanses of stagnant water. The occupation au-thorities merely contented themselves with the distribution of antimalarials.[438]

Malaria, however, became a serious problem for the nonimmune Ger-man occupying army. Mosquitoes were considered the "second enemy," af-

---

437 H. Adossidès, "Rapport de Mr. Papadopoulos et de Mme Adossidès sur leur voyage en Epire du Nord," Athens, 21 March 1944, p. 7, GR VI, Joint Relief Commission, Special Reports on Medical Supplies and Care, PAG-4/3.0.2.0.1.:2 [S-0527-0258], UN Archives.

438 Health Division Region EG History, 31, folder Greece 38, Region EG Health Division Final Report, box 36, PAG-4/4.2.:36 [S-0524-0060], UN Archives.

ter the resistance groups, and affected the fighting capability and morale of the German troops no less than the guerrilla attacks.[439] According to historian Mark Mazower, "some 25 per cent of 22 Army Corps was afflicted. In a specialist police mountain regiment which arrived in Greece after serving in Finland, the numbers of sick men rose rapidly from 30 to 400." In a practice that was also used among allied troops, German soldiers in Greece were shown the film *Feind Malaria* (Enemy malaria) to educate them on how to protect themselves from mosquito bites.[440]

The Germans made use of preexisting malaria services, as in the case of Thessaloniki and Langadas, carried out some Paris green control work, as in the case of Aidipsos in Euboea and Sparta in the Peloponnese, and created some new control stations, for instance in Molaoi and Gytheio in the southern Peloponnese, presumably to protect their troops.[441] To this end, they drew on the peacetime research on prevalence data of the Malariology Division of the Athens School of Hygiene collected between 1937 and 1939 but also conducted their own local epidemiological and entomological research between 1941 and 1943.[442]

As suggested above, Thessaloniki received some attention from the German authorities. They supplied its malaria control center with Paris green and diesel oil and retained its prewar personnel, who carried out some small-scale drainage and operated a research laboratory; this lab, in fact, carried out epidemiological surveys in some hundred towns and villages. In all, about sixty antimalarial stations in western and central Macedonia and one malaria training school in Langadas were in service, but their operation suffered from overall disorder in the last year of the occupation.[443]

---

439 Mazower, *Inside Hitler's Greece*, 202–3; Vondra, "Die Malaria," 109.

440 Mazower, *Inside Hitler's Greece*, 203. On the use of motion pictures in malaria propaganda, see Fedunkiw, "Malaria Films." With regard to civilian use, see Kardamatis, "Ai provolai," on a Greek Red Cross production in the winter of 1927.

441 See chapter 2. On incidents of German troops affected with malaria in Thessaly, see Mazower, *Inside Hitler's Greece*, 203. Combating malaria was the purpose of German medical scientific experiments on concentration camp inmates at Dachau. Ibid., 202–4.

442 Zeiss, *Seuchen-Atlas*, Map VII/4a titled "Malariavorkommen und Fiebermückenverreitung in Griechenland" indicates that German research activities extended to Crete, the Kalamata and Megalopolis area, Corinth, Attica, Euboea, Central Greece, Thessaly, the area around Ioannina, Thessaloniki, Macedonia, and Bulgarian-annexed Thrace; also, that the Italians had been active in research in the west of the country south of Albania in 1938 through 1940. I wish to thank Professor Paul Weindling for pointing out this invaluable source.

443 Health Division Region EG History, Conditions found in Greece on arrival 17 November 1944, Salonika region, 22, folder Greece 38 Region EG, Health Division Final Report, box 36, PAG-4/4.2:36 [S-0524-

To contain outbreaks of typhus epidemics in Thessaloniki, the Swiss Red Cross supplied the Greek medical authorities with small quantities of a Swiss lice-killing insecticide, dichloro-diphenyltrichloroethane (later named DDT), produced by Geigy under the Neocid and Gesarol trademarks. In the summer of 1943, Athanasios Mandekos, a 1930s RF trainee now stationed at Langadas, obtained some Neocid from the Thessaloniki representative of the Swiss Red Cross. Mandekos conducted small-scale experiments on *Anopheles* mosquitoes and discovered in Neocid an alternative method of malaria control.[444]

Thanks to the distribution policy of Geigy itself, the same chemical was being tested at the time in a number of European locations. Geigy tested it on lice in 1941 to protect Switzerland from typhus spreading from refugees and, in September 1942, supplied the Swiss Army with Neocid.[445] In late 1943, the Luftwaffe tested Gesarol near the Azov Sea coast for typhus and malaria control. Several research papers appeared, as a result, in German-language scientific journals in Germany and Switzerland in 1943 and 1944. Indeed, Gerhard Rose (1896–1992), director of the tropical medicine department at the Robert Koch Institute in Berlin, predicted that the use of this compound would revolutionize the war on vector-borne diseases. He was later convicted as a war criminal for his malaria and typhus experiments on concentration camp prisoners.[446]

At the same time, with the full support of the scientific and military capacity of the United States, the US Army conducted extensive confidential wartime experiments, unaware of the new scientific literature in German.[447] In October 1942, the Bureau of Entomology and Plant Quarantine

---

0060]; United Nations Relief and Rehabilitation Administration, Health Division, Region EG, History, Christos Damkas, Chapter X: "Malaria" 561–562, folder Greece 38, Region EG, Health Division Final Report, box 36, PAG-4/4.2.:36 [S-0524-0060], UN Archives.

444 By the end of their relief work in Greece in February 1945, the Swiss Red Cross had supplied the country with 2,665 kg of Neocid powder and another 500 kg of Neocid emulsion. Comité International de la Croix-Rouge, *Ravitaillement*, 475n1, annex III, 55. Mandekos had his paper translated into German and published in the 1944 issue of the *Deutsche Tropenmedizinische Zeitschrift*, apparently with no further impact on malaria control in Greece. Personal interview with A. Mandekos, Athens, 22 November 2003.

445 Perkins, "Reshaping," 172. Citing a company-sponsored history, Perkins notes that in 1942 Geigy "informed the diplomatic representatives of the belligerent powers in Bern about DDT and sent samples of the material to Geigy representatives outside Switzerland with instructions to approach the governments of the countries in which they were located." Perkins, "Reshaping," 172.

446 Rose, "Fortschritte," 200–201 and 211–17; Vondra, "Die Malaria," 122–23.

447 This is evident in the surprise that Fred Soper, the RF malariologist, expressed in his diary after the end of the war. F. L. Soper's diary 1944–1946, entry for 20 January 1946, box 58, RG 12.1, RAC. In a 1948 in-

of the US Department of Agriculture acquired the same substance from the Geigy office in New York and began testing it at the bureau's laboratories in Orlando, Florida. Further experiments were held in Tennessee, Arkansas, Mexico, North Africa, and the Pacific. The engineers of the Tennessee Valley Authority, who experimented with the airborne spraying of Paris green, did the same with DDT in the mid-1940s.[448]

Meanwhile, as the Allies were planning for the postwar world, Greece, already a party to the London-based Inter-Allied Committee on Post-War Requirements, was to be a beneficiary of the Middle East Relief and Refugee Administration (MERRA), set up by the British in July 1942 and was also a signatory of the agreement of 9 November 1943 that founded UNRRA. MERRA, a military organization, merged with UNRRA, a civilian agency, when the latter succeeded it under the terms of the Cairo agreement of 3 April 1944. This agreement also set up the UNRRA Balkan mission for Greece, Yugoslavia and Albania, with subordinate missions for each country. Health relief in Greece was the domain of the mission's medical division.[449]

The UNRRA staff left the Cairo Balkan Mission headquarters and landed in Greece on 23 October 1944, a mere five days after the Greek government and at the tail end of the malaria season. Its medical staff, which arrived with this first group, saw combating malaria as their top priority. UNRRA withdrew most of its staff during the fighting in Athens in December 1944, who returned on 1 April 1945.[450]

The fight against malaria was the responsibility of Daniel E. Wright, the former RF sanitary engineer in Greece, director of the sanitation section of the medical division, and a colonel in the US Public Health Service. Indeed,

terview, Daniel E. Wright noted that the first US experiments in 1942 tested the value of DDT as a moth destroyer. Written interview to the newspaper *Vradyni*, 10 May 1948, folder 4, box 1, D. E. Wright papers.

448 Stapleton, "The Dawn of DDT," 150–51. Fred Soper of the RF began testing DDT on typhus control in Algeria in August 1943. See Soper, *Ventures in World Health*, 277. In the 1930s, M. A. Barber, an RF malariologist, had found Greek Macedonia similar in climate to Tennessee. About ten years later, in 1943, while "experimenting with DDT in the streams of Tennessee and Arkansas" he "used to think of the very accessible Cyprus waters." See Barber, *A Malariologist in Many Lands*, 78 and 98.

449 For the period of military activity, UNRRA would serve as a British–US Allied Military Liaison (AML) agency. Woodbridge, *UNRRA*, vol. 1, 9, 21, 81–85, 88, and vol. 2, 130–31.

450 "Participation of UNRRA in the Balkans: Greece, Yugoslavia and Albania during the Period of Military Responsibility," UNRRA *Health Division Monthly Bulletin*, vol. 1, no. 3, November 1944, 5, box 16, PAG-4/4.2; The Balkan Mission, 13, folder Origins 16, Origins of the Balkan Mission, box 17, PAG-4/4.2, UN Archives; Close, "War, Medical Advance," 9; Alexander, *The Prelude to the Truman Doctrine*, 220.

his very reason for joining UNRRA was to defeat malaria in Greece. In August 1944, still in Cairo, he advised "UNRRA against sending malariologists into Greece on the basis that there is an adequate number of good men in the country."[451] In a 1948 interview, Wright gave the following account of his commitment to the use of DDT in Greece and of the close interconnection between military and civilian exigencies:

> There was simply no chance of obtaining supplies [of DDT] in quantity for civilian use until the needs of the army were taken care of. . . . Greece has the distinction of being the first country in the world where an effort was made on a nationwide scale to protect its civilian population. It was my experience with the use of DDT in the army, and observations made at the experimental stations at Orlando Fla. and Memphis Tenn. that convinced me, that if material could be made available and a force trained in its use DDT would solve one of the age-old curses of Greece, and every pressure that it was possible for me to exert, was brought to bear to get the program under way. In this I was fortunate in having the loyal support of the Greek people, who at my request make the largest appropriation of money in the history of the country for carrying out a program with which they were completely unfamiliar, and knew nothing except what I was able to tell them, and a few short incomplete articles, it was possible to get hold of. Most literature published up until late 1945 and early 1946 *of value*, was either restricted or confidential.[452]

Wright convinced the Greek officials and malaria specialists of his plan to conduct a DDT-based campaign "over every malarious area in Greece." His return to the familiar social environment of the Greek malariologists, as well as the limited wartime exposure of these men to the properties of Neo-

451 G. K. Strode's diary, entry for 30 August 1944, 165, RAC. In a report two years later, his deputy chief in the Sanitary Section added an interesting comment on Wright's motives in enlisting in UNRRA: "because of DDT, he joined UNRRA as their Chief Sanitary Engineer," introducing DDT to Greece on a national scale. Gordon E. Smith, Deputy Chief, Sanitation Section, UNRRA, Greece Mission, 31 August 1946, Preliminary report on the uses of DDT in Greece—1946, 1, folder Greece 22, Malaria and Sanitation, box 35, PAG-4/4.2.:35 [S-0524-0059], UN Archives.

452 Written interview to the newspaper *Vradyni*, 10 May 1948, folder 4, box 1, D. E. Wright papers; emphasis in the English original. In the same interview, he stated: "Late in 1944 and early 1945 it was possible for me through my acquaintances in the army to obtain a fairly large quantity of 10 percent DDT powder for delousing work. . . . In early 1945 pure DDT was very difficult to obtain, and only as a special favor were we able to obtain a small quantity for demonstration purposes. This was carefully and strategically used in various parts of the country for propaganda, while at the same time we were applying the old methods of oil, Paris green, drainage etc. This method of letting the people know first hand the value of DDT was of far more value than any amount of literature that might have been circulated."

cid, may have helped the initial stage of his work.[453] Clearly, the nationwide scale of the operation and airborne antilarval spraying, in disregard of medical opinion or of any initial testing phase, had been vital components in Wright's program from the outset.[454]

As soon as the UNRRA staff returned to Greece in April 1945, antimalaria work began, mainly by means of the old methods. The first 20 tons of DDT that became available in 1945 were disseminated over the entire country and used in hand spraying, with enormous propaganda effect. The government doubled its appropriation for 1946, some communities contributed voluntary labor, and UNRRA also fell into line with its support for the program. The airplane spraying program got in full swing in the late spring of 1946; the early reports on the decline of malaria incidence were encouraging. However, quite early in the day, Grigorios Livadas, the leading malariologist in Greece, who was working closely with Wright, warned against relying exclusively on the wonders of the new chemical; DDT could become the basis of the malaria program, he claimed, without replacing all other malaria control methods. Most importantly, drainage projects should be resumed, in combination with land reclamation schemes.[455]

UNRRA's DDT program in Greece consumed half of the United States's industrial production of the substance. The country received the approximate equivalent of 300 tons of pure DDT in a variety of solutions, representing the lion's share of UNRRA's total DDT shipping program for malaria control. No other country in UNRRA's program came even close to receiv-

---

453 Region ABJ, Athens 30 November 1946, 41, folder Greece 35, Health Division Historical Report, box 36, PAG-4/4.2.:36 [S-0524-0060], UN Archives.

454 In December 1944, Fred Soper, the RF authority in malaria control, with over a year of experience with DDT already, with whom Wright kept in contact, noted in his diary: "Dan Wright went into Greece leaving all medical malariologists behind explaining that Greece had Livadas and others. Then sent out one of his men with instructions to arrange purchase of 8 cub planes with equipment for spraying DDT." F. L. Soper's diary 1944–1946, entry for 29 December 1944, box 58, RG 12.1. See also F. L. Soper to G. K. Strode, 13 July 1945, folder 15, box 2, series 749 I, RG 1.1, RAC.

455 D. E. Wright, "Report on the activities of the Sanitation Section of the Health Division UNRRA from November 1944 to December 1946," 11–12, folder Greece 22, Malaria and Sanitation, box 35, PAG-4/4.2.:35 [S-0524-0059], UN Archives; Sawyer, "Achievements of UNRRA," 53–54; G. Livadas, "A Brief Review of [the] Malaria Problem and Malaria Control Activities In Modern Greece," 2 November 1945, 5, folder Greece 22, Malaria and Sanitation, box 35, PAG-4/4.2.:35 [S-0524-0059]; Francis Hennessey, "Historical Survey UNRRA Health Division F Region," 17, folder Greece 39, Region F, Health Division Historical Survey, box 36, PAG-4/4.2.:36 [S-0524-0060], UN Archives. Livadas also feared that the existing malaria service, which he headed, would lose its influence, a fear which soon proved justified when, in August 1946, the government assigned the responsibility for malaria control to the regional health centers.

ing as much.[456] At the height of its activities in 1946, the sanitary engineering section in Greece employed fifteen men and it was second in size only to that of China.[457] Besides UNRRA and the RF, the campaign also drew on the support of the Greek Army, the British Army in areas in which it had an interest, while the government invited the US Navy's 404th Epidemiological Unit to assist with epidemiological surveys.[458]

UNRRA's malaria control program in Greece was essentially in the hands of the scientists of the RF's IHD. The same was largely true of the entire division, whose director, Wilbur Sawyer, had resigned from the RF to assume the UNRRA position.[459] The attack on malaria was influenced by the idea of mosquito eradication, a program propounded by Soper, even before the advent of DDT, on the basis of his experience in Brazil and Egypt. In the eyes of the RF scientists, DDT promised to be an effective method of eradication. Their approach to the Greek case was predicated on their expectations of solving, precisely, an eradication problem. To this end, they were prepared to tolerate Wright's unorthodox procedures.[460]

For the RF, UNRRA provided a short-term administrative and logistical framework through which they could promote the foundation's health programs. However, the US government withdrew its support from UNRRA in 1946, as the Cold War unfolded, when the political climate within which

---

456 This amounted to 68 percent of its shipments of 20 percent DDT solution, used for airplane spraying; 27 percent of the total 26 percent solution, used for residual house spraying; and 37 percent of the total of pure (100 percent) DDT powder. Packard, "'No Other Logical Choice,'" 222; Sawyer, "Achievements of UNRRA," 47. The figures for Italy are 24 percent of the 26 percent solution and 28 percent of pure 100 percent DDT powder. Greece also received 3 percent of UNRRA's total DDT shipments of 10 percent DDT powder for typhus control.

457 Frederick F. Aldridge, Sanitary Engineer (R), USPHS, Chief, Sanitary Engineering Branch, Health Division, UNRRA, Washington, "The Sanitary Engineering Activities of UNRRA," 18, folder Health Division HE 5, The Sanitary Engineering Activities of UNRRA, box 16, PAG-4/4.2, UN Archives.

458 J.M. Vine, "Malaria control on a national scale—Greece, 1946," p. 13–14, Malaria and Sanitation, folder Greece #22, box 35, PAG-4/4.2.:35 [S-0524-0059], UN Archives; G. Livadas, "A Brief Review of [the] Malaria Problem and Malaria Control Activities in Modern Greece," 2 November 1945, p. 4, folder Greece 22, Malaria and Sanitation, box 35, PAG-4/4.2.:35 [S-0524-0059]; Gordon E. Smith, San. (R) USPHS, Deputy Chief, Sanitation Section, UNRRA, Greece Mission, 31 August 1946, Preliminary report on the uses of DDT in Greece—1946, 2, folder Greece 22, Malaria and Sanitation, box 35, PAG-4/4.2.:35 [S-0524-0059]; Dr. K. Robicek, Regional Medical Officer, Region D, Historical Report of UNRRA Health Division, Patra, 15 November 1946, 6–7, folder Greece 36, Health Division Historical Report, box 36, PAG-4/4.2.:36 [S-0524-0060], UN Archives.

459 Farley, *To Cast Out Disease*, 144.

460 Ibid., 142–44; F. L. Soper to G. K. Strode, 13 July 1945, folder 15, box 2, series 749 I, RG 1.1, RFA, RAC; Stapleton, "The Dawn of DDT," 152. For the circumspect use of DDT, see Mandekos, "I exafanisis ton anofelon."

UNRRA operated in Greece deteriorated. In Greece, the 31 March 1946 elections, the first in ten years, brought to power a right-wing government intent on centralizing and purging the civil service of left-wing sympathizers, exercising political patronage and cutting off the left from access to supplies. At the height of the malaria campaign, the country was on the brink of civil war. As a result, UNRRA's malaria campaign lost some of its best Greek scientists and technical staff.[461] In this new phase of its relations with UNRRA, the government, jealous of its sovereignty, handed over the operation of the antimalarial program to the Greek state authorities. Thereafter, the regional Joint Medical Supplies Committees were to assume exclusive responsibility for medical supplies and drugs at the expense of UNRRA, which withdrew from Greece in June 1947.[462]

The Civil War in Greece interfered with the DDT program in other ways as well. Wright complained that many of the pilots he had trained for aerial spraying had been drafted in the army. Thus,

> due to the revolution, we were robbed of all but six of the thirty-five spray pilots we trained, and as a result spray work this year has been badly retarded, while an effort has been made to train new men. This has resulted in a deluge of telegrams from all areas begging to have the work done. Seventy-five percent of the rural population sleep in their fields as a protection to their crops during the summer months, and while they were able to drop down any place during 46 and 47 in absolute comfort, this year they are being devoured in areas we have been unable to reach, and there is a special cry from the rice field areas.[463]

The work of residual spraying teams was subject to political disruption and was often confronted and obstructed by both government and rebel suspicion; government agents "objected to the groups going from village to village, for fear that certain members might convey messages to rebel friends," while, at the same time, rebels "were afraid that certain members of the gangs sent in for work were government agents, and use the malaria work as

461 Close, "War, Medical Advance," 10; Close and Veremis, "The Military Struggle," 101; Vassiliou, "Politics, Public Health, and Development," 198–204; Francis Hennessey, "Historical Survey UNRRA Health Division F Region," 15–18, folder Greece 39, Region F, Health Division Historical Survey, box 36, PAG-4/4.2.:36 [S-0524-0060], UN Archives.

462 "History of the Office of Public Information. UNRRA. Greece Mission, February 1947. Residual Impressions," 18, folder Greece 6, box 33, PAG-4/4.2 and Francis Hennessey, "Historical Survey UNRRA Health Division F Region," 17, folder Greece 39, Region F, Health Division Historical Survey, box 36, PAG-4/4.2.:36 [S-0524-0060], UN Archives.

463 D. E. Wright to G. K. Strode, Athens, 19 July 1948 (copy), folder 4, box 1, D. E. Wright papers.

a screen to get as much information as possible as to rebel strength etc." The problem of obstruction affected work in the villages rather than swamps and river beds, over which aerial spraying was allowed to continue.[464]

The success of the DDT program in reducing malaria incidence captured the enthusiasm of the war-weary population immediately, wherever it was applied. Without "getting caught up in other policy issues which would divert or delay attention given to malaria,"[465] Wright, who had left the country with the departure of UNRRA, arranged for his return to the Greek malaria program as a staff member of the RF within the framework of the Interim Committee of the WHO, which was implementing some of the foundation's ideas on disease control and malaria eradication in particular. Interestingly, in its early years, the WHO kept its distance from contested issues of social welfare, preferring rather to deal with politically neutral technical problems and specific diseases, an approach that favored vertical disease control programs.[466]

Like much else, the occupation shattered continuity in malaria control. As a result, malaria morbidity was far worse by the end of the war, which, however, gave rise to new international institutions and technologies in health relief, such the work of the UNRRA medical division, including in its relief baggage to Greece the revival of the RF approach and DDT, a wartime technological product of the powerful US techno-scientific complex, as well as the administration's largest DDT malaria program. The RF's influence on the use of DDT in malaria control transferred smoothly from UNRRA to the WHO framework. The same relief effort launched the invasive ideology of global disease eradication, which the WHO also inherited from UNRRA. This latter program helped the WHO to dissociate itself from broader international Cold War tensions and to offer Greece a viable peacetime solution.

---

464 [D. E. Wright], Three-page report, [1947], folder 4, box 1, D. E. Wright papers. Despite a long list of difficulties that the spraying campaign faced in 1947, the author of the document, Wright in all likelihood, noted a marked reduction in malaria cases on the basis of clinical data that seemed to point to a break in malaria transmission. "The most encouraging and convincing evidence of the successful results from the control work is found from the absence of malaria among babies a year old and under, as examination of blood smear show [sic]." Ibid.

465 Litsios, "Malaria Control," 272.

466 A. J. Warren's diary, entry for 9 December 1946, 112; entry for 13 January 1947, 5, RAC; Farley, *To Cast Out Disease*, 273 and 284–85. Several months later, in September 1947, the American Mission for Aid to Greece (AMAG) set up its Health Division in Greece. AMAG and, subsequently, the US Economic Cooperation Administration (ECA) mission in Greece took over the reorganization of the state health services and contributed funds. For their part, the members of the WHO mission worked in Greece on malaria and other specific health issues until April 1949.

CHAPTER IV

PATIENTS, DOCTORS, AND CURES

This chapter looks at the malaria patient and his relationship to treatment, physicians, and health care. The space of medical knowledge shared by doctors and their patients, the social, cultural, and epidemiological implications of the extensive use of quinine are topics also discussed. Defining who the malaria patient was in the past needs to take into account a variety of parameters. As with most older diseases, the list of modern medical designations, in the words of Christopher Hamlin, "seem to be the legacy of laborious generalization at some remote time."[1]

The terminology employed by doctors who adopted germ theory conformed to a nosological category, which corresponds to our current idea of malaria. Doctors working within the miasmatic paradigm, however, used terms that referred to a different and very broad set of fevers. This set included quotidian, tertian, and quartan intermittent, or periodic fevers, which may be interpreted effectively to also broadly correspond to our current understanding of the disease despite the fact that both the conceptual location of disease and diagnostic methods differed. As explained by Christopher Hamlin, by the eighteenth century, exposure to place added toxins to the external causes of fever.[2] Typically, in his toxicology textbook published in 1843, Xavier Landerer (1809–1885), professor of chemistry at the University of Athens and court pharmacist, wrote for his medical students about the effects of contagious substances and miasmata that, he thought, introduced poisons into the human body. The former spread infections by direct

---

1   Hamlin, *More Than Hot*, 35.
2   Ibid., 84.

or indirect physical contact with the contagious agent or was carried in the wind from infected animals, causing diseases such as syphilis, leprosy, cancer, smallpox, typhus, and plague. They were to be distinguished from the miasmata, which were airborne particles of decayed matter. Not much was known about the chemical composition of this "unknown enemy" but, as Landerer speculated, they were probably due to water and heat along with "some particular electrical condition in the atmosphere" and "fostered" epidemic diseases such as "the intermittent fever in Lamia, Karavasaras and scores of other places" and endemic diseases, that is, "those appearing almost every summer and ending in the autumn."[3]

The set also included other fever types, described by terms suggesting frequency or duration rather than periodicity, such as "remittent" and "continuous;" along with the term "typhoid fever," which was often used, that may not necessarily be reduced to malaria. In his account of fevers in 1821 Cefalonia, John Hennen associated remittent fevers with marshes, remarking that "the remittent of that year showed itself in the genuine character of the product of marsh miasmata."[4] Georgios Karamitsas later taught his miasmatic regime medical students that marshland diseases developed in five different "classes": intermittent, latent or *febris larvatae*, malignant, and remittent fevers, and marshland cachexia.[5] A. Antoniadis divided malignant fevers depending on the origin of the symptoms they produced, namely into those of the nervous, the circulatory, the respiratory, the digestive systems and of the skin. According to Dionysios Oikonomopoulos, malignant fevers were divided into those whose virulence was due to the seriousness of any one of the fever stages and those which were aggravated by a dangerous organ failure.[6] In 1908, Kardamatis criticized earlier doctors for devising a very extensive nomenclature for malaria fevers and proposed a reduced set of terms.[7]

Regarding the understanding of fevers, however, miasmatic theory was not a static explanatory framework. In the seventeenth and eighteenth cen-

---

3 Landerer, *Toxikologia*, 3–8.

4 Hennen, *Sketches*, 289.

5 Karamitsas, "Peri elodon i eleiogenon nosimaton," vol. 2, 739 and 750–53.

6 Karamitsas, "Oliga tina peri ton en Athinais dialeiponton pyreton," 140ff.; Antoniadis, "Praktikon skhediasma peri kakoithon pyreton," cited in Karamitsas, "Peri elodon i eleiogenon nosimaton," vol. 2, 754; Oikonomopoulos, "Pragmateia peri kakoithon pyreton," cited in Karamitsas, "Peri elodon i eleiogenon nosimaton."

7 Kardamatis, *Pragmateia*, 239–41 and 333–40.

turies, it underwent significant changes. When "description turned from the proximate and observable to the origins or ultimate causes of disease, invariably the discussion once more turned to physiology."[8] Explanations, thus, focused on blood circulation and consistency. Interest in various aspects of the workings of the body would now explain diseases but, as Geyer-Kordesch argues, medical consensus regarding fevers broke down completely, as doctors looked to "chemiatric, mechanistic, vitalist and other explanations."[9] Fever nomenclature indicated different fever patterns, which, in turn, denoted different fevers. They all, however, were to be attributed "to a more simple and uniform set of internal disturbances" that ought to dictate treatment.[10] As for the immediate causes of fever forms, miasmatic theory physicians held that they could be multiple and complex; fever forms could evolve from one into another and could also interact.[11] Karamitsas was unable to resolve the question how, although both were cured by quinine, simple intermittent fevers could turn malignant, but he suspected that purging and bleeding could be one of the causes which weakened the patient's body. He also drew a clear distinction between intermittent, remittent, and continuous fevers on the one hand and typhoid fever on the other, the latter of which was also endemic and likewise broke out in epidemics. These fevers may coincide and were difficult to tell apart but, he wrote, "typhoid fevers are more frequent than remittent fevers, which become more widespread only when an epidemic of intermittent fevers prevails."[12]

In this scientific context, observation raised the physical environment to prominence as one among such immediate causes of fever.[13] Karamitsas, indeed, noted that "newcomers to a place are more easily attacked by intermittent fevers than locals, who rather suffer from cachexia" and recommended that newcomers "fully observe the customs and diet of the locals."[14]

Moreover, relocating a term as a cause rather than an effect contributed further complexity to the confusion. For instance, as noted in chapter 3, for John Davy, the British physician in the Ionian Islands, "malaria"—was not a

---

8   Geyer-Kordesch, "Fevers and Other Fundamentals," 100.
9   Ibid.
10 Ibid., 106–7.
11 Karamitsas, "Peri elodon i eleiogenon nosimaton," vol. 2, 753.
12 Ibid., vol. 2, 668–69, 730–37, 772–77, and 784.
13 Bynum, "Cullen," 139–43.
14 Karamitsas, "Peri elodon i eleiogenon nosimaton," vol. 2, 737 and 795.

disease per se but the "presumed" cause of remittent and intermittent fevers and, possibly, of "the continued and ephemeral fevers also of warm climates."[15] As febrifuges were tried on fever patients indiscriminately, backward diagnosis, in other words differentiating between fevers cured by the bark or quinine and those which eluded this treatment, was not uncommon.[16] As far as nineteenth-century British doctors were concerned, it was predominantly those with overseas experience who appreciated the value of Peruvian bark in treating fever mainly thanks to the time they had served overseas.

Before Laveran, few doctors questioned miasmatic theory. Hennen, however, cited a local practitioner in Cefalonia, who attributed the July 1821 "formidable" epidemic of remittent, intermittent, and continued fevers to "the neglected state of agriculture in the Morea, owing to the political distractions of that country." Miasmatic explanations were, apparently, insufficient to account for the severity of that epidemic that "even contagion was called in."[17]

The Greek doctors who read the European medical literature translated its terminology, readily adopting the familiar Hippocratic terms.[18] Then, soon after Laveran's discovery, Karamitsas cautiously dedicated several paragraphs to it in his medical textbook. "According to the currently dominant theory, the marshland miasma is considered to be caused by a parasite. Some observers have indeed affirmed that they have found it." After describing the *Oscillaria malariae* that Laveran had witnessed and named, Karamitsas added a note of warning that the discovery may still prove false.[19] Unconvinced, however, by the vague diagnostic methodologies of contemporary internal medicine, Karamitsas looked to further advances in medical research and stated: "Clearly, if there were no doubts about the parasite of the bad air fevers and if this was found in the blood, we would need no other sign to make a diagnosis."[20]

---

15   Davy, *Notes and Observations*, vol. 2, 241.
16   See Karamitsas, "Oliga tina peri ton en Athinais dialeiponton pyreton," 149; Smith, "Medical Science," 123–24.
17   Hennen, *Sketches*, 290.
18   In 1841, Ioannis Asanis, a Greek physician trained in Padua, Vienna, and Paris, listed nineteen forms of intermittent fevers and suggested that further studies could produce an even longer list. Rubino, *Peri tou armodioterou tropou*, v–ix. See also Karamperopoulos, "Oi periodikoi i dialeipontes pyretoi," 26.
19   Karamitsas, "Peri elodon i eleiogenon nosimaton," vol. 2, 732–33. Laveran had, in fact, seen *P. falciparum* gametocytes.
20   Karamitsas, "Peri elodon i eleiogenon nosimaton," vol. 2, 785.

After 1885, when Paris-trained physician Spyridon Kanellis published a thesis on microbes, and as germ theory gained ground as the framework for understanding fevers, the need emerged, not merely for descriptive terms, but for specific causal designations that would represent the new nosological entities meaningfully in the Greek language identifying specific diseases that would not be reduced to another.[21] Terms were devised to name the causal agents of malaria *praecox* or *falciparum*, *vivax*, and *malariae* and translated as *plasmodion prooron, plasmodion zoiron* and *eloparasiton tou tetartaiou*, respectively.[22]

Some names for incidents of fever epidemics were entirely local and lay in usage. For instance, in Argos, every few years underground water levels rose causing floods; the locals called the event *trimeri* (three-day incident), which, they knew, invariably coincided with lethal fever epidemics.[23]

After decades of intensive medical experience, the terms *"elodi"* and *"eleiogeni nosimata"* (diseases generated by marshes) that associated fevers with marshes, were in circulation in the mid-1870s and 1880s, for instance, in Karamitsas's teaching and textbook. Unlike many of his contemporaries, Karamitsas was unambiguous and quite modern in his definition of this fever category as a specific disease; despite its several forms it was generated by a single cause. "The name of marsh diseases comprises many disease forms," he noted, "which are generated by the influence of *one and the same miasma*, called marshland miasma, usually appear at the same time in the same place, transform into one another, present many common pathological and anatomical phenomena and are cured by the same specific drug, quinine."[24]

The current term *"elonosia"* (marsh disease) did not exist in the Greek medical literature before the end of the nineteenth century. It took, in fact, some years of heated debating among doctors until the term *"elonosia"* came into general usage by around 1910.[25] It would, moreover, be impossible to draw a direct correspondence between the nosological entities across the divide opened by germ theory and Laveran's discovery in 1880. It is safe to say merely that some of the diagnoses of miasmatic medicine, principally those

21 Kanellis, *Ta mikrovia*; Karamperopoulos, "Oi periodikoi i dialeipontes pyretoi," 26.

22 Kardamatis, *Pragmateia*, 121ff. *Eloparasiton tou vareos therinofthinoporinou* or *tropikou pyretou* and *eloparasiton tou ipiou tritaiou* were used as alternative names for *falciparum* and *vivax* malaria.

23 Karamitsas, "Peri elodon i eleiogenon nosimaton," vol. 2, 730–31.

24 Ibid., vol. 2, 728–29; emphasis added.

25 Karamperopoulos, "Oi periodikoi i dialeipontes pyretoi," 26.

diagnosed as cases of intermittent fevers, would also be identified as malaria by doctors of the germ-theory paradigm. Likewise, physical descriptions such as enlarged spleens and cachexia are precise and consistent epidemiological indicators of endemic malaria prevalence. Thus, contemporary estimates of case mortality or other rates should be taken as nothing more than reliable indications.[26]

Lack of microscopes in diagnostic practice prevented most physicians from identifying *Plasmodia* species, led to the exclusive use of clinical diagnoses, and prolonged the use of older, pre-germ-theory, descriptive terminology from a medical cosmology before the age of the laboratory. Indeed, some publications adopted both sets of disease identifications, one based on clinical symptoms and another on *Plasmodia* species.[27]

These historical limitations set constraints on the discussion that follows. The broad picture of malaria as an extremely serious endemic public health issue remains nonetheless valid, whatever the paradigmatic context of the diagnoses and, moreover, defined the pervasive daily physical experience of the Greeks.[28]

PATIENTS

The hope to become owners of the land that covers the remains of their ancestors, who had longed for centuries for the day of independence, and of their children, who each year had been decimated by endemic fevers, was more effective in saving them from sinking into decline and total degeneracy than the presence of a priest, who performed his religious rituals mechanically and who was just as ignorant and incompetent as themselves to transmit the sacred legacy of the divine word, which elevates the spirit to disregard the ephemeral pains of this life and prepares it to enjoy the eternal benefits of the future.[29]

---

26 In 1882 Karamitsas complained about the lack of malaria statistics; data was sporadic and from hearsay. See Karamitsas, "Oliga tina peri ton en Athinais dialeiponton pyreton," 143.

27 Triantaphyllakos and Oeconomou, *Le paludisme*, 24–25 and 31–40. On the history of medical cosmology, see Jewson, "The Disappearance of the Sick-Man."

28 In 1882, Karamitsas attributed the absence of statistics to the abolition of state doctors after 1862; state doctors, he argued, should once again be reinstated and compile regular reports on diseases. Karamitsas, "Oliga tina peri ton en Athinais dialeiponton pyreton," 143–44.

29 Kalligas, *Thanos Vlekas*, 181.

The sarcastic social commentary in this passage by Pavlos Kalligas[30] suggests that the pain of the Greek peasantry at the loss of their children to fevers was a powerful experience that bound them to the land of their children's graves. In a different tone, the French author Edmond About noted how Greek parents, poor and powerful alike, took child loss in their stride.

> Mothers' emulation should have resulted in the doubling of the population of the kingdom in twenty years; however, fever has put a check on this. In the summer, children die like flies. Those who live, mostly have thin legs and bloated abdomens until the age of thirteen or fourteen. Parents save those they can and do not cry too much over the others; they know that until the age of thirteen their children's lives are provisional. One day, I asked a high-ranking official how many children he had. He counted on his fingers and replied: "Eleven or twelve, I don't know; I have seven left."[31]

The adult experience with malarial fevers survived in metaphors for fear, masterfully illustrated in the following passage, which reflects the social tensions brewing in a rural community of the Peloponnese from Kalligas's *Thanos Vlekas*: "How is it with your master? We understand the situation throughout the village was feverish, but in the cold stage, which precedes the convulsion."[32] Edmond About had also a few words to say about the universal experience of adults and their tolerance of fevers and adopted the common notion of the time that malaria was a disease of the nervous system. "Fortunately, the Greek race is so high-strung [*nerveuse*] that fevers kill only the young children: adult men have some attacks in the spring; they put a stop to the fever and forget about it until the autumn."[33]

Christopher Hamlin noted about early modern Europe that chroniclers and diarists demonstrated a "relative lack of interest in epidemics that were not plague" and, furthermore, that "fevers remained a matter of individual bodies."[34] Considering, however, the ubiquity of malaria fevers in modern Greece, it is surprising that, contrary to narratives of tuberculosis, very few direct references to malaria may be found in works of fiction. Notable ex-

---

30 Pavlos Kalligas (1814–1896), a writer, professor of law, and a leading Greek statesman, was a friend of Kharilaos Trikoupis. For a biography, see Masson-Vincourt, *Paul Calligas*.
31 About, *La Grèce contemporaine*, 168.
32 Kalligas, *Thanos Vlekas*, 206.
33 About, *La Grèce contemporaine*, 11.
34 Hamlin, *More Than Hot*, 89.

ceptions in the case of Greek literature may be found in Ioannis Kondyla-kis's *Proti agapi* (First love) and Penelope Delta's *Mystika tou valtou*. Indeed, in both works the storyline focuses on other developments: on the fear of tuberculosis in *Proti agapi*, and on heroic actions in Delta's work. A small number of other works, such as the *Zitianos* (The beggar) by Andreas Kar-kavitsas, treat malaria merely as a social backdrop. The fictitious small vil-lage of Nykhteremi in the Thessalian plain shortly after the accession of Thessaly to Greece, was a desolate place of disease, where fever "the insatia-ble ghoul, sucks human blood to the bone."[35] A possible explanation of this paradox may lie in the very banality of the malarial experience among the Greek reading public. As G. Antonakopoulos has argued convincingly, an oil painting by Theodoros Rallis (1852–1909) titled "By the Fireplace" actu-ally depicts a crouched young girl shivering with malaria by a lit fireplace, while the hot summer sun is shining through the open window.[36]

Malaria epidemics affected everyone. A fever epidemic in Cefalonia of July 1821 "extended itself to all classes, ages, and sexes," who "crowded the hospitals."[37] Malaria even struck royals. Edmond About, who was unfriendly to King Othon, attributed the king's deafness to his protracted use of quinine sulphate.[38] King Alexandros (1893–1920), who died young from an infection caused by a bite from his pet monkey, was said to have had a history of malaria according to one of the Greek physicians who treated his terminal illness.[39]

Some social groups were, however, more exposed to malaria than oth-ers. As noted in chapter 3, soldiers and military officers suffered from such exposure but had better access to medical attention and quinine. Likewise, railway employees also were afforded particular medical attention by their companies; many of the respondents to the Anti-Malaria League surveys conducted between 1905 and 1907 stated that they provided their medical services to the employees of the local lines. On some occasions, factory own-ers, notably the Retsinas family, who owned a textile industry in Piraeus, distributed quinine to their workers to keep them healthy.[40] Even a small number of landowners in Thessaly and Fthiotis were reported to have tried,

---

35 Karkavitsas, *O zitianos*, 25.
36 Antonakopoulos, "I elonosia kata zografiki apodosi Theodorou Ralli."
37 Hennen, *Sketches*, 289.
38 About, *La Grèce contemporaine*, 291.
39 Skampardonis, Skhizas, and Antonakopoulos, "To khroniko."
40 Kalopisis, "Iatrikes morfes."

at least to care for the health of their tenants and had housing built for them at a distance from the source of infection. As seen in chapter 3, the owners of the Megali Vrysis estate had housing built for some of their tenants and staff, but had failed to provide protection. The same was true about one of the successive landowners of the Dimitrias estate in Almyros. In his wartime malaria prevalence tables, Kardamatis published a list of names of large estate owners alongside the malaria prevalence figures for their estates, suggesting that they were largely responsible for the health of their tenants.[41]

Environmental factors and exposure to malaria aside, access to medical attention and medication remained the defining factor in the social impact of malaria incidence and experience. Gender moreover was important from a social perspective. As noted below, it appears that men diagnosed with intermittent fevers visited the Athens Astykliniki at higher percentages than women; it is likely that male work outdoors increased their exposure to the disease. By contrast, the widowed gleaners, or *stakhomazokhtres*, of Mani, who lay at the lower end of the social scale, exposed themselves to the hardships of gleaning after the harvest and were particularly heavily struck by malaria.[42] More generally, Kardamatis, further disagreed with his European colleagues that men were more exposed to malaria than women, arguing that Greek peasant women shared the farm work with men.[43]

Often, access to quinine determined whether some communities suffered less than others, as demonstrated in Kardamatis's nationwide statistics of 1921 and 1922. According to Kardamatis, in the immediate postwar years, when the price of quinine fluctuated heavily, access to quinine depended, to a considerable extent, on the poor rural and isolated communities being able to pay for the high price of the drug.[44]

Patients' inclination to seek medical attention may be associated with the degree of medicalization and the social construction of their own physical condition and that of their children. In the words of John Hennen, the Greeks of his day tended "to trust their diseases to nature, or at least to the most simple remedies, and rarely have recourse to a physician until their disease becomes very violent or painful."[45] When, in 1834, the refugees from

---

41 "1907," 534–43.
42 Dikaios Vagiakakos, personal communication (March 2006). See also chapter 3.
43 Kardamatis, *Pragmateia*, 63.
44 Kardamatis, "Ekthesis ton pepragmenon kata to etos 1922," 368–69.
45 Hennen, *Sketches*, 196.

Khios in Ermoupolis lost 228 infants below the age of two, Ioannis Vouros, prefecture physician to the Cyclades, noted that all over Greece fevers killed many infants "as it was not treated by doctors on account of the parents' neglect and their prejudice that medicine does not apply to infants."[46]

This, however, gradually changed. Thus, while parents rarely sought medical help for their very young children in the early days, there soon emerged a culture that medicalized childhood, initially in the towns. Several years later, in Athens, the medicalization of childhood appears quite well established, since infants were the largest age group of patients visiting the Astykliniki, the university outpatient clinic. Between 1 April and 30 June 1860 the clinic saw 314 infants, 215 youths, 101 "men," meaning adults, and 70 elderly. Of these patients, 21 infants, 24 youths, 12 adults and 8 elderly were diagnosed and treated for intermittent fevers.[47] Likewise, between 1 January and 31 March 1861 the clinic treated in all 325 infants, 167 youths, 112 adults, and 43 elderly of whom 51 infants, 27 youths, 16 adults, and 6 elderly were treated for intermittent fevers.[48] Throughout 1858, the clinic treated 312 cases of intermittent fevers out of a total of 2240 patients (14%): 174 males, 138 females, 120 children, 109 youths, 59 adults, and 24 elderly.[49] Although the age categories are vague and the terms "infants" and "children" were used inconsistently and often interchangeably, it is clear that, by the mid-nineteenth century Athenian parents had begun to seek medical help for their feverous children. In fact, in 1860, *Asklipios*, the journal of the Athens Medical Society, published an article specifically dealing with childhood intermittent fevers[50] and in 1908, Ioannis Kardamatis dedicated a full chapter to childhood malaria in his textbook.[51]

Pervasive diagnostic inconsistencies notwithstanding, the following table of cases of intermittent fevers treated at the outpatient clinic of the University of Athens between 1858 and 1860 also shows male patients consistently outnumbering females by between 9.4 and 26.2 percent.

46   Vouros, "Nosologiki katastasis," 382–83.
47   "Statistiki tis en Athinais Astyklinikis, deftera triminia tou etous 1860."
48   "Statistiki tis en Athinais Astyklinikis. I proti triminia tou etous 1861."
49   "Pinax genikos ton asthenon tis Astyklinikis tou etous 1858."
50   A. B., "Peri dialeipontos pyretou para tois paisin."
51   Kardamatis, *Pragmateia*. For an extensive treatment of the medicalization of childhood in Greece, see Theodorou and Karakatsani, *Ygieinis parangelmata*.

	July–Sept. 1858	Oct.–Dec. 1858	Jan.–Dec. 1859	April–June 1860	July–Sept. 1860	Oct.–Dec. 1860
Cases	128	82	312	65	470	209
Male	54.7%	62.2%	55.8%	63.1%	62.8%	59.8%
Female	45.3%	37.8%	44.2%	36.9%	37.2%	40.2%
Children	43%	34.1%	38.5%	32.3%	34.5%	31.6%
Youths	35.2%	36.6%	34.9%	36.9%	41.7%	40.2%
Adults	17.2%	22%	18.9%	18.5%	17.4%	18.7%
Elderly	4.7%	7.3%	7.7%	12.3%	6.4%	4.8%

Table 4.1. Malaria at Athens University outpatient clinic, 1858–60

Source: *Asklipios* (1858–1861).

Distribution by age group clearly shows that 42 percent of the patients diagnosed with intermittent fevers were younger than fifteen years old and outnumbered patients twice their age, that is, the age group between fifteen and twenty-nine.[52]

Age group	Cases	Years	Age group mean (cases/years)	Cumulative percentage
1	385	1	385	3.71
2–6	1502	5	300.40	18.19
7–14	2447	8	305.88	41.78
15–29	3863	15	257.53	79.02
30–39	956	10	95.60	88.24
40–49	653	10	65.30	94.53
50–59	357	10	35.70	97.98
60–69	171	10	17.10	99.62
70–79	33	10	3.30	99.94
80–89	3	10	0.30	99.97
90–99	3	10	0.30	100
Total	10373			

Table 4.2. Cases of intermittent fevers at Athens Astykliniki, 1860–70

Source: Karamitsas, "Peri elodon i eleiogenon nosimaton," vol. 2, 736.

---

52 Karamitsas, "Peri elodon i eleiogenon nosimaton," vol. 2, 736. General mortality data by departments and age groups collected by Clôn Stéphanos for the years 1868 to 1878 do not reveal clear distribution patterns that would associate mortality to the effects of malaria. Stéphanos, *La Grèce*, 476–77.

Interestingly, 28 percent of all cases, or 2,924 patients, visited the outpatient clinic in the epidemic year of 1865. In fact, the distribution pattern among age groups observed over the eleven-year period did not change during that epidemic outbreak.[53]

Age group	Cases	Years	Age group mean (cases/years)	Cumulative percentage
1	120	1	120	4.10
2–6	436	5	87.2	19.02
7–14	672	8	84	42.00
15–29	1049	15	69.93	77.87
30–39	253	10	25.3	86.53
40–49	217	10	21.7	93.95
50–59	103	10	10.3	97.47
60–69	57	10	5.7	99.42
70–79	15	10	1.5	99.93
80–89	0	10	0	99.93
90–99	2	10	0.2	100
Total	2,924			

Table 4.3. Cases of intermittent fevers at Athens Astykliniki, 1865

Kardamatis's Astykliniki statistics for the years between 1894 and 1903 suggest that the proportionate malaria burden of young Athenians had improved slightly after the 1860s: only one-fifth, or 20 percent, of its malaria patients were under the age of ten and one-third, or 31 percent, were below the age of fifteen.[54] However, if Kardamatis's statistics of the malaria epidemic in Athens in 1907 on the basis of 443 hospital malaria admissions are indicative, they show that the improvement was not stable and that the epidemic struck young children with particular intensity. Some 30 percent of hospital admissions were children below the age of seven, 58 percent were below the age of seventeen and almost 80 percent were patients below the age of thirty. Most of the cases belonged to the three to seven age group (20%).[55]

53 Karamitsas, "Oliga tina peri ton en Athinais dialeiponton pyreton," 146.
54 Kardamatis, *Pragmateia*, 62.
55 "I okhri panoukla." As Macdonald explained, in areas of unstable transmission the disease hits with "no marked limitation of susceptibility to the youngest age groups," who are left unprotected by immunity. Macdonald, *The Epidemiology and Control of Malaria*, 30.

Age group	Cases	Cumulative percentage
0–1	20	4.51
1–2	20	9.03
3–7	89	29.12
8–12	65	43.79
13–17	63	58.01
18–20	24	63.43
21–30	61	77.20
31–40	35	85.10
41–50	22	90.07
51–60	27	96.16
61–65	7	97.74
66–70	8	99.55
71–75	2	100
N= 443		

Table 4.4. Age distribution, malaria epidemic in Athens, 1907
Source: "I okhri panoukla."

Between 1860 and 1870 malaria cases constituted 30 percent of all admissions to the Astykliniki; this proportion varied annually between one in three and one in nine. However, as Karamitsas argued, malaria was overrepresented in these figures because "almost all patients suffering from intermittent fevers come to the establishment and are registered in its books," whereas most other patients remained at home. In all likelihood, the Astykliniki attracted malaria patients because it offered free quinine treatment. Its patients, moreover, were mostly poor peasants from the periphery of the city and surrounding villages as well as peasants from all across Attica. In other words, there was a strong inbuilt bias in the Astykliniki figures.[56]

Furthermore, the Astykliniki data comprised cases of patients, if they or their parents actively sought medical help. If some age groups were more likely than others to receive treatment at home, and, moreover, if this behavior changed over time, the proportions of these age groups would be affected. Kardamatis's data, however, from rural Oropos and Avlona, northeast of the capital, obtained during the 1905 epidemic, examined cases he

---

56 Karamitsas, "Oliga tina peri ton en Athinais dialeiponton pyreton," 144.

sought out himself. The data, nonetheless, broadly confirms the earlier age distribution pattern: 16 percent of the village inhabitants diagnosed with malaria were below the age of five, one-third, or 32 percent, were below the age of ten, and 54 percent were below the age of twenty.[57] By the age of sixteen, three out of four children in the heavily malarious village of Marathon had developed enlarged spleens and malaria cachexia, a chronic condition with severe anemia and paleness, even among breastfeeding infants. In the village of Moulki near Lake Copais, thirty-five out of fifty children between four and twelve had enlarged spleens; likewise, in Megali Vrysis, eight out of twenty-five children. Out of 108 children aged zero to twelve years with malaria cachexia, eighty-three presented heavily enlarged spleens and the others mildly enlarged spleens. Children in endemic areas who escaped this state were often seen "eating constantly and voraciously, with a piece of bread always in their hands eating nonstop"; thus "they maintain their body in a relative state of equilibrium thanks to their overfeeding."[58]

Having observed symptomless newborns with parasites in their blood in his research in Athens and Attica, Kardamatis emphasized the existence of symptomless malaria cases among infants and children with hereditary or acquired immunity and warned his readers that "these individuals constitute the greatest danger of spreading malaria. Children who appear to be in perfect health after a small number of convulsions, yet carry gametocytes in their blood, represent a similar danger; likewise, children with cachexia, in whose blood one frequently finds gametocytes and occasionally schizonts without outbreaks of fever."[59] He added that he had observed immunity to malaria even in children who had never contracted malaria and, therefore, that "we [Greeks] also have the same kind of natural immunity as the natives of tropical Africa, the Negroes, however, on a much smaller scale."[60]

Parents came to know how to help doctors save their children by rushing them to the local doctor's practice, if they failed to administer quinine themselves.[61]

---

57 Kardamatis, *Pragmateia*, 60.
58 Ibid., 622–26.
59 Ibid., 614.
60 Ibid.
61 Savvas and Kardamatis, "Apantiseis dimarkhon," 489 and 502.

Malaria became socially relevant to childhood in other ways and to such an extent that, in the interwar years, the authorities felt justified in enlisting children in the fight against malaria. Schoolchildren with their teachers' support supplemented the manpower employed in the antimalarial campaign. In the 1930s, near the lakes of Langadas, Giannitsa, and Kastoria and in the marshes of Drama, Serres, Philippi, and Lamia, schoolchildren distributed fish from the local gambusia fisheries to other locations.[62] In the mid-1930s, malariologist Konstantinos Dimissas taught a course in malariology sponsored by the Ministry of Education specifically for the benefit of schoolteachers, who were then expected to train their schoolchildren in the national antimalaria mobilization of the 1930s.[63] His course textbook covered mosquito catching methods, information for identifying *Anopheles* species, details about their habits and principles of malaria epidemiology, protection, and contemporary concepts of bonification.[64] The boys of the refugee camp in Corinth oiled mosquito breeding sites in and around Corinth under the guidance of an American nurse, Alice Carr, with the encouragement of the Corinth municipal authorities.[65] In a similar spirit, in 1938, Grigorios Livadas, head of the Malariology Division of the Athens School of Hygiene, began an experimental school program in malaria control in three villages near Drama in northern Greece. He found out though that, in the summer, his program had to compete with the parents, who needed their children back in the tobacco fields. In one of the class photographs, published by Livadas, a group of boys may be seen wearing uniforms of the Alkimoi paramilitary units, the Metaxas youth movement.[66]

Apart from its effect on the children themselves and on the buildup of population immunity, childhood malaria was, and still is, a key epidemiological index. From the time of Kardamatis's small-scale works on the Ilissos riverbed in the early twentieth century to the postwar DDT program, it measured the effects of malaria control interventions. Indeed, the success of the DDT program in reducing malaria prevalence in Greece to 1/200th of

---

62 Dimissas, *Engkheiridion*, 140.
63 Ibid., 9–10.
64 Ibid., 66, 69–71, 88, 108–10, and 124–25.
65 Morgenthau, *I Was Sent to Athens*, 284.
66 Livadas and Sfangos, *I elonosia en Elladi*, vol. 2, 273–76. For more on malaria education in schools, see Theodorou and Karakatsani, *"Ygieinis parangelmata"*, 369–70, 432, 481, and 489.

its prewar level by 1954 was based on the evidence of the WHO schoolchildren and infant parasite rates of the mid-1950s.[67]

Despite progress in combating malaria, however, even in the interwar years, peasants in large parts of the countryside were resigned to malaria. "The population endured the disease as a natural phenomenon," remarked a M. D. Mackenzie, a League of Nations expert.[68] Malaria control had clearly left these peasants out of its narrative of success.

While malaria case histories abound in nineteenth-century medical literature, accounts in the words of the patients themselves are rare. Both of the following accounts concern specialized fever cases that involved a common research question of the time: whether quinine treatment could trigger a condition called blackwater fever observed occasionally among malaria patients. Timoleon Petmezas, a medical student in 1877, told his professor, Georgios Karamitsas, his experience with fevers, quinine, and blackwater fever and his experimental use of quinine to test his own sensitivity to the drug. Petmezas remembered having his first attack of fevers at the age of ten, when he took quinine for the first time. This coincided with his move to an unspecified rural and marshy location in Akhaia. He then had multiple annual attacks, lost much of his physical stamina and tired easily when walking. He furthermore remembered that his father kept "jars full of quinine, of which generous use was made." His fevers stopped when he moved to Patras, but they resumed when he returned to the village. Neither did his occasional residence in Athens relieve him entirely. Heavy use of quinine appears to have triggered in him attacks of blackwater fever. Indeed, he offered himself to experiment with quinine to help his professor establish the connection between that condition and quinine intake.[69]

The story of E. S., a thirty-three-year-old physician, related his experience with fevers, quinine and blackwater fever, his extraordinary geographic mobility in and out of malarious places and his constant efforts to adjust his remedies. He lived for most of his childhood in malarious towns such as Aigio, Livadia, and Vonitsa, where he made continuous prophylactic and

---

67   Parasite rates had been 17.23 percent for schoolchildren and 10 percent for infants in 1940 and had dropped to 0.09 and 0.11 percent respectively by 1954. World Health Organization and the Interregional Conference on Malaria for the Eastern Mediterranean and European Regions, *Information*, 3.
68   League of Nations, Health Organisation, Health Committee, *Explanatory Memorandum*, 59.
69   Niemeyer, *Eidiki nosologia*, vol. 1, 956–58.

therapeutic use of quinine. In 1855, he visited Corfu for over a month, where he once more fell ill with intermittent fevers but had his first attack of blackwater fever after taking quinine. His visit to Corfu was cut short by a cholera epidemic. E. S. then moved to Patras to study and later to Athens, where fever attacks were less frequent. He subsequently spent over a year in a "cold town of Macedonia," during which he remained healthy. His return to Vonitsa coincided with a renewal of fever attacks. No longer wishing to take quinine for fear of triggering an attack of blackwater fever, he sought relief in sea travel and "cold showers."

Next, he spent a further three healthy years in Ottoman Macedonia only to return to the military hospital of Vonitsa in 1872 to replace a doctor on leave. After a renewal of fever attacks in October, as soon as he was allowed to escape the hardship of Vonitsa, he retreated to nearby Amphilokhikon Argos (Ampelaki), where he collapsed due to the pains and convulsions caused both by malaria and blackwater fever. He ended up in Prevesa, on the Ottoman side of the border, where he treated himself with arsenic and cold showers. Three months later, as his symptoms became less severe, he moved to the Greek garrison on the island of Lefkada, where he recovered. He then went abroad once again and spent a year in Thessaloniki, where he suffered mild fevers, which he treated with arsenic, eucalyptus extract, cold showers and even change of place if necessary. He returned to Vonitsa again in 1877; fever attacks resumed but with mild symptoms. Convinced by personal experience that his outbreaks of blackwater fever were directly related to his intake of quinine, he treated his malaria with arsenic, eucalyptus and change of place, often against the advice of his doctors.[70]

Overall, it had become established knowledge that protracted and frequent exposure to malaria produced a state of malaria cachexia, often with irregular fever outbreaks occasionally without preceding signs of a malaria attack. Only the use of a thermometer could establish the presence of such "latent" cachexias, which usually appeared toward the end of a heavy malaria season, in the autumn and winter. In his medical textbook, Karamitsas argued that the consumption of quinine after every convulsion, in the long run, often resulted in patients going through a malaria attack with no visible symptoms. Some of these patients with heavily enlarged spleens went about

---

70   Ibid., vol. 1, 959–63.

their business with no complaints. The telltale sign of malarial cachexia, however, was the patient's complexion. In Karamitsas's words:

> Patients' complexion is earthy, often resembles a suntan, has an off-yellow tending toward a jaundiced look;. . . the face is slightly bloated and melon-like; the flesh is loose; movements are sluggish, the whole body is heavy and lacking in energy; they walk slowly, and soon tire and sweat; if they stand for a while they get dizzy and tend to faint; in some cases, the hands shake when they move; their joints ache, particularly in the knees, the waist and the groin. Heavy headedness, dizziness, blocked or buzzing ears; lack of or disturbed sleep; bad tempered, sad, often depressed; with a poor appetite, they mostly refuse meat. . . . Some are constipated, others suffer from diarrhea. Some suffer pains below their left ribs, when they walk or cough and are sensitive to the touch; likewise, their chest is often sensitive or in pain under pressure without any swelling. The spleen is enlarged and often so is the liver. They are mostly without fever; some are attacked by irregular convulsions, occasionally of the tertian or quartan type with no shivers.[71]

Splenomegaly, also a distinctive feature of malaria cachexia, was socially embarrassing. Some walked and breathed with difficulty. Others, however, felt no discomfort and went about their daily work as if healthy, while children coped by eating constantly. Excessive thirst made patients drink enormous quantities of water so that popular belief attributed splenomegaly in these *dalakiarides*, as they were dubbed, to drinking too much water.[72]

Seeking medical help not only implied financial burden for peasant families; it was also regulated by their farming schedule, as illustrated in a report from 1900 Almyros:

> With all the hardships suffered by farmers at the time of threshing, they grow thin, in mid August they suffer from fevers and bone pains . . . they spend large amounts of money on doctors, castor oil, quinine and pills . . . After the time of threshing, crowds of people, men, women and children, all pale and wrapped in scarves, wait for the train in the small railway stations of the Thessaly Railway Company and scramble onto the carriages to get to the doctor in the nearest town as quickly as possible.[73]

---

71 Karamitsas, "Peri elodon i eleiogenon nosimaton," vol. 2, 785–87.
72 Kardamatis, *Pragmateia*, 305–6.
73 Klimis, *Synetairismoi*, vol. 1, 183.

DOCTORS

Despite the progress of medicalization in nineteenth-century Greek urban and rural social settings, self-medication of fever cases became easier
and more effective as the use of quinine spread in parallel with its adulteration and the price drop after 1880. As noted by D. Markopoulos, the percep-
tive physician of Petalidi, in 1905, many malaria cases received no medical
treatment, unless they ran into complications and, presumably after multiple attacks over the years, a considerable proportion became asymptomatic
carriers. Nonetheless, his practice thrived thanks to malaria: 125 of his 150
patients between August and October 1905 (83 percent) and 160 of 280 patients he saw over the entire following year (57 percent) were malaria cases.

The Greek peasantry was mainly served by private doctors, who were
paid either in cash or in kind, for instance with tobacco, wheat and other
cereals, silk cocoons, cheese, butter, and chickens and adapted their fee
to the peasants' resources. A rural doctor could also contract out his services to one or two villages for a communal fee that consisted of an annual
contribution from each peasant family. The contribution amounted to between 100 and 500 drachmas per annum and did not include medication.
This practice, the *condotta*, had been also known in Ottoman and Venetian times. The doctors, however, supplemented their income by the sale of
drugs to their patients, a practice that enabled them to offer kickbacks to
mayors, grocers, and other middlemen, who thus became part of the medical market network.[74]

Evidence on amounts spent by peasant families on medical expenses is
rare. An analysis of the annual living expenses of a five-member rural family in the 1930s in the region of Veroia, shows the family to have earmarked
300 drachmas for doctors' fees and another 300 for drugs, the same as the
amount spent on eggs. Likewise, another five-member family in Lesbos
would spend 500 drachmas on doctors and drugs.[75]

The burden of malaria encouraged a considerable number of Greek physicians to set up practice in small towns and larger villages, particularly in the
relatively prosperous Peloponnese, where there was a demand for medical

---

74 Gerakaris, "Ygeionomikoi synetairismoi eis tin ypaithron," 370.
75 Nikolaidis, "I oikonomiki simasia tis agelados Iskar," 400; Gazelas, "I perifereia Kallonis kai ai ardef-
    seis," 70.

services, as demonstrated by the distribution of the large proportion of the 777 respondents to Kardamatis's early-twentieth-century questionnaires; they constituted approximately one-third of the Greek medical body.[76] As rural wealth increased thanks to the expanding export crops and, at least in some areas as malaria prevalence and acute malaria symptoms proliferated, so did the medical market thrive. A significant proportion of doctors were drawn to rural areas, where they set up practice or continued the practice of their fathers. A study commissioned by the Agricultural Bank estimated the number of rural doctors in the 1930s at 2,500 who, generally "saw the existence of sick people in their interest, because without them they could not earn what is necessary for the doctors to make a living."[77] Venizelos's sanitary reforms of the interwar years, however, generated "great opposition on the part of the Greek medical profession." The same also happened again in the late 1940s and early 1950s, when the highly effective and popular DDT campaign spectacularly slashed malaria prevalence.[78]

By the interwar years, with malaria as their principal medical material, all physicians—indeed a large number of lay persons as well—had an opinion on the subject. As Daniel E. Wright remarked in 1930, upon his arrival in the country, "it seems that quite a large percentage of the population are malariologists, or at least lay claims to that profession."[79] In his day-to-day practice, the rural doctor often shared much of the life of a peasant. He served his patients in a private capacity and also sold quinine or provided them with free tablets. Quinine was also available in the village stores for those who could afford it. In the villages around Khalandritsa near Patras, for instance, four doctors covered fifteen villages on horseback rounds and mainly treated malaria cases. Like their patients, they owned landed property as well.[80]

Diagnosis by clinical observation remained the norm for most physicians, despite Kardamatis's teaching, in 1908, that reliable malaria diagno-

---

76 See chapter 2; also, Gardikas, "Health Policy and Private Care." Vassiliou suggests that rural doctors were suspicious of the League's work. Vassiliou, "Politics, Public Health, and Development," 60 and 77.

77 Gerakaris, "Ygeionomikoi synetairismoi eis tin ypaithron," 371–72.

78 Entry 2981 (14 May 1929), Strode diary, RFA, RAC. Vassiliou, "Politics, Public Health, and Development," 204.

79 D. E. Wright to F. F. Russell, Athens, 30 May 1930, folder 25 (Health Services) 1929–1936, 1939, box 3, 749 K, RFA 1.1, RAC.

80 League of Nations, Health Organisation, Health Committee, [Villages in District of Patra], 3–4.

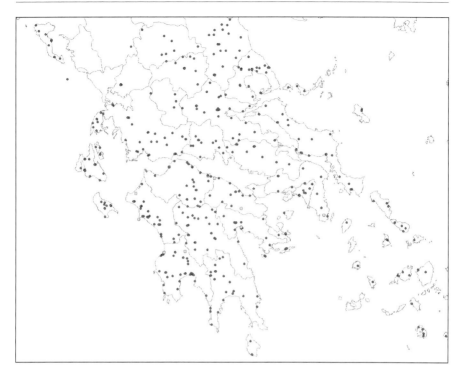

Map 4.1. Distribution of doctors, 1901–7

ses could only be confirmed by microscopy.[81] Furthermore, although they thought in terms of germ theory, when dealing with malaria, Greek physicians still used obsolete nomenclature well into the interwar years.

Cures

Before adopting quinine in the nineteenth century, lay medicine in the Greek lands fought fevers in a variety of nonspecific ways, which had been in use since antiquity, such as bleeding and sweating.[82] Some of the ancient

81 Kardamatis, *Pragmateia*, 331. Thus, case mortality of patients diagnosed with "malignant malaria," a poorly defined condition, is unreliable. For instance, microbiologist Georgios Pampoukis's case mortality figures were between 24.4 and 25.4 percent, while Typaldos's case mortality statistics from the army were 26.66. On the basis of data drawn from the malaria surveys, Kardamatis saw a drop in case mortality to 15.95 percent by 1907, which he attributed to the spread of quinine and quinine injections in particular. Ibid., 517. Doctors at the time erroneously believed that quinine injections were more effective than pills.

82 Ibid., 519. Bleeding was performed "by opening the temporal artery, by leeches and cupping." Hennen, *Sketches*, 290.

treatments had also survived in the practice of vernacular medicine. Vernacular treatments, furthermore, included magical chanting, fasting, exorcism, and marking the contours of the enlarged spleen, or *stavroma*. Muslims and Christians in the Pontus region tied a white thread around one or both their wrists. Others tied strings, ribbons, or pieces of cloth to fences, shrubs, or branches around churches of Saint John, who was particularly associated with summer fevers.[83] The practice of pouring hot water on the patient's head to rid him of fevers was sometimes replaced by the application of a chicken's head; cold patches were likewise replaced by applying a large frog on the patient's head.[84]

In nineteenth-century Crete, vernacular cures for fevers are described in Ioannis Kondylakis's novel *First Love*. The hero's mother is expected to have responded to her son's *vlavos* (harm) first by identifying it as *rigos* (shivers), and then by trying out magic, which consisted of summoning a literate person to "write out the shivers". He would write an incantation on a piece of paper and hang it around the patient's neck as a charm, or soak the paper in water and then have the patient drink the brew. If these methods failed, she would try medicinal drugs such as a decoction of wormwood or other febrifuges, and finally she might try quinine, which was hard to come by however. If the fever persisted, she would eventually "tie the shivers" to Saint John of the Shivers (Agios Giannis Rigologos) by attaching threads to the candleholders and the iconostasis of his church.[85] The practical doctor, who according to the story visited the sick man, first inquired about his birthday, then opened a book of magical signs and asked him to point his finger to a random spot on the page. From this the doctor diagnosed an attack of evil spirits. Next, his mother called for female sorcerers, both Christian and Muslim (*Romiés* and *Tourkisses*), who pronounced their religious utterances. Eventually, the sick man's fever along with centuries of magical tradition yielded to a few daily doses of quinine supplied by an acquaintance from a nearby town.[86]

---

83 Kardamatis, *Pragmateia*, 520.

84 Ibid., 521.

85 Kondylakis, *Proti agapi*, 94–95. The Greek Orthodox Church celebrates the saint's memory on 24 June; this is perhaps no coincidence, as June was the month when new infections emerged in many parts of the country. Recently, Dora Konstantellou identified a thirteenth-century fresco dedicated to St. John the Rigodioktis, or shiver chaser, in a chapel in Naxos. Dora Konstantellou, email (Athens, 28 January 2017).

86 Ibid., 95–99 and 110.

Similar beliefs are recorded from Ottoman Athens. The Athenians believed that Saint John the Healer had buried all diseases under a column. For relief from fevers, the sick should tie a silk yellow thread to the column in the church of Saint John of the Column[87]; the saint would then untie the thread, thereby curing the disease.[88]

Learned medicine had a more rational response to fevers: it used available or imported drugs or attempted to manage the Galenic nonnaturals, that is, diet, exercise, exposure to weather, sleep, excretions, and emotions.[89]

In the Ionian Islands, local doctors, many of whom had received their medical training in Italy, made use of the locally available flora.[90] In Corfu, doctors also used leeches and other methods of bleeding as well as purgatives, mostly calomel, particularly in the earlier part of the fever season. Sudorifics were administered to generate sweating and mercury in various combinations, for instance with opium.[91] With regard to the use of the bark in a variety of forms, Hennen recorded the following: "When remissions or intermissions are fairly established, it is agreed upon all hands, that the bark is a most powerful and indispensable remedy, and accordingly it is employed to a very great extent in the military hospitals of Corfu, and throughout the islands. When the powder can be borne, experience has proved it to be the best form, but it is often necessary to substitute the infusion or decoction."[92] Arsenic was administered in cases of intermittent fevers that "resisted the bark."[93]

Hennen believed that the nature of the fevers required that treatments be adapted to location, but noted that in Cephalonia chamomile and chicken broth or diluted vinegar were in use followed by the bark "in as large quantities as the stomach could bear," one physician reporting "that it alone is sufficient to cure the remittent fever of Cephalonia."[94]

Rather than the bark, a British doctor in Zante treated his fever patients "with brisk cathartics of calomel, combined with extract of colocynth or

---

87 It is one of the oldest surviving churches in Athens and lies on the right-hand side of Evripidou Street.

88 Kambouroglou, *Istoria ton Athinaion*, vol. 1, 221. The author had heard of this belief from his mother, Marianna (1819–1890), a member of the Athenian notable family of Gerontas and a writer in her own right with a keen interest in history. "Marianna Gr. Kambouroglou."

89 Hamlin, *More Than Hot*, 52.

90 Hennen, *Sketches*, 244–47.

91 Ibid., 231–33.

92 Ibid., 232.

93 Ibid., 232.

94 Ibid., 287–88.

scammony, or with calomel in simple doses, and castor oil alternately" in order to keep "the bowels open" and then administered mercurials to stimulate the liver, but avoided bleeding, particularly after the end of July.[95]

In the face of mounting numbers of malignant fever cases and deaths in October 1829 among the French soldiers in the military hospitals of Methoni, Koroni, and Navarino, Raymond Faure discovered for himself the efficacy of quinine sulphate and quinquina infusion, or the bark, against simple and pernicious intermittent as well as remittent fevers. He ascribed to the drug not merely a localized but a universal therapeutic value, and urged doctors not to be discouraged by its side effects and to administer it without delay. "It is important," he noted in a report, "to be convinced that the nervous system plays an important role in these diseases, particularly in the country, where we are situated."[96] However, the French doctors in the Peloponnese also used infusions of chamomile or of simarouba bark.[97]

Doctors associated irregular intermittent fevers with a dangerous turn in the disease that affected the nervous system and, according to Ioannis Asanis (1790–1850), treatable only with the bark, or *kina*, which he called "the heroic medium," which "extracts, so to say, the dead from Hades."[98] Along with recently isolated quinine, he reserved the bark as a last resort for dangerous cases; it could also serve to confirm the diagnosis of intermittent fevers, after the symptoms had receded.[99] Otherwise, Asanis iterated standard treatment with "bitter stimulants" such as "absynth, aloe, gentiana, cardo benedetto, chamomile."[100] Arsenic, valeriana root, ferrous sulphate, opium, sal ammoniac (ammonium chloride), and the bark of cherry, walnut, or willow trees could be useful in some cases, or even emotional stimulants and alcohol.[101] He also recommended hydrating the patient with infusions of mint, linden, or lemon juice.[102]

---

95 Ibid., 340.

96 Faure, *Des fièvres intermittentes et continues*, vol. 1, 143.

97 Roux, *Histoire*, 72.

98 Rubino, *Peri tou armodioterou tropou*, ii, xi, and xvii.

99 Ibid., xv and xviii.

100 Ibid., xii. On the use of absynth infusions for intermittent fevers and its ancient history, see Geroulanos and Skampardonis, "I elonosia stin arkhaia Ellada," 17. On the use of artemisia, see Papathanasiou, "Votanes zodion," 126. On the use of absynth, see Karamperopoulos, "Farmakeftika fyta," 242 and 249.

101 Rubino, *Peri tou armodioterou tropou*, xi–xiv. In the malaria epidemic of 1942 a group of saltpan workers in Bulgarian-held Thrace rubbed walnut husks on their wrists to fight the fevers. G. V., personal communication (Komotini, September 2006).

102 Rubino, *Peri tou armodioterou tropou*, xviii. Similar remedies were recommended in Down, *Observations*.

Some bark was occasionally available to the fighting Greeks, despite its high price. In October and November 1822, the Greek authorities in Tripolitsa placed an order for "*kina*" with their contacts in Zakynthos.[103] It was expensive and by no means widely available nor had it yet become the therapeutic norm. The state physicians who conducted the medico-statistical survey of 1838–40 recommended a variety of treatments for the seasonal fevers they observed in spring, summer, and autumn. Only a small number of these doctors called for "antiperiodic methods"[104] and occasionally alluded merely to "the suitable and known method for fevers"[105] avoiding, however, specific references to quinine or the bark. Most of the prefecture doctors, adhering to the Galenic preventive medicine of nonnaturals, advised reducing the consumption of wine or salty foods, staying away from unleavened bread,[106] unripe fruit, indigestible food, and overeating,[107] and recommended an improved diet.[108] Even much later in the 1870s, the Copaïs farm workers treated themselves with a tea of holly leaves.[109] It was even common preventive practice among peasants to add raki to kill miasmas before drinking stagnant water.[110] It is quite likely that affordability and availability rather than ignorance prolonged preference for these remedies over quinine.

QUININE

The antimalarial mechanism of quinine may still be unknown, but after over four centuries of usage around the world it has preserved its efficacy in treating malaria. Contrary to its synthetic alternatives, quinine has not gener-

---

103 *Tomos ogdoos*, 58, 63–64, and 204–5.

104 Anninos, "Iatrostatistikoi pinakes tis dioikiseos Akhaïas"; Anninos, "Iatrostatistikoi pinakes tis dioikiseos Kynaithis"; Anninos, "Iatrostatistikoi pinakes tis dioikiseos Ileias"; Velissarios, "Genikos iatrostatistikos pinax ton dimon tis dioikiseos Euboias."

105 Anninos, "Iatrostatistikoi pinakes tis dioikiseos Ileias."

106 Galatis, "Iatrostatistikoi pinakes tis dioikiseos Messinias kai tis ypodioikiseos Pylias"; Foteinos, "Iatrostatistikoi pinakes tis dioikiseos Mantineias"; Desillas, "Genikos iatrostatistikos pinax tis dioikiseos Argolidos"; Desillas, "Genikos iatrostatistikos pinax tis dioikiseos Korinthias."

107 Dekigallas, "Iatrostatistikoi pinakes tis dioikiseos Thiras"; Foteinos, "Iatrostatistikoi pinakes ton dimon tis dioikiseos Lakedaimonos."

108 Galatis, "Iatrostatistikoi pinakes tis dioikiseos Lakonias." S. Aimylios, a military doctor at the fort of Akrokorinthos, recommended warm clothing, avoiding unripe fruit, meat, and wine in the summer and treatment with febrifuge methods such as bleeding, warm applications on the abdomen, leeches, and sweating. S. Aimylios, army physician of Akrokorinthos hospital, to the War Minister, Akrokorinthos Fort, 3 August 1833, doc. 155, folder 203, subfolder Medicinalwesen, Interior Ministry, Othon's administration, GAK.

109 Belle, *Trois années en Grèce*, 135.

110 Karamitsas, "Peri elodon i eleiogenon nosimaton," vol. 2, 738.

ated *Plasmodia* resistance.[111] References to *kina* or *kina-kina* (cinchona bark) appear in Greek translations of eighteenth-century medical treatises, which were consulted by trained and some traditional doctors alike. In his 2005 study, medical historian Dimitrios Karamperopoulos lists Antonios Stratigos's (1691?–1758) translation of a work by his contemporary Venetian anatomist Giovanni Domenico Santorini (1681–1737) in 1745, Georgios Ventotis's (1757–1795) translation of a work by the Swiss physician Samuel August Tissot (1728–1797) in 1780, Georgios Zaviras's (1744–1804) translation of a work by the Viennese physician Samuel Ratz (1744–1807) in 1787, a work in Italian by Angelos Melissinos specifically on the bark, and an 1818 medical textbook by Greek physician Sergios Ioannou,[112] who extolled the properties of the bark and noted that "it should be called a gift from heaven."[113]

Travelers were advised to carry cinchona bark, while its use among the locals, although not unknown, was rare. Early in the nineteenth century, Henry Holland singled out the residents of Thessaloniki, who could purchase the drug but in adulterated form. "Much of that which is found in the shops at Salonica, and generally employed there in the treatment of agues, can by no means be relied upon for relief of this disease."[114] Use of the bark is further documented in Greek preindependence trading manuals. One such manual offers a history and botanical description of the bark and added: "As doctors believe that there is no illness without fever, and since there is no febrifuge more effective than Kina, no doubt great quantities are consumed and there is a great deal of trading; it is administered either in powder form or as an infusion, and it is also beneficial to the stomach as a tonic."[115] The Peruvian bark also appeared in a travelers' medical guide, which appeared in London in 1823. It advised travelers to Greece to carry in their medicine chest four pounds of Peruvian bark powder, a pound of "bark compound tincture," and two ounces of "bark extract" and informed them that,

---

111 Achan et al., "Quinine, an Old Anti-Malarial Drug," 144.

112 Karamperopoulos, "Oi periodikoi i dialeipontes pyretoi," 26–29.

113 Ioannou, *Pragmateias iatrikis tomos*, quoted in Karamperopoulos, "Oi periodikoi i dialeipontes pyretoi," 29. On traditional doctors, see Seriatou, "Mantzounia kai aloifes." The author publishes an eighteenth-century lay medical manuscript (manuscript 5, 18th c., Istoriko kai Palaiografiko Arkheio (IPA), Morfotiko Idryma Ethnikis Trapezis (MIET)-ELIA) a giatrosofi, in which there is clear evidence that traditional doctors were adopting contemporary European medical practices, such as the use of the bark and other compounds and drugs. On the use of the term "*kina*," see also Karamperopoulos, "Farmakeftika fyta," 238, 242, and 248–51.

114 Holland, *Travels*, 332.

115 Papadopoulos, *Ermis o kerdoos*, vol. 2, 298–99.

although they do not "understand the treatment of fever," local doctors "almost always, and at the very commencement of fevers, give the Peruvian bark, and stimulants, without ever paying attention to the secretions of the bowels, or their regular evacuation."[116]

After independence, when the country adopted Western medical institutions and education, the Bavarian military units were supplied with quinine with which civilians were also occasionally treated during the early epidemic outbreaks.[117] Moreover, both cinchona bark and quinine sulphate are listed in the first official *Greek Pharmacopeia* published in 1837 by royal order by Ioannis Vouros, Xavier Landerer, and Joseph Sartori.[118]

In the first ten years of statehood, quinine use gained ground. Although quinine had not yet come into standard practice at the time of the 1838 survey,[119] between the two fever epidemics that hit Athens in 1835 and 1842 Athenians had adopted the drug to such a degree that the amount of quinine they consumed in 1842 alone was equal to the total volume of quinine consumption since the fever epidemic of 1835.[120] Even at that early date however, the government acknowledged that quinine was "unfortunately necessary for Greece on account of the prevailing common fevers," while increased demand and a price surge as a result of a Brazilian five-year ban on bark exports called for warnings in the press against its adulteration. Indeed, in 1842, the Royal Medical Council recommended the sale of quinine at a state-controlled price.[121]

Quinine imports, sensitivity to price fluctuations, and its growing popularity should be viewed in the context of Greece's position in the internationalized market. The extensive use of quinine after the 1850s signaled a change in the popular experience of malaria. It occurred in the course of a general economic improvement and rising standards of living that accom-

---

116 Down, *Observations*, 22–23 and 75.

117 See chapter 3.

118 Vouros, Landerer, and Sartori, *Elliniki farmakopoiia*, 47–50.

119 One may well wonder whether perhaps the state physicians' reluctance to recommend the use of quinine might have been due to its limited availability in the Greek countryside and high price or to differences in medical opinion.

120 Mavrogiannis, "Protai grammai mias topografias," 542–43.

121 Landerer, "Peri nothefseos tis theiikis khininis," 81–82; Kouzis, "Ai meta tin idrysin tou Vasileiou tis Ellados," 74–75; G. Glarakis, Interior Minister, to Othon, "On quinine sulphate," Athens, 30 December 1839, doc. 137, folder 191, Interior Ministry, Othon's administration, GAK; Karamperopoulos, "Oi periodikoi i dialeipontes pyretoi," 29.

panied increased cash exports.[122] Quinine, however, remained expensive for the rural masses. Indeed, particularly in heavily malarious areas, it was always in short supply.[123] The first direct state intervention to organize supply occurred in October 1854, when the Interior Ministry requested all departmental and prefecture doctors to report on the quinine requirements of every municipality in their jurisdiction, in order to prepare stocks of the drug for delivery to pharmacists, doctors, and patients in anticipation of the next epidemic of lethal intermittent fevers.[124] The first government attempt to intervene, however, came to nothing. Nonetheless, the success of the British and French military forces at the time of protecting their troops with quinine proved an educational experience for the Greek military and civilian doctors. A civilian doctor practicing in malaria-ridden Sparti was convinced about the efficacy of quinine thanks to his medical experience in the army in Lamia in 1856.[125]

In 1858 in Athens, the university outpatient clinic, which was required by its founding decree of August 1856 to provide the poor with free medicines, treated intermittent fevers with quinine sulphate, sometimes in combination with iron. In severe cases, however, the clinic's doctors still applied leeches and cool compresses and administered laxatives along with large doses of quinine.[126]

By the 1870s, the Greek peasantry had adopted quinine for relief from suffering into their daily lives as a staple so extensively that Clôn Stéphanos wrote that the Greek peasants themselves had rejected bleeding and purging as ineffectual and harmful and "held quinine to be equal to bread."[127] Likewise, Karamitsas's informant, Petmezas, and his family always had jars of quinine available at home.[128] Doctors even prescribed quinine for other

122 Petmezas, "Agrotiki oikonomia," 110.

123 In Copaïs, Henri Belle suspected the farm boss for stealing the quinine packets Belle had left for the Albanian migrant laborers. Belle, *Trois années en Grèce*, 135.

124 Ypourgeion Esoterikon, *Peri promitheias kininou*; ELIA 290/D190; Velonakis, *Syllogi apanton ton nomon*, 196. A decree issued in December of the same year placed the sale of quinine under government regulation. Ibid., 197.

125 *Asklipios*, Period II, 1, no. 12 (June 1857): 590. See chapter 3 on the use of quinine in 1854 by the British and French occupying forces.

126 "Statistiki tis en Athinais Astyklinikis. Triti triminia tou etous 1858"; Velonakis, *Syllogi apanton ton nomon*, 249–56.

127 Stéphanos, *La Grèce*, 502.

128 Niemeyer, *Eidiki nosologia*, vol. 1, 956.

complaints such as sore throats,[129] while it was also used during a typhus epidemic in Athens in 1868.[130]

Once convinced of the merits of quinine, the Greeks self-medicated extensively. For instance, villagers in Akarnania at the end of the nineteenth century, "always use their own judgment about the amount of quinine they are to take and never weigh it."[131] Usually self-medicating peasants took insufficient doses; sometimes they decided to take it if they were alarmed when fevers became irregular.[132]

Physicians and peasants alike relied on quinine as a lifesaver to such a degree that, often "even upon the slightest indisposition of a family member, they have recourse to it as toward a safe and secure anchor of salvation." Villagers therefore depended on the availability of doctors for a guaranteed supply of good quinine.[133] Indeed, quinine consumption had become so essential among the Greek peasantry that M. C. Balfour remarked in the 1930s: "Free government quinine is by many years' tradition an inalienable right of Greek citizenship. Those who know Greece will fully comprehend that remark. Not to take quinine in the summer would seem as unreasonable to the majority as to omit bread from the diet."[134]

Supply was never equal to demand. Thus, when villagers encountered malariologists conducting malaria research, "they were always willing to offer a drop of blood, not for drachmas but for tablets of quinine," wrote M. A. Barber about his experience in the 1930s.

> So we needed no persuasion other than tablets of quinine to collect the people for examination; they knew the value of quinine and were eager for it. During the periods when the schools were in session, children were always available; but scarcely less so during vacations. Then we had only to ring the school bell, and within a half-hour or less we had plenty of children, some alone and some carried by their mothers or led by hand. Once when we gave

---

129 Ibid., vol. 1, 966.

130 Ibid., vol. 2, 667n2 and 669n1.

131 Kardamatis, "Peri elodon pyreton kakoithous morfis," 494.

132 Triantaphyllakos and Oeconomou, *Le paludisme*, 16 and 23.

133 Savvas and Kardamatis, "Apantiseis dimarkhon," 489 and 502.

134 Balfour further explained sympathetically: "Even though quinine may be a palliative, it is necessary, under the conditions of malaria endemicity in Greece, to prevent deaths and to reduce the severity of the disease." [M. C. Balfour], "Quinine Distribution Service of Ministry of Health, Greece," [October 1933], 5820, 903, R6164, 8C, League of Nations Archives.

some children their choice of sweetmeats or quinine tablets, they chose the quinine. Like Oliver Twist, they were always ready for more.[135]

During the German occupation, in Thessaly in 1943, quinine was hoarded and used as barter currency, so it soon disappeared from circulation. Atabrine, on the other hand, circulated on the black market, from where it was purchased by doctors in the resistance, who also obtained medical materials by bribing or stealing from the Germans. Scarcity of both quinine and Atabrine inevitably led to their adulteration.[136] After the occupation, reports from Greece emerged of "the pathetic expressions of the people asking for medicinal products, especially for the fight against malaria. Only next to this need come those for food and clothing. British soldiers found that Atabrine tablets used by the allied armies in place of quinine were the best means of currency. Peasants would gladly exchange a turkey or chicken for four tablets of Atabrine and a piece of chocolate."[137]

There is evidence of episodes of adulteration as early as the mid-1830s. In 1836, in fact, pharmacologist Xavier Landerer published an article in *Asklipios* specifically on this subject titled "On the Adulteration of Quinine."[138] The Royal Medical Council soon mobilized and ordered a study of means to control quinine adulteration in September 1839.[139]

The popularity of quinine signified a spectacular cultural transfer of medical knowledge among professionals and lay population. The introduction of quinine to Greece easily undermined the lay therapeutic tradition despite its ancient history. Quinine in various adulterated forms became available at local groceries and shops, whose owners offered advice on its

---

135 Barber, *A Malariologist in Many Lands*, 85–86.

136 Report Greece, Medical, General summary [date of information:] March 1944, 10 May 1944, p. 3, folder Health Division, Intelligence Reports, Greece #43, box 36, PAG-4/4.2.:36 [S-0524-0060], UN Archives; The Hygienic and Social Welfare Problems of Greece, Report Greece, Medical Summary, 30 July 1944, pp. 1–2, folder Greece #42, box 36, PAG-4/4.2:36 [S-0524-0060], UN Archives.

137 Excerpt from Confidential report to General Director of Welfare and Hygiene, April [1948], cited in: A four-year program for public health in Gr. by ECA [Economic Cooperation Administration, Washington, DC] mission to Greece, 10 November 1948, p. 7, folder 4, box 1, 749 I, Projects Series 749 Greece, RG 1.1, RAC.

138 See p. 291, note 121 in this chapter. Quinine was being adulterated with "magnesium sulphate, calcium sulphate, sodium sulphate, magnesium carbonate, stearin, margarine, cetin and sugar" and salicin, a febrifuge in its own right extracted from willow bark that was produced by several European industries. Landerer, "Peri nothefseos tis theiikis khininis," 81–82; Landerer, "Peri nothefseos tis theiikis khininis me salikinin," 328. On adulterated quinine in the 1900s, see Kardamatis, *Pragmateia*, 523–24.

139 Kouzis, "Ai meta tin idrysin tou Vasileiou tis Ellados," 74–75.

use.[140] If a village was fortunate to have a resident doctor, then its peasants could be confident that they had access to quinine.[141]

As medical professionals became concerned about the adulteration of the drug Ioannis Kardamatis, with the backing of the Anti-Malaria League, campaigned passionately to have quinine imports and sale placed under

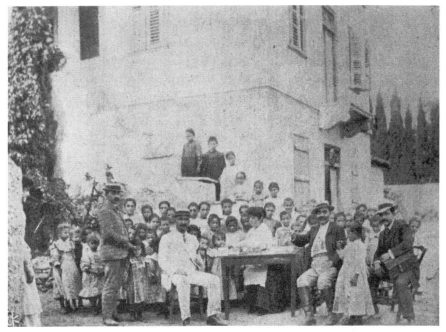

Figure 4.1. The Anti-Malaria League distributing quinine to a school
in Marathon, 1908
Source: Kardamatis, *Pragmateia*, 585.

state regulation and argued his case in the press against opposition from doctors, pharmacists, and importers.[142] The outcome of his campaign, Law 3252 of 13 March 1908, was a compromise between his own views in favor of a state monopoly on quinine imports and the interests of private importers. The state would import processed quinine from the Italian state quinine factory in Turin, but private imports remained legal. The sale of state quinine would occur at a regulated price through the Chemical Laboratory

---

140 Asklipios 12, no. 2 (1874): 122.
141 Savvas and Kardamatis, "Apantiseis dimarkhon," 489 and 502.
142 Vassiliou, "Politics, Public Health, and Development," 55 and 76–77. "O loimos." See also letters of protest by the Patras Chamber of Commerce and concerned citizens of Pyrgos in *Athinai* 5:147 (17 March 1907):1. I wish thank Helen Gardikas Katsiadakis for bringing this to my attention.

of the Finance Ministry, the tax and customs offices, post and telegraph offices, schoolteachers, and other state authorities appointed by law. Local authorities were responsible for ensuring adequate amounts of state quinine, particularly in the summer and autumn months. State services and charities were obliged to use exclusively state quinine. Privately imported and sold quinine would be subject to state laboratory control. Also heavily malarious municipalities were required to earmark funds for the purchase of state quinine for free distribution to their indigent citizens.[143]

Before the 1908 law, effectively there had been no regulation on the sale of quinine.[144] Thus, a corollary of the reliability of therapeutic results after the 1908 law was that confidence in quinine grew. During the Balkan Wars the administration of quinine to soldiers became obligatory.[145]

The Greeks followed the early Italian model of "intensive quinine therapy," about which Lewis Hackett wrote disapprovingly in words that could apply to the Greeks as well: "Considering how best to spend their limited funds, the Italians had fallen back on intensive quinine therapy, a time-honored resource with a history of 300 years of continual defeat." Indeed, even before going to Italy, Hackett criticized the Italians for developing "an elaborate machinery for taking care of the sick individual, but no provision is made for the study of the local causes of malaria or the control of *Anophelene* mosquitoes." However, with Paris Green, which he had tested "on the quiet" in Sardinia, Hackett believed he had "another weapon up [his] sleeve." As he reminisced years later: "We had no doubt from the first that it would put quinine out of the running as an antimalaria measure." Indeed, the result of a competition between two Sardinian villages treated either with quinine or Paris green, ensured the triumph of Hackett's program.

> The Sardinian demonstration put our modest Malaria Experiment Station on the map, nationally and internationally. I was appointed Vice President of the Malaria Commission of the League of Nations, a purely ornamental job if there ever was one, but indicating the change in attitude, and Prof. Missiroli was at last able to obtain the ear of his government, whose authority

---

143 Law 3532, On the Sale of Quinine, *FEK* 1908, A: 60 (18 March 1908); Decree on the Implementation of Law 3532, *FEK* 1908 A: 150 (9 June 1908). The Turin factory, which imported its raw material from Java, was recommended by the Anti-Malaria League. At the time, world production amounted to 940,000 lbs of quinine, the output of some twenty factories worldwide. Kardamatis, *Pragmateia*, 523.

144 *Asklipios* 12, no. 2 (1874): 122.

145 Vassiliou, "Politics, Public Health, and Development," 86.

was then concentrated in the person of Mussolini. It transformed the official malaria-control measures in Italy, and the use of Paris green spread around the world. The attack on the mosquito now had a decided edge over the attack on the parasite, which it has never lost.[146]

The Greeks copied more than just the Italian model for combating malaria. Konstantinos Savvas published a pamphlet in 1903 to promote Angelo Celli's ideas on malaria control.[147] On a visit to Rome in 1904, he was inspired by the *Società per gli studi sulla malaria* founded by Celli and went on to create the Greek Anti-Malaria League the following year in Athens.[148] Savvas and the League turned again to Italy and the Italian malariologists after the war, in 1927, two years before Savvas's death and the demise of the League, and arranged for an extensive training visit for K. Dimissas the following year. It was there that Dimissas became acquainted with the work of the Italian malariologist Alberto Missiroli, the RF's work in Italy, and with Lewis Hackett's research.[149]

State interventions, international trade, war, peace, and epidemics all affected the availability and price of quinine. Writing in 1933, Phokion Kopanaris, secretary general of the Health Ministry, argued that, considering the country's economic difficulties, at the time quinine was the most effective means to control malaria until more radical control measures became feasible. Kopanaris estimated the country's annual quinine requirements at forty tons, second only to Russia's 68 tons.[150] Like in the international community of malariologists, however, this policy was not without criticism in Greece. To demonstrate how pointless the policy of free quinine was, G. Alivisatos argued that to protect the two million Greeks at risk the government required 100 tons of quinine annually, a quantity that was beyond the reach of even the wealthiest states with uncertain results at that.[151]

The two figures below reflect the amounts of quinine imported between 1891 and 1940 and price fluctuations during the same period. It is worth noting that before 1908, when the government began importing state controlled quinine from the Italian state factory in Turin, about three-fourths

146 See Hackett, "Once Upon a Time," 110–11.
147 Tsiamis, Piperaki, and Tsakris, "The History of the Greek Anti-Malaria League," 64.
148 Vassiliou, "Politics, Public Health, and Development," 52.
149 Tsiamis, Piperaki, and Tsakris, "The History of the Greek Anti-Malaria League," 69–71.
150 Kopanaris, *I dimosia ygeia en Elladi*, 219–20.
151 Comments by G. Alivisatos in Iatriki Etairia Thessalonikis, *Praktika*, 326–27.

were purchased from Germany. After the 1908 law, an equivalent proportion of the imports came from Italy. After the First World War, when the Kina Bureau in Amsterdam assumed monopolistic control over the world supply of quinine, more than half of Greece's imports arrived from the Netherlands.[152] In fact, until 1923 the Greek government imported manufactured quinine first from Italy and then Holland. To reduce cost, in 1923, Greece decided to import the raw material for local private industries to process, still under the control of the Ministry of Finance. Thus, the position of the state monopoly was further compromised.[153]

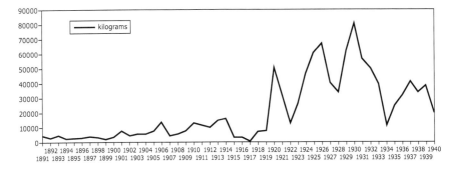

Figure 4.2. Quinine imports (kg), 1891–1940

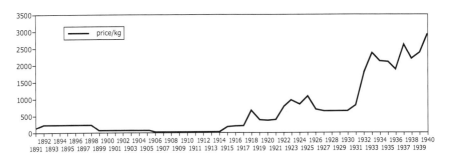

Figure 4.3. Quinine price per kilogram, 1891–1940

152 Data on quinine imports for 1891–1940 were drawn from the official series on Greece's foreign trade: Ypourgeion Oikonomikon, Statistikon Grafeion, *Emporion tis Ellados*; Elliniki Dimokratia, Ypourgeion Ethnikis Oikonomias, Diefthynsis Statistikis, *Statistiki*; also "Diati apo deftero kheri," *Akropolis* 23: 6073 (2 March 1908): 1. The article argued in favor of German imports and claimed that at the time Greece obtained 90 percent of its quinine from Germany. On the interwar quinine trade from Amsterdam, see chapter 1. On the success of the Kina Bureau in maintaining high prices for quinine on the international market between 1914 and 1938, see Van der Hoogte and Pieters, "Quinine, Malaria, and the Cinchona Bureau," 17–19.

153 Vassiliou, "Politics, Public Health, and Development," 140.

In addition to regular imports, some of the Greek interwar quinine was due to a provision in the Treaty of Versailles that allowed for part of the German wartime cash reparations to be commuted to reparations in-kind, specifically to output from the German chemical industries.[154] Additionally, substantial amounts of quinine were imported by the American and the British Red Cross and the Refugee Settlement Commission for their own projects.[155]

In the midst of escalating demand and following a quinine adulteration scandal, in June 1931, the government changed the 1908 law and placed the total responsibility for the import, packaging, and sale of quinine under state monopoly under the jurisdiction of the Health Ministry. Free state quinine was to be provided to state services and to the indigent.[156] Even though the state promised to distribute free quinine to the poor, there was a fair amount of corruption with free quinine ending up with people of influence and their clientele.[157]

About 60 percent of government imports under the new law were sold on the market. Quinine finally reached the malaria patients, who purchased it from doctors, pharmacists, teachers, priests, mayors, post office and tax officials, agronomists, kiosks, and railway staff. This extensive and heterogeneous network constituted the retail end of the quinine market. For most peasants at risk, however, the cost of quinine tablets remained prohibitive. According to a League of Nations memorandum, the cost of fifty tablets in 1929 was sixteen drachmas, while rural doctors received no more than one-fifth of the free quinine they had requested for distribution to their indigent patients.[158] Georgios Ioakeimoglou (1887–1979), professor of pharmacology at the University of Athens, believed in substituting the synthetic drug tota-

---

154 Treaty of Versailles, Article 244, Annex vi.1.

155 Kopanaris estimated that in the five years between 1924 and 1928 Greece received more than 234 tons of quinine from various sources; in the months between August 1931 and February 1933 the country imported more than 70 tons. Kopanaris, *I dimosia ygeia en Elladi*, 222.

156 Law 5043 on the establishment of a state quinine monopoly (20 June 1931), *FEK* 1: 170 (27 June 1931), 1188–89. On the quinine adulteration affair of 1930, a political scandal which contributed to the downfall of the Venizelos cabinet, see Dafnis, *I Ellas metaxy dyo polemon*, vol. 2, 31–33; Vassiliou, "Politics, Public Health, and Development," 139–46.

157 For a criticism of the inadequacy, waste, and corruption involved in distributing some 5 tons of free quinine annually, see comments by G. Alivisatos in Iatriki Etairia Thessalonikis, *Praktika*, 326–27. On the quantities of free quinine, see Balfour, "Some Features," 9.

158 Kopanaris, *I dimosia ygeia en Elladi*, 500; Law 5043 on the Establishment of a State Quinine Monopoly (20 June 1931), *FEK* 1: 170 (27 June 1931), 1188–89; League of Nations, Health Organisation, Health Committee, *Explanatory Memorandum*, 59.

quina for quinine in order to reduce the government's expense for free quinine. To investigate this possibility, he visited the League of Nations in Geneva and the Italian state quinine laboratory in Turin in 1934.[159]

Reliance on quinine extended to Crete, which benefitted from its close ties with the kingdom even before its accession to Greece in 1913. The Agricultural Society of Georgioupolis, which was founded in 1906, purchased quinine from the Greek government for free distribution to the peasants, while after 1908 the Greek government began sending quinine over free of charge.[160]

Overall, estimates set the average Greek imports of quinine in the interwar years to between one-fifth and one-quarter of global production.[161] Clearly, the only feasible course for Greece, namely quinine distribution, was proving, nonetheless, inadequate. Whatever medical thinking had favored the Italian sanitization program before the First World War, blanket distribution of quinine to social groups instead of medical examination of individual patients was no longer a policy either of prophylaxis or of control; it aimed merely at relieving suffering and reducing the number of malaria deaths but was only available to a fraction of the population. "All we want from quinine is to reduce the days of sickness and to limit the number of deaths," wrote K. Dimissas in 1937.[162]

Even M. C. Balfour, a proponent of malaria control work, realistically conceded that the therapeutic use of quinine would remain the backbone of relief for most of the country for years.[163] Thus, quinine became part of the sanitary culture of the Greeks, a daily concern and a citizen's right. It

---

159 Georgios Ioakeimoglou to Frank Boudreau, 16 June 1934, doc 9857, dossier 9837, box R 6110, 8A (Health-General), C (1933–1940), League of Nations Archives; G. Ioakhimoglou to Emilio Pampana, Athens 11 June 1934, doc 11597, dossier 1025, box R 6163, 8C (Health-Malaria), C (1933–1940), League of Nations Archives.

160 Simandiraki, *Georgioupoli*, 68.

161 "A four-year program for public health in Greece," ECA [Economic Cooperation Administration, Washington, DC] mission to Greece, 10 November 1948, folder 4. box 1, 749 I, Projects Series 749 Greece. RG 1.1, RAC; Stavrianos, Greece, 192. Livadas estimated the average annual consumption of quinine before the Second World War at 29,981 kilograms. Livadas, "A Brief Review of [the] Malaria Problem and Malaria Control Activities in Modern Greece," 2 November 1945, Malaria and Sanitation, folder Greece #22, box 35, PAG-4/4.2.:35 [S-0524-0059], UN Archives. According to another estimate for the period before the First World War, in 1909, Old Greece consumed 8,456 kilograms of quinine. Konstantinos Moutoussis's statement at Conférence de l'échange entre personnels sanitaires spécialisés dans la lutte contre le paludisme, Procès verbal provisoire de la 1ère séance tenue à Genève le jeudi 14 juin 1923, CH/EPS/PV1, p. 20, document 28980, dossier 25944, box R 849,12B (Social-Health), A (1919–27), League of Nations Archives.

162 Dimissas, *Engkheiridion*, 99–100.

163 Balfour, "Some Features," 9.

saved lives and provided relief from the life-degrading symptoms of all types of malaria.

Quinine distribution in interwar Greece conformed more to the League of Nations model than the Italian *bonifica* model.[164] Universal access to quinine transcended simple patient–doctor relationships, and developed into a social epidemiological reality that the lay public could understand. Indeed, as K. Dimissas noted in the 1930s in his malariology textbook, the large numbers afflicted by malaria at the same time made it impossible for physicians to examine and treat patients individually and therefore required the administration of quinine to entire social groups. The state, according to Dimissas, should ensure free quinine to the poor. He had come to believe that both malaria control and malaria sanitization by quinine were beyond the state's means. It could only alleviate the suffering among the indigent.[165]

Before the arrival of the RF team in Greece in 1930 and the environmental control model it introduced, quinine distribution on a mass scale had become a substitute for costly malaria control work. Through state intervention and management, the financial burden for quinine was more easily distributed over the years among several agents and, more importantly, had immediate effect, whereas malaria control had proven expensive and in need of costly maintenance.[166] Moreover, reliance on quinine persisted as though the scientific paradigmatic shift of germ theory had never happened. It thus required no mental adaptation on the part of the Greek peasantry.

Quinine remained popular even after the introduction of synthetic drugs in the 1930s, whose high toxicity required medical surveillance. Therefore, synthetic antimalarials did not lend themselves to consumption on a mass scale.[167]

---

164 Similarly, in interwar Spain, between 1924 and 1934, Gustavo Pittaluga, the Spanish member of the League of Nations Malaria Commission, objected to the Italian *bonifica* and its social engineering model and preferred the enforced treatment of affected individuals with free quinine. At the same time, however, he encouraged the state malaria service to serve in a consulting capacity on all major irrigation and land reform. See Rodriguez-Ocaña, "International Health Goals," 266.

165 Dimissas, *Engkheiridion*, 99–100.

166 Reducing the cost of control work was in the minds of the RF team members, who advocated an entomological approach. They recommended a narrowly focused experiment targeting *P. falciparum* in August and September, the most virulent parasite in the months of its greatest transmission. It should begin with attacking its most effective vector, *A. sacharovi*, in its preferred environment, the brackish lagoon waters. The proposal took into account the greater vulnerability of *P. falciparum* to environmental interventions than *P. vivax*. Vassiliou, "Politics, Public Health, and Development," 152–53.

167 Dimissas, *Engkheiridion*, 149. Testing of Atabrine and Plasmochin was performed in Aigio and Drama by the RF team in 1932. Balfour, "Some Features," 9–12.

After over more than a century of intensive usage in Greece, quinine did not generate any significant *Plasmodium* resistance. Nevertheless, it was unsuitable for the blanket application endorsed by those who believed in malaria sanitization since it failed to kill the most dangerous of *Plasmodia* life-forms, the *falciparum* gametocytes. Nor did it prevent relapses of *vivax* malaria due to the latent phase of *P. vivax* in the human liver. Given, therefore, that *vivax* and *falciparum* malaria were the two main sources of malaria epidemics, quinine usage had its epidemiological limitations. Treatment with quinine merely relieved individual cases and reduced mortality but did not prevent carriers from infecting mosquitoes.[168]

Exclusive reliance on quinine for malaria control in the decades before the 1930s was doomed to fail for yet another reason; as MacDonald demonstrated in 1958, provided they survive the hostilities of control work, the population size of *Anopheles* mosquitoes and their biting frequency are more critical factors in efficiently propagating the disease than the amount of *Plasmodia*.[169]

How did this massive, very often indiscriminate, consumption of quinine affect the epidemiology of malaria in Greek society? Writing about modern-day definitions of endemicity, Socrates Litsios has noted that "too many people have 'interfered' with the evolution of their natural immunity by means of self-treatment."[170] Is this confirmed by the evidence in the case of Greece? The question, however, had not been asked before eradication. In the absence of longitudinal case records, such epidemiological implications are hard to assess retrospectively. In fact, with their circumstantial comments contemporary physicians point to contradictory directions. For instance, for Karamitsas, long-term quinine intake resulted in the suppression of malaria symptoms.[171] To further complicate the translation of observations according to current ideas of immunity, cachexias, the result of long-term acquired

---

168 By 1900 it was already known that quinine did not kill *falciparum* gametocytes. Harrison, *Mosquitoes, Malaria, and Man.*

169 See chapter 1.

170 Litsios, *The Tomorrow of Malaria*, 128. For a coevolutionary approach to immunity responses to *falciparum* malaria, see Mackinnon and Read, "Immunity." The authors conclude that "virulence in malaria is an unavoidable consequence of natural selection maintaining the transmission-related advantages of high asexual multiplication" and, furthermore, that "what matters to virulence evolution are the fitness consequences of virulence variation at the level of the whole parasite, and their impact on the whole parasite population." This may mean that, even though quinine does kill asexual-stage *falciparum* parasites, by doing so it may place adaptive pressure on the parasite and drive it toward greater virulence.

171 Karamitsas, "Peri elodon i eleiogenon nosimaton," vol. 2, 785–86.

immunity, were an ill-defined condition, unevenly distributed across malarious regions, and impossible to associate either with *Plasmodium* species or with quinine intake. The broad range of proportions on the basis of available figures are not very illuminating. Thus, according to statistics from Athens hospitals, two cachexias corresponded to every hundred patients with intermittent fevers; according to information collected from the provinces, the proportion was 17 percent, while according to data on 144,709 cases studied by the Anti-Malaria League the proportion was 1.95 percent.[172]

Even so, one may wonder whether the Greek practice of continuous quinine intake might have interfered with the build-up of acquired immunity from an early age. If this were so, the culture of quinine certainly reduced case mortality but could have added to a vicious circle of suffering, cure, and increased wretchedness and susceptibility to malaria where the disease was already entrenched. It is furthermore difficult to isolate the effects of other contributing factors such as fragmented geography and erratic climate from the probable effects of degraded acquired immunity. Nor is it possible to answer the question whether quinine contributed more to the suppression of one *Plasmodium* species at the expense of another, favoring, for instance, *vivax*, by failing to prevent relapses, over *falciparum* malaria, by failing to kill its gametocytes.

In heavily malarious Elos, for instance, infants with multiple infections were treated with quinine. General mortality was relatively high according to the local doctor, but mostly followed intestinal diseases, in cases of children, and pneumonia in adults. In 1900 none of the 600 inhabitants of Elos died between June and August. They attributed their salvation to the effects of self-treatment with quinine, mostly only when they observed alarming symptoms, or with the first onset of irregular fevers, and usually with insufficient dosage.[173] On the effect of popular quinine consumption, the two Athenian physicians visiting Elos observed: "Ever since quinine appeared in the closets of private homes, pernicious fevers have diminished considerably, and, whereas in the past comatose fevers of the entire body were more widespread, currently spasmodic fevers predominate, depending on the individual's predisposition, and choleric fevers."[174]

---

172 Kardamatis, *Pragmateia*, 289–99.
173 Triantaphyllakos and Oeconomou, *Le paludisme*, 16 and 23.
174 Ibid., 24–25.

Although this description of malaria prevalence is more consistent with intense, unstable, epidemic malaria than with stable endemicity sustained through constant exposure, it is impossible to draw conclusions on the epidemiological effects of quinine from the language used in such evidence. Even less so than in Elos, in the case of malaria prevalence in Sopoto and its surrounding area, where there appears to have existed little if any acquired immunity, it would be impossible retrospectively to distinguish the effects of quinine consumption on immunity from other contributing factors to the high degree of malaria instability.

As noted in chapter 2, when mountain villagers lost their acquired immunity by remaining healthy, they became more vulnerable when the *Anopheles* population increased and offered *Plasmodia* a large pool of susceptible individuals—that also included newborns, young children, and migrants—to set off an epidemic.[175] Thus, the local history of immunity and age structure regulate the "state of balance" of the disease. However, as Macdonald pointed out, in areas of irregular malaria transmission such as many of the landscapes portrayed in this study "there is no marked limitation of susceptibility to the youngest age groups, the extent to which it occurs depending on the length and regularity of the period of transmission." Thus, cases would multiply "unfettered by immunity" among parts of a community that had no resistance to malaria. Immunity would eventually set in and, soon enough, reduce the amount of gametocytes. The immunity emerging from such epidemic circumstances that are abnormal for the area "is considerably more than is necessary to limit the normal degree of transmission." Subsequently, therefore, "an abnormal reduction of the disease, under some conditions" may even lead to its "local elimination."

Thus, serious malaria epidemics may be followed by a malaria-free period, sometimes only local in extent and interspersed with residual foci of transmission, as well as "a patchwork condition" with transmission in some areas and none in others. The disease recedes for a while until it "flares up ultimately into an epidemic to be again followed by the same sequence of events," Macdonald wrote.[176]

---

175   Barber and Rice, "Malaria Studies in Greece: The Infection Rate," 19, folder 18, 749 I, RF 1.1, RFA; Barber, *A Malariologist in Many Lands*, 85.
176   Macdonald, *The Epidemiology and Control of Malaria*, 28–31.

CONCLUSION

Malaria disappeared from Greece in the mid-1970s after successful programs of control and eradication. The narratives of this success and of its protagonists have been related by historians and by the protagonists themselves. This study, however, has been an attempt to reconstruct a different story, that of the precarious lives of peasants, townspeople, and soldiers in their daily encounters with their physical environment and to historicize a shared, banal experience of pain. Yet, the interactions that this encounter generated were a complex matter that I have broken down into two social environments: peace and wartime.

The stories of malaria suffering and death were mediated mostly by the doctors involved, who not only related case histories and accounts, produced statistics, and advocated campaigns, but transferred advances in Western science to a responsive local audience, that is, colleagues, patients, and administrators, and participated in a medical marketplace that had, in fact, been inflated by malaria. Often their writing was in itself an act of empathy.

Malaria remained the country's primary sanitary concern from the early days of statehood until after the Second World War. In the intervening century and a half, a considerable proportion of endemic malaria sites yielded largely to the beneficial effects of agriculture without, however, becoming malaria-free. Epidemic malaria appears to have become an ever-threatening prospect as it spread to areas of intensive, modern economic, and military activity. It is not easy to compare and infer an increase in malaria prevalence in the years after independence. The Greek lands before statehood were medically unexplored territory, while subsequent malaria prevalence figures, which were usually rounded, were at best rough estimates of mostly detectable cases that failed to include symptomless cases. Symptomless cases were in fact no less infective and therefore very much part of the story. Moreover, to further complicate any comparative approach, the intervening paradigm shift from miasmatic to germ theory generated a new nosological entity in malaria out of the old generic "fevers." Nevertheless, the evidence suggests that whatever the imputed amount of malaria prevalence, the experience of malaria epidemics increasingly produced recordable and overwhelming suffering. Interestingly, however, this universally shared experience, so prominent in Greek medical literature, rarely appeared in contemporary works of fiction, and when it did, it was more often as a metaphor or a backdrop.

The initial questions concerning the dynamics of the disease after independence have been explored but the answers are indirect or inconclusive. If, as the amount of existing accounts suggests, there was indeed a rise in malaria prevalence in its epidemic configuration, this would be consistent with a number of factors related to socioeconomic pressures and choices after independence as they played out in the country's highly fragmented geographical context and proverbially unstable climatic regime.

Throughout the nineteenth century, the new market-driven agricultural landscape of export crops, primarily currants, which invited the mountain populations to colonize the plains, not only transformed the Greek countryside but increased population densities and mobility within, out of, and into the Peloponnese and created a favorable environment for malaria. These developments accelerated after the mid-1860s until the currant boom crashed in the 1890s. Road and railway communications constructed to serve the new economy increased mobility and facilitated the transfer of infections. Apart from economic developments, nation-building reforms throughout southeastern Europe created conditions that enhanced the chances of mosquitoes and *Plasmodia*: the military reforms of the 1880s in Greece included conscription that exposed troops to a homogenized environment of infectious diseases, which they consistently transferred to the civilian population. Likewise, the large numbers of displaced persons and refugees generated by nationalist persecution, which intensified in the first quarter of the twentieth century, present another source of malaria epidemic outbreaks.

It is against this socioeconomic background that the particular nature of immunity to malaria played its defining role. Hereditary immunity apart, malaria infections produce in their victims a degree of short-lived acquired immunity that requires maintenance with constant reinfections. This fact introduces an epidemiological dilemma, normally resolved in favor of short-term cure and relief at the expense of maintaining one's immunity.

In the epidemiological context summarized above, *falciparum* malaria, the only life-threatening type of malaria, was of particular importance. Although it was the malarial disease most vulnerable to adverse circumstances and was the first to respond to control measures, its prevalence surged under epidemic conditions. Thus, although its existence emerges from early descriptive evidence, it is highly likely that it acquired its subsequent dominance, relative to *vivax* malaria, a milder, though life-degrading disease, thanks to the rise of epidemic malaria and the failure of control measures.

Responses to socioeconomic pressures and the pursuit of health were developments prescribed by a large degree of determinism. Public health choices, however, were available particularly after the causation of the disease was clarified in 1898. The Greek authorities followed the early-twentieth-century Italian example in relying on the consumption of quinine. In fact, they opted merely for one aspect of the broader program of social interventions, further developed and propounded by the League of Nations Malaria Commission. The alternative approach, mosquito control, would require prohibitively costly, large-scale environmental interventions, principally drainage schemes and repetitive oiling and Paris greening. Drainage schemes had, indeed, been and continued to be executed nonetheless, with variable degrees of success and presupposed economic returns, such as reclamation of agricultural lands. Public health dividends alone could not make them viable. Finally, however, interwar and postwar foreign technical and economic aid, loans, and DDT spraying in all its triumphal modernity transformed Greece into a malaria-free country with nascent scientific infrastructures.

The level of quinine consumption in Greece and its fusion with local culture were, indeed, unique. It had begun to spread in the mid-nineteenth century; soon the Greek peasantry was taking quinine *"comme du pain"* in the words of a Greek physician. Imports of the drug had become affordable to a significant part of the population, largely thanks to the success of the country's currant and other exports. In the interwar years, following the humanitarian crisis of the refugees of 1922, though reliant on foreign aid, Greece had come to consume approximately one-fifth of the global quinine production. Quinine did not appear to have produced *Plasmodium* resistance. On the contrary, it appears to have reduced case mortality. If, however, by successfully mitigating the serious symptoms of malaria, it interfered with the build up of acquired immunity in the population—an unproven hypothesis—it would have further contributed to the severity of the epidemic outbreaks and a vicious cycle of suffering.

To conclude on a personal note, thanks to the centrality of the malaria experience in Greece, pieces of written and oral evidence emerge constantly. They may accumulate and they are still disturbing all the same. Very recently, the story of the women of Epirus fleeing to the marshes from the destruction caused by the Germans in 1944 was brought home to me with renewed intensity, when my friend A. D. spoke of her mother, at the time a young teacher in Epirus, who lost a son to malaria under the same harsh conditions.[1]

---

1   A. D., personal communication (Athens, 13 January 2012).

APPENDIX I

Kardamatis's Description of Malaria Symptoms[1]

We shall give a detailed analysis of the three-stage symptoms of this fever, which is referred to as rare, with an exact representation, as far as possible, since we had the misfortune to see this rare illness eight times within six years in our own family and witness at first hand its entire development.

Stage I. As soon as the individual is first attacked by this fever, he may experience a distinct foreboding of the imminent convulsion, since a feeling of fatigue prevails, a general failing of strength, the body becomes sluggish, the muscles loose, a sluggishness replaces the earlier liveliness, and yawning is followed by stretching. As the convulsions approach, fatigue changes to be succeeded by a sensation of heat, a burning, so to say, of the long bones, particularly of the legs, and pains in all the joints, especially in the joints of the phalanges of each finger and both ends of the joints of the metacarpals. An aura encircles the entire body, the limbs become cold, the finger nails become blackish, a slight paleness prevails in the face, the lips become whitish, a feeling of irritation begins, while the shivers succeed each other.

Stage II. The patient goes to bed, is agitated, shivers even before his teeth begin to chatter, and we have the flinging of the limbs and the tossing of the body on the mattress; always with the first shiver begins the pain, which foremost and principally is located at a finger's width above and below the navel, that is exactly the area around the navel which can be covered by a five franc piece. The shivers increase, no matter how many hot water bottles

---

1   Kardamatis, "Peri elodon pyreton kakoithous morfis," 430–33. Translated from the Greek original.

he may receive beneath his feet, the patient tosses, folds his legs and bends them against his abdomen, buries his head under the heavy blankets, curves his body with his head against his chest, joins his hands between his legs, and forms a circle, so to say.

To this curling is contributed not only severe shivering but also pain, which develops in parallel, and reaches at times a medium degree, most often though a maximum, and radiates from the area around the navel toward the entire abdomen.

The pain is stabbing, burning in intensity as if from a scorching piece of iron, rarely medium or small, mostly intensive and, by the account of those who have suffered, exceeding the labor pains. Its intensity lasts about an hour, and it then begins to recede. It does not retreat easily to dosages of narcotics, but eases slightly and retreats, without us being able to attribute its retreat even to quinine itself. Already respiration becomes shortened, body temperature rises, the patient is afraid to speak, the shivers begin to retreat after an hour, and always at the same time and in parallel we say that the pain retreats and the patient, as his throat begins to become dry, whispering, asks for some iced water. He brings his head out of the blankets and already his face appears flushed, his conjunctiva is reddish, and the head shakes on account of the shivers. Half an hour goes by and the shivers along with the pain persist, but with less intensity, while as these symptoms recede, so increases the dryness of the mouth, the throat, and the esophagus, there is an astringent feeling as if from pure hyperchloride ferrum, indeed perhaps this is the reason why the patient is seen to avoid speaking. He drinks cold water insatiently and immediately feels nauseous, he then emits choleric vomitus, initially in great volume, then with difficulty and trouble, but once the patient has vomited several times a choleric and occasionally greenish vomitus, he relaxes, while, if he fails to vomit three to four times within two hours, his nausea is not settled, despite any pharmaceutical or scientific assistance you may wish to oppose. With every rising from the bed the patient experiences vertigo, he instantly loses consciousness, delirium is not rare, while there also exist disturbing dreams. We once observed a case of asphyxia of a female patient who abruptly rose from her bed to breath upright, such was her discomfort. By this time the patient has a burning sensation, throws of his blankets, and the more he previously held to them curling under them, the more he now shakes them off violently, he kicks them and gathers them below his feet. He feels discomfort, flings his arms and legs to and fro, however, he is no longer in pain and is soothed by applications of cool pads on his head, and after a few hours of more heat, he falls into the stage of laxness, and a long profusion of sweat ends the entire scene.

Stage III. During this stage of laxness, we always have profuse sweating, the more extensive the symptoms or the heavier the convulsion, the more lasting and profuse the sweating stage. The bed becomes soaked with sweat, which falls in drops from the face and forehead. An exhausting sense of fatigue prevails, with a great laxness of forces, the recovering patient unable to stand upright, he feels the need to rest for more hours in his bed. His head and arms shake slightly at every move. His mouth has a dull, foul, bitterish taste; he rejects any substance from entering his stomach, however, he drinks iced lemonade with pleasure. His nervous system is very excited, the slightest noise and the smallest clatter causes unrest, whereas he is satisfied in isolation and in absolute quiet.

The temperature never rises above 40.5° C, indeed three times it reached up to 39°C. High temperature lasted between five and eight hours including the period of shivers, while a great degree of analogy and parallel development was observed between the symptoms. On three occasions the pain and the shivers did not rise in intensity steeply; on these same occasions the temperature did not exceed 39°C nor did it last longer than five hours including the period of shivers. Again on eight occasions the shivers and the pain reached such an intensity as to produce tears; on these occasions the temperature exceeded 40°C and lasted eight hours including the period of shivers. The maximum height of the temperature curve lasted between half an hour and an hour, but never longer.

APPENDIX II

*C. M. Wenyon's Description of the Macedonian Landscape
around Lakes East of Thessalloniki*[2]

Of the front line the Doiran-Vardar section was an exception to the general rule that the line was in low-lying swampy valleys. Except to the south of Lake Doiran where there was a good deal of marsh but not nearly as extensive as around the other lakes, the line passed over the low hills between the lake and the Vardar River.

. . .

The small valleys and gullies between the hills remained green and often contained trees and brushwood which concealed the water running beneath them. In every gully there was a stream which was a rapid torrent in the winter or during sudden storms of summer but which soon became a mere trickle, forming rocky pools green with algae, or little reedy marshes according to the nature of the ground. A typical hill stream in Macedonia commenced as a spring high up near the summit of some mountain two or three thousand feet above the sea. Such a spring was often converted into a fountain by the natives as a water supply for some neighbouring village or for the convenience of shepherds or other wanderers. The overflow from the spring or fountain, the built-in part of which frequently harboured mosquito larvae, especially A. *bifurcatus*, as well as frogs and newts, formed the source of the stream. Around the fountain there was generally an overgrown marshy patch of ground in which larvae and frogs abounded. The stream

---

2   Wenyon, "Malaria in Macedonia," 12–16.

trickled away between the rocks, forming the numerous tiny grass-grown pools in which larvae thrived. It was quickly joined by other tiny streams and gradually became larger. It would flow across a comparatively level stretch of grass forming marshy patches of various sizes or little reed-bordered ponds swarming with frogs, snakes, water boatmen and *Culex* and *Anopheles* larvae. Further on it would pass through dense brush and be followed only with the greatest difficulty. Here in the deep shade *Anopheles* larvae and other living creatures were not as plentiful as in the open reaches. Lower down, the stream would break in a small cataract in stony ground or fall over a ledge into some deep rocky pool. In the shade the rocks were overgrown with moss and ferns and the pool would harbour the ubiquitous frog, many species of which abound everywhere, snakes and even fish, all of which lived in harmony with the ever-present mosquito larvae. Below the pool the stream would restart on its course again, always joined by others on either side. On sandy or gravelly soil, it would suddenly disappear completely below the ground and only be traced again a hundred yards or more lower down the gully. In the interval pools and marshy patches might still indicate its presence. Finally, it would become large enough to receive such a name as the Gumus dere, Orljak dere, Copachi dere, regular little rivers which broke from the hills on the plain. In the wintertime and in the spring and early summer these rivers continued their course across the valley into the Struma River, not omitting, however, to spread out over the plain into extensive marshes. As the summer advanced the hills dried up and less and less water descended. The streams were reduced to tiny trickles and when the valley was reached the water disappeared underground and only reappeared in the plain in the swamps and marshes, which were helped in their formation, in many places, by the level of the valley being below that of the river itself. High up in the hills in the summertime water still appeared at the source and the endless ramifications of the tiny stream system still persisted, with its small pools and marshes always harbouring frogs and mosquito larvae, even as high up as 4,000 feet above the sea.

APPENDIX III

Statistical Association between Malaria Prevalence (1908),
Sickle-cell Trait and β-thalassemia (1971)

The purpose of the analysis was to test the null hypothesis that the relationship between, on the one hand, ranked levels of malaria prevalence derived from a malaria map of Greece of 1908 compiled on the basis of the surveys of the Anti-malaria League, the independent variable, and on the other, frequencies in β-thalassemia and the sickle-cell trait published in 1971 by Skhizas and his coauthors, the dependent variables, are random.

Only data for Old Greece were included. The Anti-malaria League map gives departmental-level percentages whereas the data of the dependent variables are at the prefecture level. Therefore, with regard to the dependent variables, each department assumed the data of from the prefecture to which it belonged. The classes of the independent variable were given ranked values derived from the midpoint of the respective range for each category; for instance, the class with the lowest malaria incidence, which ranged between 0 and 10 percent, assumed the value 5 percent. The statistical technique used was the Kruskal Wallis test in SAS 9.2.

After a preliminary analysis, Corfu was excluded as an outlier; so was Crete, which was still under Ottoman sovereignty in 1908. The results indicated that the null hypothesis cannot be rejected in the case of the relationship between levels of malaria prevalence (malaria08) and the sickle-cell trait (HS%). It must be rejected though in the case of β-thalassemia (Hb%). In other words, the relationship between levels of malaria prevalence and β-thalassemia is nonrandom ($p < .0001$).

One-Way Analysis of Variance
Results
The ANOVA Procedure
Class-Level Information

Class	Levels	Values[3]
malaria08	6	5 15 25 35 45 75

Number of Observations 66

Results
The ANOVA Procedure
Dependent Variable: Hb%[4]

Source	DF	Sum of Squares	Mean Square	F Value	Pr > F
Model	5	119.3271035	23.8654207	6.45	<.0001
Error	60	221.9286495	3.6988108		
Corrected Total	65	341.2557530			

R-Square	Coeff Var	Root MSE	Hb% Mean		
0.349671	20.53170	1.923229	9.367121		
Source	DF	Anova SS	Mean Square	F Value	Pr > F
malaria08	5	119.3271035	23.8654207	6.45	<.0001

Results
The ANOVA Procedure
Dependent Variable: HS%[5]

Source	DF	Sum of Squares	Mean Square	F Value	Pr > F
Model	5	6.30200693	1.26040139	1.25	0.2955
Error	60	60.28845519	1.00480759		
Corrected Total	65	66.59046212			

R-Square	Coeff Var	Root MSE	HS% Mean		
0.094638	97.24895	1.002401	1.030758		
Source	DF	Anova SS	Mean Square	F Value	Pr > F
malaria08	5	6.30200693	1.26040139	1.25	0.2955

---

3   Percentage of population.
4   Percentages of β-thalassemia carriers.
5   Percentage of sickle-cell trait carriers.

BIBLIOGRAPHY

"1905. Ai peri tis kata topous elonosias pliroforiai ton iatron" [1905: Doctors' information about malaria by places]. In *I elonosia en Elladi kai to pepragmena tou syllogou*, ed. Konstantinos Savvas and Ioannis P. Kardamatis, 412–61. Athens: Typografeion Paraskeva Leoni, 1907.

"1907 [Apantiseis iatron kai dimarkhon]" [1907: Doctors' and mayors' responses]. In *I elonosia en Elladi kai ta pepragmena tou Syllogou*, ed. Konstantinos G. Savvas and Ioannis P. Kardamatis, 235–554. Athens: Typografeion Paraskeva Leoni, 1908.

About, Edmond. *Greece and the Greeks of the Present Day*. London, 1855.

———. *La Grèce contemporaine* [Contemporary Greece]. 11th ed. Paris: Hachette, 1897.

A. B. "Peri dialeipontos pyretou para tois paisin" [On childhood intermittent fever]. *Asklipios*, Period II, 5, no. 1 (August 1860): 25–28.

Achan, J., et al. "Quinine, an Old Anti-Malarial Drug in a Modern World: Role in the Treatment of Malaria." *Malaria Journal* 10, no. 1 (2011): 144.

Afentoulis, Theodoros. *Farmakologia, itoi peri fyseos kai dynameos kai khriseos farmakon* [Pharmacology, or on the nature, potency and usage of drugs]. 3 vols. Athens: Paliggenesia, 1890–1891.

Alcock, Thomas. *Travels in Russia, Persia, Turkey and Greece in 1828–9*. London: E. Clarke, 1831.

Alexander, G. M. *The Prelude to the Truman Doctrine: British Policy in Greece, 1944–1947*. Oxford: Clarendon Press, 1982.

Alexander, J. C. *Toward a History of Post-Byzantine Greece: The Ottoman Kanunnames for the Greek Lands, circa 1500–circa 1600*. Athens, 1985.

Alivizatos, Babis V. "I georgiki Ellas kai i exelixis tis" [Agrarian Greece and its development]. *Deltion Agrotikis Trapezis*, 4 (1939): 291–380.

Alvanitis, Aristomenis K. "Peri profylaxeon apo tis fymatioseos kai tis elonosias" [On protection from tuberculosis and malaria]. In *Praktika tou en Kerkyra Protou Panioniou Synedriou (20–22 Maïou 1914) kai ai en afto anakoinoseis*, 138–40. Athens, 1915.

Anagnostopoulos, N. I. "O Kampos ton Serron" [The plain of Serres]. *Deltion Agrotikis Trapezis Ellados* 1, no. 4-6 (1936): 381–414, 492–518, 596–630.

Anastasopoulos, A. K., G. Kapanidis, and M. Dimitriou. "Ai elodeis nosoi en to dimo Marathonos kata to 1906" [Malarial diseases in the municipality of Marathon in 1906]. In *I Elonosia en Elladi kai ta Pepragmena tou Syllogou*, ed. Konstantinos G. Savvas and Ioannis P. Kardamatis, 277–86. Athens: Typografeion Paraskeva Leoni, 1907.

Anderson, Warwick. *Colonial Pathologies: American Tropical Medicine, Race, and Hygiene in the Philippines*. Durham: Duke University Press, 2006.

Angel, J. L. "Ecology and Population in the Eastern Mediterranean." *World Archaeology* 4 (1972): 88–105.

———. "Porotic Hyperostosis, Anemias, Malaria and Marshes in the Prehistoric Eastern Mediterranean." *Science*, no. 153 (1966): 760.

Anninos, A. "Iatrostatistikoi pinakes tis dioikiseos Akhaïas" [Medico-statistical tables of the administration of Akhaia]. *Ellinikos Takhydromos* Supplement, no. 32 (1839).

———. "Iatrostatistikoi pinakes tis dioikiseos Ileias" [Medico-statistical tables of the administration of Ileia]. *Ellinikos Takhydromos* Supplement, no. 29 (1839).

———. "Iatrostatistikoi pinakes tis dioikiseos Kynaithis" [Medico-statistical tables of the administration of Kynaithi]. *Ellinikos Takhydromos* Supplement, no. 47 (1839).

Antonakopoulos, Georgios N. "I elonosia kata zografiki apodosi Theodorou Ralli" [Malaria according to the pictorial representation by Theodoros Rallis]. *Deltos*, no. 30 (December 2005): 86–89.

———. "Klon Stefanos (1854–1915). I zoi kai to ergo tou protou ellina anthropologou" [Clôn Stéfanos (1854-1915): Life and work of the first Greek anthropologist]. In *Praktika imeridas Istorias tis Iatrikis, "I Iatriki sta nisia tou Arkhipelagous"*, 40–42. Khios, 2004.

———. "The Royal Medical Council of Greece, 1834–1922." In *Deltos: Private and Public Medical Traditions in Greece and the Balkans*, ed. Marius Turda, 33–36. 2012.

Antoniadis, A. "Praktikon skhediasma peri kakoithon pyreton" [Practical outline on malignant fevers]. *Asklipios* 2, no. 6 (1861).

"Apantiseis ton k. Iatron epi ton Ypovlithenton aftois Erotimaton ypo tis Epitropis" [Doctors' responses to the questions submitted to them by the Committee]. In *I Elonosia en Elladi kai ta Pepragmena tou Syllogou*, ed. Konstantinos G. Savvas and Ioannis P. Kardamatis, 198–263. Athens: Typografeion Paraskeva Leoni, 1907.

Armand-Delille, P. *Malaria in Macedonia: Clinical and Haematological Features and Principles of Treatment*. Ed and preface by Ronald Ross, with a preface by Alphonse Laveran, trans. J. D. Rolleston. London: University of London Press, 1918.

Armand-Delille, P., G. Paisseau, and H. Lemaire. "Le paludisme de première invasion observé en Macédoine pendant l'été 1916" [Primary malaria observed in Macedonia during the summer, 1916]. *Archives de Médecine et de Pharmacie Militaires* 66 (1916).

Armand-Delille, P., P. Abrami, G. Paisseau, and Henri Lemaire. *Le paludisme macédonien* [Macedonian malaria]. Paris: Masson, 1917.

Arrowsmith, John. *Greece and the Ionian Islands*. London, 1844.

Ayala, F. J., A. A. Escalante, and S. M. Rich. "Evolution of *Plasmodium* and the Recent Origin of the World Populations of *Plasmodium Falciparum*." In "The Malaria Challenge after One Hundred Years of Malariology," ed. Mario Coluzzi and David Bradley, special issue, *Parassitologia* 41, no. 1–3 (September 1999): 55–68.

Baldwin, Peter. *Contagion and the State in Europe, 1830–1930*. Cambridge: Cambridge University Press, 1999.

Balfour, A. "The Medical Entomology of Salonika." *Wellcome Bureau of Scientific Research* (1916).

Balfour, M. C. "Malaria Studies in Greece: Measurements of Malaria, 1930–33." *American Journal of Tropical Medicine* 15 (1935): 301–30.

———. "Some Features of Malaria in Greece and Experience with Its Control." Offprint from *Rivista di Malariologia* 1, no. 2 (1936): 114–31.

Barber, M. A. *A Malariologist in Many Lands*. Lawrence: University of Kansas Press, 1946.

Barber, M. A., and J. B. Rice. "Malaria Studies in Greece: The Infection Rate in Nature of Certain Species of *Anopheles* of Macedonia." *Annals of Tropical Medicine and Parasitology* 29, no. 3 (1935): 329–48.

———. "Malaria Studies in Greece. The Seasonal Variation of the Malaria Parasite, Anemia and Spleen Indices of a Group of Villages in Macedonia." A preliminary report. With the cooperation of B. Valaoras, D. Messinezy, and J. Sphangos, 1934.

Belle, Henri. *Trois années en Grèce* [Three years in Greece]. Paris: Hachette, 1881.

Bhatt, S., et al. "The Effect of Malaria Control on *Plasmodium Falciparum* in Africa between 2000 and 2015." *Nature* 526, no. 7572 (8 October 2015): 207–11. doi:10.1038/nature15535.

Biris, Kostas I. *Ai Athinai apo tou 19ou eis ton 20on aiona* [Athens from the nineteenth to the twentieth century]. Athens: Melissa, 1995. (Original publication date: 1966.)

Blanc, Georges, and Ferdinand Heckenroth. "Répartition du paludisme dans la région de Koritza (Basse Albanie), Carte des indices spléniques" [Distribution of malaria in the region of Koritza (Lower Albania), map of splenic indices]. In "Travaux et résultats de la Mission Antipaludique à l'Armée d'Orient," special issue, *Bulletin de la Société de Pathologie Exotique* 11, no. 6 (1918): 470–83.

Blanchard, Raphaël. "Le danger du paludisme et de la fièvre jaune en France, moyens de l'éviter." *Bulletin de l'Académie Médecine*, 3rd series, vol. 77 (May 1917): 657–69.

Bory de Saint-Vincent, J. B. G. M. *Relation du voyage de la commission scientifique de Morée dans le Péloponnèse, les Cyclades et l'Attique* [Account of the voyage of the scientific commission of the Morea in the Peloponnese, the Cyclades and Attica]. 2 vols. Paris, 1836–38.

Bradley, D. J. "Watson, Swellengrebel and Species Sanitation: Environmental and Ecological Aspects." *Parassitologia* 36, no. 1–2 (August 1994): 137–47.

Braudel, Fernand. *The Mediterranean and the Mediterranean World in the Age of Philip II*. London: Harper & Row, 1976.

Brown, Peter J. "Malaria, Miseria, and Underpopulation in Sardinia: The 'Malaria Blocks Development' Cultural Model." *Medical Anthropology* 17 (1997): 239–54.

Bruce-Chwatt, Leonard Jan, and Julian de Zulueta. *The Rise and Fall of Malaria in Europe: A Historico-Epidemiological Study*. Oxford: Oxford University Press, 1980.

Bruce-Chwatt, Leonard Jan, C. C. Draper, D. Avramidis, and O. Kazandzoglou. "Sero-Epidemiological Surveillance of Disappearing Malaria in Greece." *Journal of Tropical Medicine and Hygiene* 78 (1975): 194–200.

Brullé, Gaspar Auguste. *Section des sciences physiques. Zoologie. Des animaux articulés* [Section of physical sciences. Zoology. On the articulated animals]. Vol. 3, part 1, section 2, *Expédition scientifique de Morée*. Paris: Levraux, 1832.

Bussière, Fr. "Paludisme et drainage. Travaux exécutés dans la région d'Eksissu, Macédoine occidentale" [Malaria and drainage: Works executed in the region of Eksissu, West Macedonia]. In "Travaux et résultats de la Mission Antipaludique à l'Armée d'Orient," special issue, *Bulletin de la Société de Pathologie Exotique* 11, no. 6 (1918): 517–30.

Buttimer, Anne. "Airs, Waters, Places: Perennial Puzzles of Health and Environment." In *Medical Geography in Historical Perspective*, ed. Nicolaas Rupke, 211–16. London: Wellcome Trust Centre for the History of Medicine at UCL, 2000.

Bynum, W. F. "Cullen and the Study of Fevers in Britain, 1760–1820." In *Theories of Fever from Antiquity to the Enlightenment*, ed. W. F. Bynum and V. Nutton. Medical History Supplement, no. 1, 135–47. London: Wellcome Institute for the History of Medicine, 1981.

———. "An Experiment That Failed: Malaria Control at Mian Mir." *Parassitologia* 36, no. 1–2 (1994): 107–20.

Carter, Richard, and Kamini N. Mendis. "Evolutionary and Historical Aspects of the Burden of Malaria." *Clinical Microbiology Reviews* 15, no. 4 (October 2002): 564–94.

Celli, Angelo. *Storia della malaria nell'agro Romano* [History of malaria in the Agro Romano]. Città di Castello, 1925.

Christakis, J., et al. "A Comparison of Sickle Cell Syndromes in Northern Greece." *British Journal of Haematology* 77 (1991): 386–91.

Close, David H. "The Changing Structure of the Right, 1945–1950." In *Greece at the Crossroads: The Civil War and Its Legacy*, ed. John O. Iatrides and Linda Wrigley, 122–56. University Park: Pennsylvania State University Press, 1995.

———. "War, Medical Advance and the Improvement of Health in Greece, 1944–53." *South European Society and Politics* 9, no. 3 (Winter 2004): 1–27.

Close, David H., and Thanos Veremis. "The Military Struggle, 1945–1949." In *The Greek Civil War (1943–1950): Studies of Polarization*, ed. D. H. Close, 97–128. London: Routledge, 1993.

Coluzzi, M. "The Clay Feet of the Malaria Giant and Its African Roots: Hypotheses and Inferences about Origin, Spread and Control of *Plasmodium Falciparum*." *Parassitologia* 41 (1999): 277–83.

———. "Malaria and the Afrotropical Ecosystems: Impact of Man-Made Environmental Changes." *Parassitologia* 36 (1994): 223–27.

Comité International de la Croix-Rouge. *Actions de Secours* [Relief actions]. Vol. III, *Rapport du Comité international de la Croix-Rouge sur son activité pendant la seconde guerre mondiale (1er septembre 1939–30 juin 1947)*. Geneva, 1948.

———. *Ravitaillement de la Grèce pendant l'occupation 1941–1944 et pendant les premiers cinq mois après la libération. Rapport final de la Commission de Gestion pour les Secours en Grèce sous les auspices du Comité International de la Croix-Rouge* [Relief supplies of Greece during the 1941–1944 occupation and during the first five months after liberation. Final report of the Distribution Commission for the Relief in Greece under the auspices of the International Committee of the Red Cross]. Athens: Imprimérie de la "Société Hellénique d'Éditions," 1949.

Cormier, Loretta A. *The Ten-Thousand Year Fever: Rethinking Human and Wild-Primate Malaria.* Walnut Creek, CA: Left Coast Press, 2011.

Cousinéry, M. E. M. *Voyage dans la Macédoine, contenant des recherches sur l'histoire, la géographie et les antiquités de ce pays.* 2 vols. Paris: Imprimérie Royale, 1831.

Crumley, Carole L. "Foreword." In *Advances in Historical Ecology,* ed. William Ballé, ix–xiv. New York: Columbia University Press, 2006.

Dafnis, Grigorios. *I Ellas metaxy dyo polemon, 1923–1940* [Greece between two wars, 1923–1940]. Athens: Ikaros, 1955.

Davidson, A. *Geographical Pathology: An Inquiry into the Geographical Distribution of Infectious and Climatic Diseases.* 2 vols. London, 1892.

Davis, Jack L. "Prosper Baccuet and the French Expédition Scientifique de Morée: Images of Navarino in the Gennadius Library." In "Hidden Treasures at the Gennadius Library," ed. Maria Georgopoulou and Irini Solomonidi, special issue, *The New Griffon* 12 (2011): 57–70.

Davy, John. *Notes and Observations on the Ionian Islands and Malta with Some Remarks of Constantinople and Turkey, and on the System of a Quarantine as at Present Conducted.* 2 vols. London: Smith, Elder, 1842.

Dekigallas, I. "Iatrostatistikoi pinakes tis dioikiseos Thiras" [Medico-statistical tables of the administration of Thira]. *Ellinikos Takhydromos* Supplement (1839).

Delamare, Gabriel, and Robin. "Carte du paludisme des confins albano-macédoniens" [Malaria map of the Albania-Macedonia borders]. In "Travaux et résultats de la Mission Antipaludique à l'Armée d'Orient," special issue, *Bulletin de la Société de Pathologie Exotique* 11, no. 6 (1918): 483–503.

Delta, Penelope. *Ta mystika tou Valtou* [Secrets of the swamp]. Athens: Estia, 1937.

Dertilis, G. B. *Istoria tou ellinikou kratous, 1830–1920* [History of the Greek state, 1830–1920]. Athens: Hestia, 2005.

Desillas, D. "Genikos iatrostatistikos pinax tis dioikiseos Argolidos" [General medico-statistical table of the administration of Argolis]. *Ellinikos Takhydromos* Supplement, no. 58 (1839).

———. "Genikos iatrostatistikos pinax tis dioikiseos Korinthias" [General medico-statistical table of the administration of Korinthia]. *Ellinikos Takhydromos* Supplement, no. 65 (1839).

De Zulueta, J. "Forty Years of Malaria Eradication in Sardinia." *Parassitologia* 32 (1990): 231–36.

———. "Insecticide Resistance in *Anopheles Sacharovi.*" Geneva: World Health Organization, 1959. WHO/Mal/217. http://whqlibdoc.who.int/malaria/WHO_Mal_217.pdf.

———. "Malaria and Ecosystems: From Prehistory to Posteradication." *Parassitologia* 36, no. 1–2 (August 1994): 7–15.

———. "Malaria and Mediterranean History." *Parassitologia* 15 (1973): 1–15.

Diligiannis, T., and G. K. Zinopoulos. *Elliniki nomothesia* [Greek legislation]. Athens: Typografeion Ioannou Angelopoulou, 1853–76.

Dimakopoulos, G. D. "I epi tou Agonos yper tis Dimosias Ygeias Kyvernitiki Politiki" [Government public health policy during the Revolution]. *Epistimoniki Epetiris tis Panteiou Anotatis Skholis Politikon Epistimon tou Akadimaïkou Etous 1971–1972* (1972): 247–92.

Dimissas, K. A. "Eisigisis epi tis epidimiologias tis elonosias en Makedonia kai Thraki" [Papers on malaria epidemiology in Macedonia and Thrace]. In *Praktika tou protou synedriou ton iatron tis Voreiou Ellados me monon thema "I elonosia en Makedonia kai Thraki",* 15–53. Thessaloniki: Iatriki Etairia Thessalonikis, 1933.

—–. "Ekthesis peri tis eis tas perifereias tis Ipeirou anthelonosiakis apostolis" [Report on the antimalaria mission in the region of Epirus]. In *I Elonosia en Elladi kai ta Pepragmena tou Syllogou (1914–1928),* vol. 5, ed. Konstantinos G. Savvas and Ioannis P. Kardamatis, 39–53. Athens: Syllogos pros Peristolin ton Elodon Noson, 1928.

———. *Engkheiridion praktikis elonosiologias* [Textbook of practical malariology]. Athens: Typografeion E. D. Alexiou, 1937.

Dobson, Mary. "Bitter-Sweet Solutions for Malaria: Exploring Natural Remedies from the Past." *Parassitologia* 40 (1998): 69–81.

———. *Contours of Death and Disease in Early Modern England*. Cambridge: Cambridge University Press, 2002.

Down, John Sommers. *Observations on the Nature and Treatment of the Fevers and Bowel Complaints Which Travellers in Greece Are Exposed to, Including Remarks on Climate, Mal Aria, the Safest Period of the Year for Travelling and Hints for the Preservation of Health*. London: Rowland Hunter, 1823.

Durham, William H. *Coevolution: Genes, Culture and Human Diversity*. Stanford: Stanford University Press, 1991.

Eckart, W. U., and H. Vondra. "Malaria and World War II: German Malaria Experiments 1939–45." *Parassitologia* 42, no. 1–2 (June 2000): 23–58.

Elliniki Dimokratia, Ypourgeion Ethnikis Oikonomias, Diefthynsis Statistikis. *Statistiki tou eidikou emporiou tis Ellados meta ton xenon epikrateion* [Statistics of the special commerce of Greece with foreign countries]. Athens: Imprimérie Nationale, 1924–40.

Evans, H. "European Malaria Policy in the 1920s and 1930s: The Epidemiology of Minutiae." *Isis* 80 (March 1989): 40–59.

Fantini, B. "Anophelism without Malaria: An Ecological and Epidemiological Puzzle." *Parassitologia* 36 (1994): 85–106.

———. "The Concept of Specificity and the Italian Contribution to the Discovery of the Malaria Transmission Cycle." *Parassitologia* 41, no. 1–3 (September 1999): 39–47.

———. "Malaria and the First World War." In *Die Medizin und der Erste Weltkrieg*, ed. W. U. Eckart and C. Gradmann, 241–72. Pfaffenweiler: Centaurus, 1996.

Farley, John. *To Cast Out Disease: A History of the International Health Division of the Rockefeller Foundation (1913–1951)*. Oxford: Oxford University Press, 2004.

Farr, Ian. "Medical Topographies in 19th Century Bavaria." In *Health and Medicine in Rural Europe (1850–1945)*, ed. J. L. Barona and S. Cherry, 231–48. Valencia: Seminari d'estudis sobre la ciència, 2005.

Fatouros, Giorgos. *Limnon periigisis* [A tour of the lakes]. Athens: Patakis, 2006.

Faure, Raymond. *Des fièvres intermittentes et continues* [On intermittent and continuous fevers]. Paris: Germer-Baillière, 1833.

Fedunkiw, Marianne. "Malaria Films: Motion Pictures as a Public Health Tool." *American Journal of Public Health* 93, no. 7 (July 2003): 1046–56.

Filotis. "Ekvoles Evrota" [Evrotas estuary]. http://filotis.itia.ntua.gr/biotopes/c/GR2540003/

———. "Limnothalassa Antinioti (Kerkyra)" [Antinioti lagoon (Kerkyra)]. http://filotis.itia.ntua.gr/biotopes/c/GR2230001/

Finke, Leonhard Ludwig. "On the Different Kinds of Geographies, but Chiefly on Medical Topographies, and How to Compose Them." Intro. and trans. by George Rosen. *Bulletin of the History of Medicine* 20, no. 4 (1946): 527–38.

———. *Versuch einer allgemeinen medicinisch-praktischen Geographie, worin der historische Theil der einheimischen Völker- und Staaten-Arzeneykunde vorgetragen wird* [Attempt at a general medical practical geography, in which is presented the historical part of the indigenous peoples' and country's medicine]. Leipzig: Weidmann, 1792–95.

Fortner, Robert. "Drug Resistant Malaria Takes New Ground, Raising Fears of Global Spread." *Ars Technica*, 22 March 2012. http://arstechnica.com/science/2012/03/drug-resistant-malaria-takes-new-ground-raising-fears-of-global-spread/.

Foteinos, N. A. "Iatrostatistikoi pinakes tis dioikiseos Mantineias" [Medico-statistical tables of the administration of Mantineia]. *Ellinikos Takhydromos* Supplement, no. 22 (1839).

———. "Iatrostatistikoi pinakes ton dimon tis dioikiseos Lakedaimonos" [Medico-statistical tables of the administration of Lakedaimon]. *Ellinikos Takhydromos* Supplement, no. 82 (January 1840).

Franghiadis, Alexis. "Peasant Agriculture and Export Trade: Currant Viticulture in Southern Greece, 1830–1893." PhD thesis, European University Institute, 1990.

Galatis, E. "Iatrostatistikoi pinakes tis dioikiseos Messinias kai tis ypodioikiseos Pylias" [Medico-statistical tables of the administration of Messinia and the subadministration of Pylia]. *Ellinikos Takhydromos* Supplement, no. 80 (August 1839).

Galatis, I. "Iatrostatistikoi pinakes tis dioikiseos Lakonias" [Medico-statistical tables of the administration of Lakonia]. *Ellinikos Takhydromos* Supplement, no. 42 (1839).

Gardikas, Katerina. "Dystopika topia kai i dynamiki tous" [Dystopian landscapes and their dynamics]. Paper presented at Conference *Istoriko kai politistiko topio: paremvaseis kai diakheirisi, proslipsi kai metaskhimatismoi*, Athens, 3–4 November 2016.

———. "Health Policy and Private Care: Malaria Sanitization in Early Twentieth Century Greece." In *Health, Hygiene and Eugenics in Southeastern Europe to 1945*, ed. Christian Promitzer, Sevasti Trubeta, and Marius Turda, 127–42. Budapest: Central European University Press, 2011.

———. "Relief Work and Malaria in Greece, 1943–1947." *Journal of Contemporary History* 43, no. 3 (2008): 493–508.

Gavaris, P. "Peri epidimias ikterodous aimatourikou pyretou en Sparti" [On an epidemic of bilious haemoglobinuria fever in Sparta]. In *Praktika tis en Athinais Synodou ton Ellinon Iatron (1882) ekdidomena en onomati tou grafeiou*, ed. N. Makkas and Kh. G. Rallis, 158–63. Athens: Typografeion Adelfon Perri, 1883.

Gavroglou, Kostas, Vangelis Karamanolakis, and Khaido Barkoula. *To Panepistimio Athinon kai i istoria tou (1837–1937)* [The University of Athens and its history (1837–1937)]. Irakleio: Panepistimiakes Ekdoseis Kritis, 2014.

Gazelas, D. "I perifereia Kallonis kai ai ardefseis" [The region of Kalloni and irrigation]. *Deltion Agrotikis Trapezis Ellados* 4, no. 1 (1939): 42–76.

Georgiou, Evangelos. "I elonosia en to metalleio Larymnis eparkhias Lokridos" [Malaria in the mine of Larymna in the district of Locris]. In *I Elonosia en Elladi kai ta Pepragmena tou Syllogou*, ed. Konstantinos G. Savvas and Ioannis P. Kardamatis, 315–23. Athens: Typografeion Paraskeva Leoni, 1907.

Gerakaris, M. K. "Ygeionomikoi synetairismoi eis tin ypaithron" [Sanitary cooperatives in the countryside]. *Deltion Agrotikis Trapezis* 1, no. 4 (1936): 369–80.

Geroulanos, Stefanos, and Grigorios I. Skampardonis. "I elonosia stin arkhaia Ellada" [Malaria in ancient Greece]. *Deltos*, no. 30 (December 2005): 13–18.

Geyer-Kordesch, Johanna. "Fevers and Other Fundamentals: Dutch and German Medical Explanations, c. 1680 to 1730." In *Theories of Fever from Antiquity to the Enlightenment*, ed. W. F. Bynum and V. Nutton. Medical History Supplement, no. 1, 99–120. London: Wellcome Institute for the History of Medicine, 1981.

Giannuli, Dimitra. "'Repeated Disappointment': The Rockefeller Foundation and the Reform of the Greek Public Health System, 1929–40." *Bulletin of the History of Medicine* 72, no. 1 (1998): 47–72.

Goudas, Anastasios. "Erevnai peri iatrikis khorografias kai klimatos Athinon" [Research on the medical topography and climate of Athens]. Reprint from *Iatriki Melissa* 6 (1858).

Greene, Lawrence S., and Maria Enrica Danubio, eds. *Adaptation to Malaria: The Interaction of Biology and Culture*. Amsterdam: Gordon and Breach Publishers, 1997.

———. "Adaptation to Malaria: The Interaction of Biology and Culture." In *Adaptation to Malaria: The Interaction of Biology and Culture*, ed. Lawrence S. Greene and Maria Enrica Danubio, 367–95. Amsterdam: Gordon and Breach Publishers, 1997.

Greenwood, David. "Conflicts of Interest: The Genesis of Synthetic Antimalarial Agents in Peace and War." *Journal of Antimicrobial Chemotherapy* 36, no. 5 (1995): 857–72.

Grigorakis, Gr. "Peri eleiogenon pyreton en Gytheio" [On malarial fevers in Gytheio]. In *Praktika tis en Athinais Synodou ton Ellinon Iatron (1882) ekdidomena en onomati tou grafeiou*, ed. N. Makkas and Kh. G. Rallis, 166-170. Athens: Typografeion Adelfon Perri, 1883.

Grmek, Mirko Drazen. "La malaria dans la Méditérranée orientale préhistorique et antique"

[Malaria in the prehistoric and ancient eastern Mediterranean]. *Parassitologia* 36, no. 1–2 (August 1994): 1–6.

———. *Les maladies à l'aube de la civilisation occidentale* [Diseases at the dawn of Western civilization]. Paris: Payot, 1983.

Hackett, L. W. "Distribution of Malaria." In *Malariology*, ed. M. F. Boyd, vol. 1, 722–35. Philadelphia: W. B. Saunders, 1949.

———. *Malaria in Europe: An Ecological Study*. Oxford: Oxford University Press, 1937.

———. "Once Upon a Time: Presidential Address." *American Journal of Tropical Medicine and Hygiene* 9 (1960): 105–15.

Hadjimichalis, M., and Jean P. Cardamatis. "Report on the Work of the Greek Antimalaria League during the Year 1907." Reprint from the *Annals of Tropical Medicine and Parasitology* 2, no. 2 (June 1908).

Hadjinicolaou, J., and B. Betzios. "Biological Studies on *Anopheles Sacharovi* Favr in Greece." Geneva: World Health Organization, 1972. WHO/MAL/72.787, WHO/VBC/72.409. http://whqlibdoc.who.int/malaria/WHO_MAL_72.787.pdf.

———. "Gambusia Fish as a Means of Biological Control of *Anopheles Sacharovi* in Greece." Geneva: World Health Organization, 1973. WHO/MAL/73.818, WHO/VBC/73.463. http://whqlibdoc.who.int/malaria/WHO_MAL_73.818.pdf.

———. "Resurgence of *Anopheles Sacharovi* Following Malaria Eradication." *Bulletin of the World Health Organization* 48 (1973): 699–703.

Haldane, J. B. S. "The Rate of Mutation of Human Genes." *Proceedings of the Eighth International Congress of Genetics. Hereditas* 35 (1949): 267–73.

Hamlin, Christopher. *More Than Hot: A Short History of Fever*. Baltimore: Johns Hopkins University Press, 2014.

Hardin, Garrett. "The Tragedy of the Commons." *Science* 162, no. 3859 (13 December 1968): 1243–48.

Harrison, Gordon A. *Mosquitoes, Malaria, and Man: A History of the Hostilities since 1880*. London: J. Murray, 1978.

Harrison, Mark. *The Medical War: British Military Medicine in the First World War*. Oxford: Oxford University Press, 2010.

———. "Medicine and the Culture of Command: The Case of Malaria Control in the British Army during the Two World Wars." *Medical History* 40 (1996): 437–52.

Hartl, Daniel L. "The Origin of Malaria: Mixed Messages from Genetic Diversity." *Nature Reviews. Microbiology* 2, no. 1 (January 2004): 15–22.

Hatzianastassiou, N., B. Katsoulis, J. Pnevmatikos, and V. Antakis. "Spatial and Temporal Variation of Precipitation in Greece and Surrounding Regions Based on Global Precipitation Climatology Project Data." *Journal of Climate* 21, no. 6 (March 2008): 1349–70.

Hay, S. I., C. A. Guerra, A. J. Tatem, A. M. Noor, and R. W. Snow. "The Global Distribution and Population at Risk of Malaria: Past, Present, and Future." *The Lancet Infectious Disease* 4, no. 6 (June 2004): 327–36.

Hennen, John. *Sketches of the Medical Topography of the Mediterranean Comprising an Account of Gibraltar, the Ionian Islands, and Malta to Which Is Prefixed, a Sketch of a Plan for Memoirs on Medical Topography*. London: Thomas and George Underwood, 1830.

Hionidou, Violetta. "The Demographic System of a Mediterranean Island: Mykonos, Greece 1859–1959." *International Journal of Population Geography* 1 (1995): 1–22.

———. *Famine and Death in Occupied Greece, 1941–1944*. Cambridge: Cambridge University Press, 2006.

Hirsch, August. *Handbook of Geographical and Historical Pathology*. Trans. Charles Creighton. London: The New Sydenham Society, 1883.

Holland, Henry. *Travels in the Ionian Isles, Albania, Thessaly, Macedonia Etc. During the Years 1812 and 1813*. London: Longman, 1815.

Holland, Thomas D., and Michael J. O'Brien. "Parasites, Porotic Hyperostosis, and the Implications of Changing Perspectives." *American Antiquity* 62, no. 2 (April 1997): 183–93.

Honigsbaum, Mark. *The Fever Trail: In Search of the Cure for Malaria*. London: Macmillan, 2001.

Horden, Peregrine, and Nicholas Purcell. *The Corrupting Sea: A Study of Mediterranean History*. Oxford: Blackwell, 2000.

Humphreys, Margaret. *Malaria: Poverty, Race, and Public Health in the United States*. Baltimore: Johns Hopkins University Press, 2001.

Iatriki Etairia Thessalonikis. *Praktika tou protou synedriou ton iatron tis Voreiou Ellados me monon thema "I elonosia en Makedonia kai Thraki"* [Proceedings of the first congress of the doctors of northern Greece with single subject "Malaria in Macedonia and Thrace"]. Thessaloniki, 1933.

I istoria tis elonosias stin Ellada [The history of malaria in Greece]. Special issue, *Deltos* 30 (December 2005).

Imerys Metallurgy Division. "World Locations. History." http://www.imerys-additivesformetallurgy.com/imerys-metallurgy-division/history/.

Ioannou, Sergios. *Pragmateias iatrikis tomos protos periekhon epitomon istorian tis iatrikis tekhnis* [Volume one of a medical study that includes a concise history of the art of medicine]. Constantinople, 1818.

"I okhri panoukla. Posous etherise eis tin Athina kai poson vyzainei to aima" [Pale plague: How many has it reaped in Athens and of how many has it sucked the blood]. *Akropolis* 23, no. 6066 (23 February 1908): 2.

Jewson, N. D. "The Disappearance of the Sick-Man from Medical Cosmology, 1770–1870." *International Journal of Epidemiology* 38, no. 3 (2009): 622–33.

Jones, W. H. S., and E. T. Withington. *Malaria and Greek History: To Which Is Added the History of Greek Therapeutics and the Malaria Theory*. Manchester: Manchester University Press, 1909.

Jones, W. H. S., Ronald Ross, and G.G. Ellett. *Malaria, a Neglected Factor in the History of Greece and Rome*. Cambridge: Macmillan & Bowes, 1907.

Joy, D. A., Jianbing Mu, Hongying Jiang, and Xinzhuan Su. "Genetic Diversity and Population History of *Plasmodium Falciparum* and *Plasmodium Vivax*." *Parassitologia* 48, no. 4 (December 2006): 561–66.

Kalafatis, Thanasis. *Agrotiki pisti kai oikonomikos metaskhimatismos sti V. Peloponniso: Aigialeia teli 19ou aiona* [Agrarian credit and economic transformation in northern Peloponnese: Aigialeia at the end of the nineteenth century]. Athens: Morfotiko Idryma Ethnikis Trapezis, 1990.

Kalligas, Pavlos. *Thanos Vlekas*. Athens: Nefeli, 1987. (Originally published in 1855.)

Kalogeropoulos, N. "Iatrostatistikoi pinakes tis dioikiseos Voiotias" [Medico-statistical tables of the administration of Voiotia]. *Ellinikos Takhydromos* Supplement, no. 17 (1839).

Kalopisis, Th. I. "Iatrikes morfes: Georgios P. Loulos (1837–1921)" [Medical personalities: Georgios P. Loulos (1837–1921)].

Kambouroglou, Dimitrios Gr. *Istoria ton Athinaion. Tourkokratia, periodos proti 1458–1687* [History of the Athenians: Turkish rule, first period, 1458–1687]. Athens, 1889.

Kaminopetros, I. *I erythrovlastiki anaimia ton laon tis anatolikis Mesogeiou* [Erythroblastic anemia of the peoples of the eastern Mediterranean]. Series: Pragmateiai tis Akadimias Athinon, vol. 6, no. 3. Athens: Akadimia Athinon, 1937.

Kanellis, Spyridon I. *Ta mikrovia en skhesei pros tas nosous* [Microbes in relation to diseases]. Athens: Spyridon Kousoulinos, 1885.

Karadimou-Gerolympou, Aleka. "Poleis kai ypaithros: metaskhimatismoi kai anadiarthroseis sto plaisio tou ethnikou khorou" [Towns and the countryside: Transformation and restructuring within the national space]. In *Istoria tis Elladas tou 200u aiona*, vol. B. 1, ed. Khristos Khatziiosif, 59–105. Athens: Vivliorama, 2002.

Karamperopoulos, Dimitrios A. "Farmakeftika fyta sta entypa ellinika vivlia tis epokhis tou Neoellinikou Diafotismou (1745–1821)" [Pharmaceutical plants in Greek printed books from the period of the modern Greek Enlightenment (1745–1821)]. In *Farmakeftika kai aromatika fyta. Paradosiakes khriseis kai dynatotites axiopoiisis tous*, 237–61. Athens: Politistiko Tekhnologiko Idryma ETBA, 1997.

———. "Oi periodikoi i dialeipontes pyretoi kata tin proepanastatiki epokhi" [Periodic or intermittent fevers in the pre-Revolutionary period]. *Deltos* 30 (2005): 26–30.

Karamitsas, G. "Oliga tina peri ton en Athinais dialeiponton pyreton" [A few words on the intermittent fevers in Athens]. In *Praktika tis en Athinais Synodou ton Ellinon Iatron (1882) ekdidomena en onomati tou grafeiou*, ed. N. Makkas and Kh. G. Rallis, 142–54. Athens: Typografeion Adelfon Perri, 1883.

———. "Peri elodon i eleiogenon nosimaton" [On malarial diseases]. In Niemeyer, Felix von. *Eidiki nosologia kai therapeftiki: syntetagmeni kat'anaforan idios pros tin fysiologian kai pathologikin anatomian*, trans. Georgios Karamitsas, vol. 2, 728–800. Athens: Varvarrigos, 1879 [1885].

Kardamatis, Ioannis P. *Ai aparkhai tis exygiaseos tou khoriou Moulki para tou diefthyntou tis Etaireias Kopaidos k. Daniel Steele* [The beginning of sanitization of the village of Moulki by the director of the Copais Company, Mr. Daniel Steele]. Athens, 1909.

———. *Ai Athinai elonosopliktoi* [Malaria-stricken Athens]. Athens, 1927.

———. "Ai provolai tis epi tis elonosias kinimatografikis tainias E. E. Stavrou" [The viewings of the motion picture of the Hellenic Red Cross on malaria]. In *I Elonosia en Elladi kai ta Pepragmena tou Syllogou (1914–1928)*, vol. 5, ed. Konstantinos G. Savvas and Ioannis P. Kardamatis, 226–27. Athens: Syllogos pros Peristolin ton Elodon Noson, 1928.

———. "Ekthesis peri tis en to Fthiotiko pedio elonosias kai ton meson exygiaseos aftou. To elos Megali Vrysis kai skhesis aftou pros tin ygieinin tis poleos Lamias" [Report on malaria in the plain of Fthiotis and on the sanitization measures. The Megali Vrysi marsh and its relation to the health of the town of Lamia]. In *Vathmiaia exygiasis ton Athinon. Epireia ton en Iliso exygiastikon ergon. Metra exygiaseos synoikismou Averofeiou. To elos Megali Vrysis kai i elonosia en to Fthiotiko pedio. Peri exygiaseos ton Loutron Ypatis kai Kyllinis kai diaforoi allai meletai*, 19–29. Athens, 1908.

———. "Ekthesis peri ton en Volo, Almyro kai Amaliapolei epidhmion eleiogenon pyreton metaxy ton prosfygon kata to theros tou 1907" [Report on the epidemics of malarial fevers among the refugees in Volos, Almyros and Amaliapolis in the summer of 1907]. In *I elonosia en elladi kai ta pepragmena tou Syllogou*, ed. Konstantinos G. Savvas and Ioannis P. Kardamatis, 217–23. Athens: Typografeion Paraskeva Leoni, 1908.

———. "Ekthesis ton pepragmenon pros peristolin tis elonosias kata to etos 1922" [Report of the proceedings for malaria control in 1922]. In *I elonosia en Elladi kai ta pepragmena tou Syllogou (1914–1928)*, ed. Konstantinos G. Savvas and Ioannis P. Kardamatis, 307–84. Athens: Syllogos pros Peristolin ton Elodon Noson, 1928.'

———. "Ekthesis ton pepragmenon pros peristolin tis elonosias kata to etos 1924" [Report of the proceedings for malaria control in 1924]. In *I elonosia en Elladi kai ta pepragmena tou Syllogou (1914–1928)*, ed. Konstantinos G. Savvas and Ioannis P. Kardamatis, 402–19. Athens: Syllogos pros Peristolin ton Elodon Noson, 1928.

———. *I apostoli tou Syllogou en ti Lavreotiki kata to ear tou 1909* [The mission of the League in the Lavreotiki district in the spring of 1909]. Athens, 1909.

———. "I elonosia en Athinais apo ton arkhaiotaton khronon mekhri simeron" [Malaria in Athens from antiquity to the present]. In *I elonosia en Elladi kai ta pepragmena tou Syllogou*, ed. Konstantinos G. Savvas and Ioannis P. Kardamatis, 109–61. Athens: Typografeion Paraskeva Leoni, 1907.

———. "I elonosia en Elladi kata to 1905" [Malaria in Greece in 1905]. In *I elonosia en Elladi kai ta pepragmena tou Syllogou*, ed. Konstantinos G. Savvas and Ioannis P. Kardamatis, 184–91. Athens: Typografeion Paraskeva Leoni, 1907.

———. "I elonosia en to nomo Attikis" [Malaria in the prefecture of Attica]. In *I Elonosia en Elladi kai ta Pepragmena tou Syllogou*, ed. Konstantinos G. Savvas and Ioannis P. Kardamatis, 264–76. Athens: Typografeion Paraskeva Leoni, 1907.

———. "I kata to theros tou 1907 endimoepidimia eleiogenon pyreton en Athinais" [Endemoepidemic of malarial fevers in Athens in the summer of 1907]. In *Vathmiaia exygiasis ton Athinon. Epireia ton en Iliso exygiastikon ergon. Metra exygiaseos synoikismou Averofeiou. To elos Megali Vrysis kai i elonosia en to Fthiotiko pedio. Peri exygiaseos ton loutron Ypatis kai Kyllinis kai diaforoi allai meletai*, 1–15. Athens, 1908.

———. "Peri elodon pyreton kakoithous morfis" [On malarial fevers of malignant type]. *Galinos,* Period II, 15 (1893): 429–33, 445–450,461–466, 477–83, 493–97.

———. "Peri elodon pyreton kakoithous morfis" [On malarial fevers of malignant type]. Reply to I. Theophanidis. *Galinos,* Period II, 15 (1893): 661–63.

———. "Peri tis par'imin sykhnotitos ton eloparasiton kat'eidos, kath'oran tou etous kai kata mina kata tas imeteras paratiriseis epi tis teleftaias dekaetias 1900–1910" [On the frequency of malaria: Malaria parasites by species, season, and month, according to our observations of the past decade, 1900–10]. In *Ai exygiastikai ergasiai en Athinais kai Marathoni. Peri tis en ti Lavreotiki kai ti Kopaïdi elonosias. I simasia tis diadoseos tis kininis tou kratous. Statistiki klinikon kai mikroskopikon paratiriseon epi tis elonosias. Poia i kat'etos sykhnotis ton par'imin eloparasiton k.t.l.,* 62–63. Athens, 1910.

———. "Peri tou para tin Pylon ikhthyotrofeiou, exetazomenou apo ygieinis apopseos" [On the Pylos fishery from a sanitary perspective]. In *I Elonosia en Elladi kai ta Pepragmena tou Syllogou (1914–1928),* vol. 5, ed. Konstantinos G. Savvas and Ioannis P. Kardamatis, 573–78. Athens: Syllogos pros Peristolin ton Elodon Noson, 1928.

———. *Pragmateia peri eleiogenon noson* [Study on malarial diseases]. Athens: Typografeion Paraskeva Leoni, 1908.

———. *Statistikoi pinakes ton elon kai tis sykhnotitos tis elonosias en Elladi* [Statistical tables of the marshes and the frequency of malaria in Greece]. Athens: Ypourgeion Syngkoinonias, Tmima Ygeionomikon, 1924.

———. *Ta pepragmena pros peristolin tis elonosias en to kratei kata to 1922* [Proceedings for the control of malaria in the country in 1922]. Athens: Ypourgeion Syngoinonias. Tmima Ygeionomikon, 1923.

———. *Vathmiaia exygiasis ton Athinon. Epireia ton en Iliso exygiastikon ergon. Metra exygiaseos synoikismou Averofeiou. To elos Megali Vrysis kai i elonosia en to Fthiotiko pedio. Peri exygiaseos ton loutron Ypatis kai Kyllinis kai diaforoi allai meletai* [Gradual sanitization of Athens. The effect of the sanitary measures of Ilissos. Sanitization measures of the Averof district. The Megali Vrysi marsh and malaria in the plain of Fthiotis. On the sanitization of the Ypati and Kyllini baths and various other studies]. Athens, 1908.

[Kardamatis, Ioannis P.]. *Eortasmos ogdoikontaetiridos 1859–1939, pentikontaetiridos 1889–1939* [Celebration of the eightieth anniversary, 1859–1939, fiftieth anniversary, 1889–1939]. Athens, 1939.

Karkavitsas, A. *O zitianos* [The beggar]. Athens: Estia, 2003.

Kastorkhis, D. E. "Eli–Fylakai" [Marshes prisons]. *Estia* 11: 4689 (22 February 1907).

Kazamias, G. "Turks, Swedes and Famished Greeks: Some Aspects of Famine Relief in Occupied Greece, 1941–44." *Balkan Studies* 33, no. 2 (1992): 293–307.

KEELPNO. "Ekthesi epidimiologikis epitirisis. Elonosia stin Ellada, etos 2015 eos 16/10/2015" [Epidemiological surveillance report. Malaria in Greece, year 2015 to 16/10/2015]. Athens 2015.

Khoremis, K. and Spiliopoulos, I. "Peri tis aitiologias kai therapeias tis anaimas typou Jaksch-Cooley" [On the etiology and treatment of type Jaksch-Cooley anemia]. *Iatrika Khronika* (February 1936): 83.

King, Gary, Robert O. Keohane, and Sidney Verba. *Designing Social Inquiry: Scientific Inference in Qualitative Research.* Princeton: Princeton University Press, 1994.

King, Helen. *The Disease of Virgins: Green Sickness, Chlorosis, and the Problems of Puberty.* London: Routledge, 2004.

Kitzmiller, James B. *Anopheline Names: Their Derivations and Histories.* College Park, MD: Entomological Society of America, 1982.

Klados, A.I. *Efetiris (Almanach) tou Vasileiou tis Ellados dia to etos 1837* [Almanach of the Kingdom of Greece for 1837]. Athens: Vasiliki Typografia kai Lithografia, 1837.

Klimis, A.N. *Oi synetairismoi stin Ellada* [Cooperatives in Greece]. 3 vols. Athens: I. Pitsilos; PASEGES, 1985-1991.

Koliopoulos, Giannis. *Listes. I kentriki Ellada sta mesa tou 19ou aiona* [Brigands: Central Greece in the mid-nineteenth century]. Athens: Ermis, 1979.

Kondylakis, Ioannis. *Proti agapi* [First love]. 1919. Athens: Nefeli, 1988.

Kontogiorgi, Elisabeth. "I katastasi tis dimosias ygeias sti Thessaloniki kai oi protaseis tis Epitropis Organosis Ygeias tis Koinonias ton Ethnon gia tin anadiorganosi ton ygeionomikon ypiresion (1922–1932)" [The condition of public health in Thessaloniki and the proposals of the League of Nations Health Committee for the reorganization of the health services (1922–1932)]. In *Thessaloniki, protevousa ton prosfygon. Oi prosfyges stin poli apo to 1912 mekhri simera*, 182–99. Thessaloniki: Adelfoi Kyriakidi, 2013.

———. *Population Exchange in Greek Macedonia: The Rural Settlement of Refugees, 1922–1930*. Oxford: Clarendon Press, 2006.

Kontos, Vas. "I nisos Ios" [The island of Ios]. *Deltion Agrotikis Trapezis Ellados* 4, no. 5 (1939): 450–66.

Kopanaris, Phokion. *I dimosia ygeia en Elladi* [Public health in Greece]. Athens, 1933.

Kostis, Kostas. *Ta kakomathimena paidia tis istorias: I diamorfosi tou neoellinikou kratous, 18os–21os aionas* [The spoilt children of history: The formation of the modern Greek state, eighteenth–twenty-first centuries]. Athens: Polis, 2013.

Kourti, Paraskevi. "Oi prosfygikoi synoikismoi tis 'dytikis pleyras' kai i anadysi mias neas topikotitas" [The refugee settlements of the "western side" and the emergence of a new local identity]. In *Thessaloniki, protevousa ton prosfygon. Oi prosfyges stin poli apo to 1912 mekhri simera*, Istoriko Arkheio Prosfygikou Ellinismou Dimou Kalamarias, 530–42. Thessaloniki: Adelfoi Kyriakidi, 2013.

Kousoulis, Antonis A., et al. "Malaria in Laconia, Greece, Then and Now: A 2500-Year-Old Pattern." *International Journal of Infectious Diseases* 17, no. 1 (January 2013): e8–e11.

Kouzis, Aristotelis P. "Ai meta tin idrysin tou Vasileiou tis Ellados protai par'imin arkhai ygieionomikis politikis kai organoseos tis dimosias ygeias epi ti vasei ton anekdoton xeirografon praktikon tou Iatrosynedriou" [Our first principles of sanitary policy and the organization of public health after the foundation of the Greek Kingdom on the basis of the unpublished manuscript proceedings of the Medical Council]. *Praktika tis Akadimias Athinon* 21 (1946): 61–91.

———. Ethnikon kai Kapodistriakon Panepistimion Athinon. *Istoria tis Iatrikis Skholis* [History of the Medical School]. Series: Ekatontaetiris 1837–1937 [Centenary 1837–1937]. Athens: Pyrsos, 1939.

———. "Tina peri eleiogenon pyreton kata tous arkhaious Ellinas iatrous" [About malaria fevers according to the ancient Greek doctors]. In *I Elonosia en Elladi kai ta Pepragmena tou Syllogou*, ed. Konstantinos G. Savvas and Ioannis P. Kardamatis, 97–108. Athens: Typografeion Paraskeva Leoni, 1907.

Kyriopoulos, Giannis, ed. *Dimosia ygeia kai koinoniki politiki: o Eleftherios Venizelos kai i epokhi tou* [Public health and social policy: Eleftherios Venizelos and his era]. Athens: Papazisis, 2008.

Laiou-Thomadakis, A. "The Politics of Hunger: Economic Aid to Greece, 1943–1945." *Journal of the Hellenic Diaspora* 7 (1980): 27–42.

Landerer, Xavier. "Peri nothefseos tis theiikis khininis" [On the adulteration of quinine sulphate]. *Asklipios* II (1 September 1836): 81–82.

———. "Peri nothefseos tis theiikis khininis me salikinin" [On the adulteration of quinine sulphate with salicin]. *Asklipios* IX (1 April 1837): 328.

———. *Toxikologia: engkheiridion dia iatrous, farmakopoious, dikastikous kai astynomikous ypallilous* [Toxicology: Textbook for doctors, pharmacists, judges, and police officials]. Athens: Antoniadis, 1843.

Lappas, Kostas. *Panepistimio kai foitites stin Ellada kata ton 19o aiona* [University and students in Greece during the nineteenth century]. Athens: Kentro Neoellinikon Erevnon E.I.E., 2004.

Laskaratos, I. "I katastasi tis ygeias kai i perithalpsi sto Ionio kratos" [Health and health care in the Ionian state]. In *To Ionio: perivallon, koinonia, politismos*, 143–58. Athens: Kentro Meleton Ioniou, 1984.

League of Nations. Health Organisation. Health Committee. I *The Prefecture of Cavalla*, II *The Prefecture of Drama*. By Dr. McLaughlin. C.H./Greece/8 (Vol. 359). Geneva, 1929.

———. *Explanatory Memorandum on the Documentation Collected by the Commission Together with a Subject Index*. By M. D. Mackenzie. C.H./Greece/4 (Vol. 359). Geneva, 1929.

———. *Health and Hospital Survey of Salonica*. By Dr. McLaughlin. C.H./Greece/18 (Vol. 360). Geneva, 1929.

———. *Hospital and Health Survey of Athens and Piraeus*. Part I. By Prof. Haven Emerson. C.H./Greece/13 (Vol. 360). Geneva, 1929.

———. *Patras*. By Dr. Park. C.H./Greece/28 (Vol. 360). Geneva, 1929.

———. *Rapport sur les travaux de la commission des épidémies depuis janvier 1923* [Report on the works of the epidemics commission since January 1923]. C.H./84 (Vol. 287). Geneva, 1923.

———. [Villages in District of Patra]. By M. D. Mackenzie. C.H./Greece/12 (Vol. 360). Geneva, 1929.

———. *Visite à l'île de Corfou* [Visit to the island of Corfu]. By Dr. Borcic. C.H./Greece/22 (Vol. 360). Geneva, 1929.

———. *Visite dans la province d'Épire* [Visit to the province of Epirus]. By Dr. Borcic. C.H./Greece/9 (Vol. 359). Geneva, 1929.

Leake, William Martin. *Travels in Northern Greece*. 4 vols. London: J. Rodwell, 1835.

———. *Travels in the Morea*. 3 vols. London: John Murray, 1830.

Leconte, Casimir. *Etude économique de la Grèce, de sa position actuelle, de son avenir* [Economic study of Greece, its current situation, and its future]. Paris: Firmin Didot, 1847.

Lee, Wenn-Chyau, et al. "Hyperparasitaemic Human *Plasmodium Knowlesi* Infection with Atypical Morphology in Peninsular Malaysia." *Malaria Journal* 12, no. 88 (2013).

Legroux, René. "Présentation du matériel de prophylaxie anti-paludique destiné à l'Armée d'Orient" [Presentation of the antimalarial prophylactic material destined for the Armée d'Orient]. *Bulletin de la Société de Pathologie Exotique* 10, no. 6 (1917): 421–26.

Leivadaras, N.E. "To proto nosokomeio tis epanastatimenis kai eleftheris Elladas stin Ermoupoli Syrou, 1825" [The first hospital in revolutionary and free Greece in Ermoupolis of Syros, 1825]. Medical School, Aristotle University of Thessaloniki, 2012. http://ikee.lib.auth.gr/record/130146/files/GRI-2012-9437.pdf.

Liakos, Antonis. *Ergasia kai politiki stin Ellada tou mesopolemou* [Labor and politics in Greece in the interwar years]. Athens: Idryma Erevnas kai Paideias tis Emporikis Trapezas tis Ellados, 1993.

Litsios, Socrates. "Malaria Control, the Cold War and the Post-War Reorganization of International Assistance." *Medical Anthropology* 17, no. 3 (1997): 255–78.

———. *The Tomorrow of Malaria*. Wellington, NZ: Pacific Press, 1997.

Liu, Weimin, et al. "African Origin of the Malaria Parasite *Plasmodium Vivax*." *Nature Communications* 5 (21 February 2014): article number: 3346.

Livadas, G., and D. Athanassatos. "The Economic Benefits of Malaria Eradication in Greece." *Rivista di Malariologia* 42, no. 4–6 (1963): 177–87.

Livadas, Grigorios A. "Araiosis kai exafanisis ton epipolazonton en Attiki anofelikon eidon synepeia tou efarmosthentos anthelonosiakou programmatos (1946–1949)" [Rarefaction and disappearance of *Anopheles* species in Attica on account of the antimalarial program applied (194649)]. *Elliniki Iatriki* 19, no. 3 (1950).

———. "Malaria Vector Resistance to Insecticides." Inter-Regional Conference on Malaria for the Eastern Mediterranean and European Regions (1956: Athens, Greece). Geneva: World Health Organization, 1956. WHO/Mal/166. http://whqlibdoc.who.int/malaria/WHO_Mal_166.pdf.

Livadas, Grigorios A., and G. Georgopoulos. "Development of Resistance to DDT by *Anopheles Sacharovi* in Greece." WHO Expert Committee on Malaria. Geneva: World Health Organization, 1953. WHO/Mal/80; WHO/Mal/80 Add.1. http://whqlibdoc.who.int/malaria/WHO_MAL_80.pdf; http://whqlibdoc.who.int/malaria/WHO_MAL_80_Add.1.pdf.

Livadas, Grigorios A., and Ioannis K. Sfangos. *I elonosia en Elladi 1930–1940: erevna, katapolemisis* [Malaria in Greece 1930–40: Research, control]. Athens: Pyrsos, 1940.

———. *Malaria in Greece, 1930–1940*. Athens: Pyrsos, 1941.

Livadas, Grigorios A., Athanasios P. Kanellakis, and V. G. Valaoras. "Paratiriseis epi tis aima-tologikis eikonos en ti elonosia" [Observations on the hematological picture in malaria]. *Akadimaiki Iatriki*, March 1939.

Livieratos, Spyridon G. "I elonosia kai i fymatiosis en Eptaniso" [Malaria and tuberculosis in the Ionian Islands]. In *Praktika tou en Kerkyra Protou Panioniou Synedriou (20–22 Maïou 1914) kai ai en afto anakoinoseis*, 163–97. Athens, 1915.

Lombard, Henri Clermond. *Traité de climatologie médicale, comprenant la météorologie médicale et l'étude des influences physiologiques, pathologiques, prophylactiques et thérapeutiques du climat sur la santé* [Treatise on medical climatology, comprising a medical meteorology and the study of physiological, pathological, prophylactic, and therapeutic influences of climate on health]. Paris: Baillère, 1877–80.

Lonie, Iain M. "Fever Pathology in the Sixteenth Century: Tradition and Innovation." In *Theories of Fever from Antiquity to the Enlightenment*, ed. W. F. Bynum and V. Nutton. Medical History Supplement, no. 1, 19–44. London: Wellcome Institute for the History of Medicine, 1981.

Loukopoulos, Dimitris. "Hemoglobin Variants and Thalassemia in Greece." In *Hemoglobin Variants in Human Populations*, ed. William P. Winter, vol. 1, 165–80. Boca Raton, FL: CRC Press, 1986.

Louloudis, Leonidas. "Georgikos eksynkhronismos kai metaskhimatismos ton agrotikon domon. I periptosi tis koinotitas Anthilis" [Agricultural modernization and transformation of agrarian structures. The case of the Anthili community]. Agricultural University of Athens, 1990.

Macdonald, G. *The Epidemiology and Control of Malaria*. Oxford: Oxford University Press, 1957.

Mackinnon, Margaret J., and Andrew F. Read. "Immunity Promotes Virulence Evolution in a Malaria Model." *PLoS Biol* 2, no. 9 (2004): 1286–92.

———. "Virulence in Malaria: An Evolutionary Viewpoint." *Philosophical Transactions of the Royal Society. B Biological Sciences* 359 (2004): 965–86.

Makkas, N., and Kh. G. Rallis, eds. *Praktika tis en Athinais Synodou ton Ellinon Iatron (1882) ekdidomena en onomati tou grafeiou* [Proceedings of the Athens conference of Greek doctors (1882) published in the name of the office]. Athens: Typografeion Adelfon Perri, 1883.

Malaria and Quinine. Amsterdam: Bureau for Increasing the Use of Quinine, 1927.

Mandekos, A. G. "I ex asiteias kai elonosias thnisimotis eis Thessalonikin kai agrotikas periokhas tis Makedonias (1940–1943)" [Famine and malaria mortality in Thessaloniki and the agricultural regions of Macedonia (1940–1943)]. *Praktika tis Akadimias Athinon* 19 (1944): 75–87.

———. "I exafanisis ton anofelon kai tis elonosias en Elladi einai katorthoti dia tis khrisimopoiiseos tou DDT?" [Is the disappearance of *Anopheles* and malaria in Greece achievable with the use of DDT?]. *Praktika tis Akadimias Athinon* (1946), 292–304.

Mandyla, Maria, et al. "Pioneers in the Anti-Malaria Battle in Greece (1900–1930)." *Gesnerus* 68, no. 2 (2011): 180–97.

Manousos, P. "Idiaiteros pinax ton dimon Trifylias" [Separate table of the municipalities of Trifylia]. *Ellinikos Takhydromos* Supplement, no. 36 (1839).

Manoussakis, E. *To elonosiakon provlima. Erevnai kai efarmogai en Thessalia. O oloklirotikos agon kata tis elonosias* [The malarial problem: Research and applications in Thessaly: Total struggle against malaria]. Larissa, 1939.

Marciniak, Stephanie, et al. "*Plasmodium Falciparum* Malaria in 1st–2nd Century CE Southern Italy." *Current Biology* 26, no. 23 (5 December 2016): R1220–22. doi:10.1016/j.cub.2016.10.016.

"Marianna Gr. Kambouroglou," *Poikili Stoa* 9, no. 1 (1891): 181–82.

Mariolopoulos, E. G., and Livathinos A. N. *Atlas climatique de la Grèce* [Climatic atlas of Greece]. Athens: National Observatory of Athens, 1935.

Mariolopoulos, Elias G. *To klima tis Ellados* [The climate of Greece]. Athens: Athan. A. Papaspyrou, 1938.

Martini, E. *Berechnungen und Beobachtungen zur Epidemiologie und Bekämpfung der Malaria auf Grund von Balkanerfahrungen* [Accounts and observations on the epidemiology and control of malaria on the basis of the Balkan experience]. Hamburg: W. Gente, 1921.

Masson-Vincourt, Marie-Paule. *Paul Calligas (1814–1896) et la fonction de l'état grec* [Paul Calligas (1814–1896) and the function of the Greek state]. Paris: L'Harmattan, 2000.

Maurer, Georg Ludwig von. *Das griechische Volk in öffentlicher, kirchlicher und privatrechtlicher Beziehung vor und nach dem Freiheitskampfe bis zum 31. Juli 1834* [The Greek people in public, church, and civil law relationship before and after the struggle for independence until 31 July 1834]. Heidelberg: Akademische Buchhandlung, 1835.

Mavrogiannis, K. "Paratiriseis epi ton klimaton tis Ellados" [Observation on the climates of Greece]. *Evropaikos Eranistis* 2, no. 3, 4 (1840): 211–32, 341–73.

———. "Protai grammai iatrikis topografias kai katastatikis tis Peloponnisou" [First lines of a medical topography and an account of the Peloponnese]. *Evropaïkos Eranistis* 1, no. 5 (1842): 293–325.

———. "Protai grammai mias topografias kai katastatikis tis Peloponnisou. Topografiki diastixis ton nosodon meron tis Peloponnisou" [First lines for a topography and an account of the Peloponnese: Scattered topography of the unhealthy parts of the Peloponnese]. *Eranistis* 1, no. 8 (1843): 535–54.

Mazower, Mark. *Inside Hitler's Greece: The Experience of Occupation, 1941–1944*. New Haven, CT: Yale University Press, 1993.

McCann, James C. *Historical Ecology of Malaria in Ethiopia: Deposing the Spirits*. Athens, Ohio: Ohio University Press. Kindle edition, 2015.

McLay, Kenneth. "Part III. Haematological Investigations on Malaria in Macedonia." In *Malaria in Macedonia, 1915–1919, Part I.–Part V.*, ed. C. M. Wenyon, A. G. Anderson, K. McLay, T. S. Hele, and J. Waterston, 93–105. London, 1921–22.

McManus, Kimberly F., et al. "Population Genetic Analysis of the DARC Locus (Duffy) Reveals Adaptation from Standing Variation Associated with Malaria Resistance in Humans." *PLOS Genetics* 13, no. 3 (10 March 2017): e1006560. doi:10.1371/journal.pgen.1006560.

McNeill, John Robert. *Mosquito Empires: Ecology and War in the Greater Caribbean, 1620–1914*. Cambridge: Cambridge University Press, 2010.

———. *The Mountains of the Mediterranean World: An Environmental History*. Cambridge: Cambridge University Press, 1992.

———. *Something New under the Sun: An Environmental History of the Twentieth-Century World*. New York: Norton, 2000.

McNeill, William H. *The Metamorphosis of Greece since World War II*. Chicago: University of Chicago Press, 1978.

———. *Plagues and Peoples*. Garden City, NY: Anchor Press, 1976.

Migliani, R., J.-B. Meynard, J.-M. Milleliri, C. Verret, and C. Rapp. "Histoire de la lutte contre le paludisme dans l'armée française: de l'Algérie à l'Armée d'Orient pendant la Première Guerre mondiale" [History of the antimalarial struggle in the French Army: From Algeria to the Armée d'Orient during the First World War]. *Médecine et Santé Tropicales* 24 (2014): 349–61.

Mikanowski, Jacob. "Dr Hirszfeld's War: Tropical Medicine and the Invention of Sero-Anthropology on the Macedonian Front." *Social History of Medicine* 25, no. 1 (February 2012): 103–21.

Mitman, G., and R. L. Numbers. "From Miasma to Asthma: The Changing Fortunes of Medical Geography in America." *History and Philosophy of the Life Sciences* 25, no. 3 (2003): 391–412.

Morgan-Forster, Antonia H. "Climate, Environment and Malaria during the Prehistory of Mainland Greece." Department for the History of Medicine, Medical School, University of Birmingham, 2010. http://etheses.bham.ac.uk/1579/1/MorganForster11PhD.pdf.

Morgenthau, Henry. *I Was Sent to Athens*. Garden City, NY: Doubleday, 1929.

Mueller, Ivo, et al. "Key Gaps in the Knowledge of *Plasmodium Vivax*, a Neglected Human Malaria Parasite." *The Lancet Infectious Diseases* 9, no. 9 (September 2009): 555–66.

Nájera, José A. "Epidemiology in the Strategies for Malaria Control." *Parassitologia* 42 (2000): 9–24.

———. "Malaria Control: Achievements, Problems and Strategies." *Parassitologia* 43, no. 1–2 (June 2001): 1–89.

Nájera, José A., and Joachim Hempel. *The Burden of Malaria*. Geneva: World Health Organization, 1996. http://www.rollbackmalaria.org/cmc_upload/0/000/009/511/burden_najera.pdf.

Nerlich, Andreas G., Bettina Schraut, Sabine Dittrich, Thomas Jelinek, and Albert R. Zink. "*Plasmodium Falciparum* in Ancient Egypt." *Emerging Infectious Diseases* 14, no. 8 (2008): 1317–19.

Niclot, M. "Le paludisme en Grèce, en Macédoine et à l'Armée d'Orient" [Malaria in Greece, Macedonia and in the Armée d'Orient]. *Archives de Médecine et de Pharmacie Militaires* 66, no. 6 (December 1916): 753–74.

Nicolaidy, B. *Les Turcs et la Turquie contemporaine. Itinéraire et compte-rendu de voyages dans les provinces ottomanes* [The Turks and contemporary Turkey: Itinerary and travel account in the Ottoman provinces]. Paris: F. Sartorius, 1859.

Niemeyer, Felix von. *Eidiki nosologia kai therapeftiki: syntetagmeni kat'anaforan idios pros tin fysiologian kai pathologikin anatomian* [Special nosology and therapeutics: Compiled with particular reference to physiology and pathology]. Trans. Georgios Karamitsas. 2 vols. Athens: Varvarrigos, 1879.

Nikolaidis, Kik. "I oikonomiki simasia tis agelados Iskar" [The economic significance of the Iskar breed cow]. *Deltion Agrotikis Trapezis Ellados* 3, no. 4 (1938): 378–403.

Numbers, Ronald L. "Medical Science before Scientific Medicine: Reflections on the History of Medical Geography." In *Medical Geography in Historical Perspective*, ed. Nicolaas Rupke, 217–20. London: Wellcome Institute for the History of Medicine, 2000.

Oikonomopoulos, D. "Pragmateia peri kakoithon pyreton" [Study on malignant fevers]. *O Iatros tou Laou* 2, no. 13 (1862).

"O loimos" [The epidemic]. *Estia* 11, no. 4684 (19 February 1907): 1.

Osborne, M. "Resurrecting Hippocrates: Hygienic Sciences and the French Scientific Expeditions to Egypt, Morea and Algeria." In *Warm Climates and Western Medicine*, ed. D. Arnold, 80–98. Amsterdam: Rodopi, 1996.

Packard, R. M. *The Making of a Tropical Disease: A Short History of Malaria*. Baltimore, MD: Johns Hopkins University Press, 2007.

———. "'No Other Logical Choice': Global Malaria Eradication and the Politics of International Health in the Post-War Era." *Parassitologia* 40 (1998): 217–29.

Pallis, A. V. "Periergos therapeia noserou idrotos" [Strange cure of an unhealthy sweat]. *Asklipios* 4 (1 November 1836): 129–133.

Panagiotopoulos, Dimitris. *Petros Kananginis. I symvoli tou stin anamorfosi tou perivallontos tis ypaithrou ston Mesopolemo* [Petros Kananginis: His contribution to the environmental transformation of the countryside in the interwar years]. Athens: Estia, 2013.

Panagiotopoulos, Vasilis. *Plithysmos kai oikismoi tis Peloponnisou, 13os–18os aiona* [Population and settlements of the Peloponnese, thirteenth–eighteenth centuries]. Athens: Istoriko Arkheio Emporikis Trapezas tis Ellados, 1985.

Papadimitriou, Dimitrios Gr. *Emmanuel Manoussakis (1896–1968)*. Athens: Athanasopoulos, Papadamis, 1993.

Papadopoulos, Nikolaos. *Ermis o kerdoos itoi emporikh egkyklopaideia* [Hermis Kerdoos, or commercial encyclopedia]. Athens: Politistiko Tekhnologiko Idryma ETBA, 1989.

Papadopoulos, Titos. "Physiologia tis Voiotias kai idios tis Eparkhias Thivon" [The physiology of Boeotia and especially of the province of Thebes]. *Asklipios* 5, no. 10 (30 May 1861): 440–60.

Papaioannou, Khristos. "Georgooikonomiki erevna tis komopoleos Arnaias" [Agrarian economic research in the town of Arnaia]. *Deltion Agrotikis Trapezis Ellados* 5, no. 2 (1940): 146–87.

Papastefanaki, Lida. "Dimosia Ygeia, Fymatiosi kai Epangelmatiki Pathologia stis Ellinikes Poleis stis Arkhes tou 20ou Aiona: i Antifatiki Diadikasia tou Astikou Eksyngkhronismou" [Public health, tuberculosis, and occupational medicine in Greek cities in the beginning of the twentieth century: The conflicting processes of bourgeois modernisation]. In *Eleftherios Venizelos kai Elliniki Poli: Poleodomikes Politikes kai Koinonikopolitikes Anakatataxeis*, 155–70. Athens: Ethniko Idryma Erevnon kai Meleton "Eleftherios K. Venizelos"; Eptalofos, 2005.

———. *I fleva tis gis. Ta metalleia tis Elladas, 19os–20os aionas* [The vein of the earth. The ores of Greece, 19th–20th centuries]. Athens: Vivliorama, 2017

Papathanasiou, Maro K. "Votanes zodion kai planiton se kheirografa ton 14ou–16ou aionon"

[Herbs of signs and planets in fourteenth- and sixteenth-century manuscripts]. In *Farmakeftika kai aromatika fyta. Paradosiakes khriseis kai dynatotites axiopoiisis tous*, 113–27. Athens: Politistiko Tekhnologiko Idryma ETBA, 1997.

Pentogalos, Gerasimos. *Skholeia iatrikis paideias stin Ellada. 1. Iatrokheirorgikon Skholeion (1835–1837). 2. Kheirourgiki Skholi (1838–1840)* [Schools of medical education in Greece. 1. School of medicine and surgery (1835–1837). 2 School of surgery (1838–1840)]. Epistimoniki Epetirida tou Tmimatos Iatrikis tis Skholis Epistimon Ygeias. Supplement. Thessaloniki: Aristoteleio Panepistimio Thessalonikis, 1991.

"Peri dimosiou ygeias apo 1 Oktovriou 1858 mekhri protis Ianouariou 1859" [On public health from 1 October 1858 to 1 January 1859]. *Asklipios*, Period II, 3 (March 1859): 429–431.

"Peri tis dimosiou ygeias tou kratous apo 1 Iouniou mekhri 31 Dekemvriou 1860" [On state public health from 1 June to 31 December 1860]. *Asklipios*, Period III, 5, no. 6 (30 January 1861): 286–87.

Perkins, John H. "Reshaping Technology in Wartime: The Effect of Military Goals on Entomological Research and Insect-Control Practices." *Technology and Culture* 19, no. 2 (April 1978): 169–86.

Petmezas, Socrates. "Agrotiki oikonomia" [Agrarian economy]. In *I Anaptyxi tis Ellinikis Oikonomias kata ton 19o Aiona (1830–1914)*, ed. Kostas Kostis and Socratis Petmezas, 103–52. Athens: Alexandreia, 2006.

———. *I elliniki agrotiki oikonomia kata ton 19o aiona. I perifereiaki diastasi* [Greek agrarian economy in the nineteenth century: The regional dimension]. Irakleio: Panepistimiakes Ekdoseis Kritis, 2003.

Piel, Frederic B., et al. "Global Distribution of the Sickle Cell Gene and Geographical Confirmation of the Malaria Hypothesis." *Nature Communications* 1, no. 104 (2 November 2010).

"Pinax genikos ton asthenon tis Astyklinikis tou etous 1858" [General table of the patients of Astykliniki in the year 1858]. *Asklipios*, Period II, 3 (June 1859): page following 592.

Piperaki, Evangelia-Theofano, et al. "Assessment of Antibody Responses in Local and Immigrant Residents of Areas with Autochthonous Malaria Transmission in Greece." *American Journal of Tropical Medicine and Hygiene* 93, no. 1 (July 2015): 153-158.

Politis, P. G. "To agrotikon zitima. Ai Thessalikai kliroukhiai. I enkatastasis ton prosfygon" [The agrarian issue: The Thessalian allotments]. *Empros* 11: 3753 (1 April 1907).

"Praktika tis en Athinais ypo tin prostasian tis A.M. Iatrikis Etairias, Synedriasis tis 22 Noemvriou 1861" [Proceedings of the meeting of 22 November 1861 of the Athens Medical Society, which operates under His Majesty's patronage]. *Asklipios*, Period III, 6, no. 6 (January 1862): 272–73.

Prugnolle, F., et al. "African Great Apes Are Natural Hosts of Multiple Related Malaria Species, Including *Plasmodium Falciparum*." *Proceedings of the National Academy of Sciences of the United States of America* 107, no. 4 (26 January 2010): 1458–63.

République Hellénique. Ministère de l'Économie Nationale. Statistique Générale de la Grèce. *Résultats statistiques du recensement de la population de la Grèce du 15–16 mai 1928. Population de fait et de droit. Réfugiés*. Athens: Imprimérie Nationale, 1933.

———. *Recensement de la population de la Grèce au 19 décembre 1920/1 janvier 1921. Résultats statistiques généraux* [Population census of Greece on 19 December 1920/1 January 1921. General statistics results]. Athens: Imprimerie Nationale, 1928.

Rich, S. M. "The Unpredictable Past of *Plasmodium Vivax* Revealed in Its Genome." *Proceedings of the National Academy of Sciences* 101, no. 44 (2 November 2004): 15547–48.

Rich, S. M., and F. J. Ayala. "Progress in Malaria Research: The Case for Phylogenetics." *Advances in Parasitology* 54 (2003): 255–80.

———. "Population Structure and Recent Evolution of *Plasmodium Falciparum*." *Proceedings of the National Academy of Science* 97, no. 13 (June 2000): 6994–7001.

Rich, S. M., et al. "The Origin of Malignant Malaria." *Proceedings of the National Academy of Sciences of the United States of America* 106, no. 35 (1 September 2009): 14902–7.

Rich, Stephen M., Monica C. Licht, Richard R. Hudson, and Francisco J. Ayala. "Malaria's Eve:

Evidence of a Recent Population Bottleneck throughout the World Populations of Plasmodium Falciparum." *Proceedings of the National Academy of Science* 95 (1998): 4425–30.

Rizopoulos, D. "Nosologiki katastasis tis eparkhias Fthiotidos" [The disease situation in the province of Fthiotis]. In *Praktika tis en Athinais Synodou ton Ellinon Iatron (1882) ekdidomena en onomati tou grafeiou*, ed. N. Makkas and Kh. G. Rallis, 499–522. Athens: Typografeion Adelfon Perri, 1883.

Rodriguez-Ocaña, Esteban. "International Health Goals and Social Reform: The Fight against Malaria in Interwar Spain." In *Facing Illness in Troubled Times:. Health in Europe in the Interwar Years, 1918–1939*, ed. Iris Borowy and Wolf D. Gruner, 247–76. Frankfurt am Main: Peter Lang, 2005.

Rose, G. "Fortschritte in der Bekämpfung des Läuse-Fleckfiebers und der Malaria" [Progress in the fight against typhus and malaria]. *Acta Tropica* 1 (1944): 193–218.

Ross, Ronald. "Malaria in Greece." In *The Smithsonian Report for 1908*, 697–710. Washington, DC: Smithsonian, 1909.

———. *Memoirs, with a Full Account of the Great Malaria Problem and Its Solution*. London: J. Murray, 1923.

Roux, Guillaume Gaspard. *Histoire médicale de l'armée française en Morée: pendant la campagne de 1828* [Medical history of the French Army of the Morea: During the 1828 campaign]. Paris: Méquignon, 1829.

Royaume de Grèce and Ministère de l'Intérieur. *Resultats statistiques du recensement de la population de 17–18 octobre 1896* [Statistical results of the population census of 17–18 October 1896]. Athens: Imprimerie et Lithographie Nationale, 1897.

Rubino, Pietro. *Peri tou armodioterou tropou eis to na empodizontai ai ypostrofai ton periodikon pyreton afou idi koposi me tin kinan* [On the most appropriate way to avoid relapses of intermittent fevers once they have been stopped with cinchona]. Trans. Ioannis Asanis. Constantinople: K. A. Kolonellos, 1841.

Ruisinger, Marion Maria. *Das griechische Gesundheitswesen unter Koenig Otto (1833–1862)* [Greek health service under King Otto (1833–62)]. Frankfurt: Peter Lang, 1997.

Rupke, Nicolaas. "Humboldtian Medicine." *Medical History* 40 (1996): 293–310.

Russell, Paul Farr. *Man's Mastery of Malaria*. London: Oxford University Press, 1955.

———. "World-Wide Malaria Distribution, Prevalence, and Control." *American Journal of Tropical Medicine and Hygiene* 5, no. 6 (1956): 937–65.

Sallares, Robert. *Malaria and Rome: A History of Malaria in Ancient Italy*. Oxford: Oxford University Press, 2002.

———. "Role of Environmental Changes in the Spread of Malaria in Europe during the Holocene." *Quaternary International* 150, no. 1 (June 2006): 21–27.

Sallares, Robert, Abigail Bouwman, and Cecilia Anderung. "The Spread of Malaria to Southern Europe in Antiquity: New Approaches to Old Problems." *Medical History* 48 (2004): 311–28.

Savvaidis, Paraskevas. "Thessalonki: poli ton stratopedon, poli ton prosfygon" [Thessaloniki: City of camps, city of refugees]. In *Thessaloniki, protevousa ton prosfygon. Oi prosfyges stin poli apo to 1912 mekhri simera*, Istoriko Arkheio Prosfygikou Ellinismou Dimou Kalamarias, 509–29. Thessaloniki: Adelfoi Kyriakidi, 2013.

Savvas, K. *Peri tis en Elladi kai Kriti sykhnotitos tis elonosias* [On the frequency of malaria in Greece and Crete]. Athens: Typographeion Paraskeva Leoni, 1909.

Savvas, K., and I. Kardamatis. "Apantiseis dimarkhon tou kratous os pros ta en ti perifereia tou dimou ton eli" [Responses of the country's mayors about the marshes in the area of their municipality]. In *I Elonosia en Elladi kai ta Pepragmena tou Syllogou*, vol. 3, ed. Konstantinos G. Savvas and Ioannis P. Kardamatis, 235–554. Athens: Typografeion Paraskeva Leoni, 1908.

Savvas, K., I. Kardamatis, and Sp. Dasios. "1906. Ai peri tis kata topous elonosias pliroforiai ton iatron" [1906: Doctors' information about malaria in their respective districts]. In *I Elonosia en Elladi kai ta Pepragmena tou Syllogou*, ed. Konstantinos G. Savvas and Ioannis P. Kardamatis, 462–641. Athens: Typografeion Paraskeva Leoni, 1907.

Sawyer, Wilbur A. "Achievements of UNRRA as an International Health Organization." *American Journal of Public Health* 37, no. 1 (January 1947): 41–58.

Seriatou, Pinelopi. "Mantzounia kai aloifes. Syntages iasis tis laikis iatrikis se ena giatrosofi tou 18ou ai" [Herbal cures and ointments: Prescriptions of popular medicine in a lay medical text of the eighteenth century]. MA thesis, University of Athens, 2013.

Service, Mike W., and Harold Townson. "The *Anopheles* Vector." In *Essential Malariology*, ed. David A. Warrell and Herbert M. Gilles, 59–84. London: Arnold, 2002.

Setzer, Teddi J. "Malaria Detection in the Field of Paleopathology: A Meta-Analysis of the State of the Art." *Acta Tropica* (2014), 97–104.

Shanks, G. Dennis, and Nicholas J. White. "The Activation of *Vivax Malaria* Hypnozoites by Infectious Diseases." *The Lancet Infectious Diseases* 13, no. 10 (2013): 900–906.

Sharp, Paul M. "*Plasmodium Vivax* in African Apes." Abstract from the New York Academy of Sciences Conference "Advances in *P. Vivax* Malaria Research," Barcelona, 28–29 May 2013. http://www.nyas.org/Events/Detail.aspx?cid=97552a13-4718-4a31-8239-51b62d13f52e.

Simandiraki, Zakharenia. *Georgioupoli. Maties stin istoria tis* [Georgioupoli: Glances at its history]. Khania: Koinofeles Idryma "Agia Sophia," 1994.

Sinden, Robert E., and Herbert M. Gilles. "The Malaria Parasite." In *Essential Malariology*, ed. David A. Warrell and Herbert M. Gilles, 8–34. London: Arnold, 2002.

Skampardonis, Grigorios, Georgios N. Antonakopoulos, and Nikolaos Skhizas, eds. *Iatriki Efimeris tou Stratou (1890–1897). Katalogos periekhomenon kai epilogi arthron* [The Medical Journal of the Greek Army (1890–97): Catalogue of contents and selected articles]. Athens: Parisianou, 2001.

Skampardonis, Grigorios, Nikolaos Skhizas, and Georgios N. Antonakopoulos. "To khroniko tis astheneias kai tou thanatou tou vasileos Alexandrou (17 Sept.–12 Okt. 1920), symfona kai me skhetiki anekdoti epistoli tou kathigitou Konstantinou Savva" [The chronicle of the disease and death of king Alexandros (17 Sept.–12 Oct. 1920), according to an unpublished letter of professor Konstantinos Savvas]. *Deltos* 12, no. 23 (June 2002): 5–15.

Skhizas, Nikolaos D., and Grigorios I. Skampardonis. "I elonosia stin Ellada sta khronia tis tourkokratias. Opos tin eidan oi xenoi taxidiotes" [Malaria during the Turkish rule, as seen by foreign travelers]. *Deltos*, no. 30 (December 2005): 19–25.

Skhizas, N., et al. "Sykhnotis kai katanomi mesogeiakis anaimias kai pathologikon aimosfairinon eis ton ellinikon khoron. Erevnai epi 15,500 neosyllekton" [Frequency and distribution of thalassemia and hemoglobinopathies in Greece: Research on 15,000 army recruits]. *Iatriki Epitheorisis Enoplon Dynameon* 11, no. Supplement 1 (1977): 197–209.

Skouzes, Panagis. *Apomnimonevmata: I tyrannia tou Khatzi-Ali Khaseki stin tourkokratoumeni Athina (1772–1796)* [Memoirs: The tyranny of Khatzi Ali Khaseki in Turkish-ruled Athens (1772–96)]. Ed. Thanasis Kh. Papadopoulos. Athens: Kedros, 1975.

Small, Jennifer, Scott J. Goetz, and Simon I. Hay. "Climatic Suitability for Malaria Transmission in Africa, 1911–1995." *Proceedings of the National Academy of Sciences* 100, no. 26 (2003): 15341–45.

Smith, Dale C. "Medical Science, Medical Practice and the Emerging Concept of Typhus in Mid-Eighteenth-Century Britain." In *Theories of Fever from Antiquity to the Enlightenment*, ed. W. F. Bynum and V. Nutton. Medical History Supplement, no. 1, 121–34. London: Wellcome Institute for the History of Medicine, 1981.

———. "Quinine and Fever: The Development of the Effective Dosage." *Journal of the History of Medicine and Allied Sciences* 31 (1976): 343–67.

Snow, Robert W., and Herbert M. Gilles. "The Epidemiology of Malaria." In *Essential Malariology*, ed. David A. Warrell and Herbert M. Gilles, 85–106. London: Arnold, 2002.

Snowden, Frank M. *The Conquest of Malaria. Italy, 1900–1962*. New Haven, CT: Yale University Press, 2006.

Society for Ecology and Development and la Documentazione e l'Educazione Ambientale Agenzia per la Ricerca. *Programme for the Creation of a Nature Park in the Area of Mount Kandili in Euboea. Final Report*. Athens: Commission of the European Communities, 1990. http://www.noel-baker.co.uk/kandili.html.http://www.noel-baker.co.uk/kandili.html.

Soper, Fred Lowe. *Ventures in World Health: The Memoirs of Fred Lowe Soper*. Washington, DC: Pan American Health Organization, Pan American Sanitary Bureau, Regional Office of the World Health Organization, 1977.

Soutsos, Ioannis. *Dokimion peri ton Oikonomikon Metarrythmiseon*. Athens, 1863.

Stamatoyannopoulos, G., and P. Fessas. "Thalassaemia, Glucose-6-Phosphate Dehydrogenase Deficiency, Sickling, and Malarial Endemicity in Greece: A Study of Five Areas." *British Medical Journal* 1, no. 5387 (April 1964): 875–79.

Stapleton, D. H. "The Dawn of DDT and Its Experimental Use by the Rockefeller Foundation in Mexico, 1943–1952." *Parassitologia* 40 (1998): 149–58.

———. "Internationalism and Nationalism: The Rockefeller Foundation, Public Health and Malaria in Italy, 1923–1951." *Parassitologia* 42, no. 1–2 (2000): 127–34.

"Statistiki tis en Athinais Astyklinikis. Triti triminia tou etous 1858" [Statistics of the Athens Astykliniki. Third trimester of the year 1858]. *Asklipios*, Period II, 3 (November–December 1858): 210–211.

"Statistiki tis en Athinais Astyklinikis, deftera triminia tou etous 1860" [Statistics of the Athens Astykliniki, second trimester of the year 1860]. *Asklipios*, Period III, 5, no. 2 (November 1860): 69–70.

"Statistiki tis en Athinais Astyklinikis. I proti triminia tou etous 1861" [Statistics of the Athens Astykliniki. First trimester of the year 1861]. *Asklipios*, Period III, 5, no. 12 (30 July 1861): 551–552.

Stavrianos, Leften Stavros. *Greece: American Dilemma and Opportunity*. Chicago: H. Regnery, 1952.

Stavropoulos, A.K. "I nosologia tis Messinias kai i iatriki kata tin Epanastasi. To epistimoniko ergo ton giatron tou Gallikou ekstratefikou somatos ston Moria (1828–1833)" [Diseases in Messinia and medicine during the Revolution: The scientific work of the doctors of the French expeditionary force in the Morea (1828–33)]. *Deltos* 8 (December 1994): 4–7.

Stéphanos, Clôn. *La Grèce au point de vue naturel, ethnologique, anthropologique, démographique et médical: Extrait du* Dictionnaire Encyclopédique des Sciences Médicales [Greece from a natural, ethnological, anthropological, demographic, and medical perspective: Extract from the *Dictionnaire Encyclopédique des Sciences Médicales*]. 363–580. Paris: G. Masson, 1884.

Sufian, Sandra M. *Healing the Land and the Nation: Malaria and the Zionist Project in Palestine, 1920–1947*. Chicago: University of Chicago Press, 2007.

Tadmouri, Ghazi Omar, et al. "History and Origin of [Beta]-Thalassemia in Turkey: Sequence Haplotype Diversity of [Beta]-Globin Genes." *Human Biology* 73, no. 5 (2001): 661–74.

"Ta filika telmata" [Friendly marshes]. *Athinai* 5: 154 (3 April 1907): 1.

"Ta mekhri 1906 ypo tou kratous dapanithenta khrimatika posa pros apoxiransin elon k.l.p" [State expenditure for marsh drainage etc. until 1906]. In *I elonosia en Elladi kai ta pepragmena tou Syllogou*, ed. Konstantinos G. Savvas and Ioannis P. Kardamatis, 72–76. Athens: Typografeion Paraskeva Leoni, 1908.

The National Archives. "War Office: The Macedonian Mule Corps in World War I." http://discovery.nationalarchives.gov.uk/details/r/C16161.

Theodoridis, A. G. "Paratiriseis tines epi tis elomianseos en tais eparkhiais tis Kritis" [Some observations on malaria in the provinces of Crete]. In *I elonosia en Elladi kai ta pepragmena tou Syllogou*, vol. 3, ed. Konstantinos G. Savvas and Ioannis P. Kardamatis, 506–26. Athens: Typografeion Paraskeva Leoni, 1908.

Theodorou, Vasiliki, and Despoina Karakatsani. "Health Policies in Interwar Greece: The Intervention by the League of Nations Health Organisation." *Dynamis* 28 (2008): 53–75.

———. *"Ygieinis parangelmata": iatriki epivlepsi kai koinoniki pronoia gia to paidi tis protes dekaeties tou 200u aiona* ["Hygiene commands": Childhood welfare and medical supervision in the first decades of the twentieth century]. Athens: Dionikos, 2010.

Thiersch, Frédéric. *De l'état actuel de la Grèce et des moyens d'arriver à sa restauration* [The current situation of Greece and the means for its restoration]. 2 vols. Leipzig: Brockhaus, 1833.

Thomadakis, S. "Black Markets, Inflation and Force in the Economy of Occupied Greece." Ed. J. Iatrides. In *Greece in the 1940's: A Nation in Crisis*, 61–80. Hanover, NH: University Press of New England, 1981.

To ergon tis kyverniseos Venizelou kata tin tetraetian 1928–1932 [The works of Venizelos's government during the four-year period, 1928–32]. Athens, 1932.

Tognotti, E. "The Spread of Malaria in Sardinia: An Historical Perspective." In *Adaptation to Malaria: The Interaction of Biology and Culture*, ed. Lawrence S. Greene and Maria Enrico Danubio, 237–47. Amsterdam: Gordon and Breach Publishers, 1998.

Tomos ogdoos. Lyta engrafa etous 1822. Meros III: Engrafa oikonomikou periekhomenou. Vol. 15, iii, *Archeia tis Ellinikis Paliggenesias, 1821–1832. Lyta engrafa A' kai B' vouleftikis periodou* [Eighth volume. Loose documents of 1822. Part III: Financial documents. Vol. 15, iii, Archives of the Greek Regeneration, 1822–32. Loose documents of the first and second parliamentary period]. Athens: Vivliothiki tis Voulis ton Ellinon, 1997.

"Travaux et résultats de la mission antipaludique à l'armée d'Orient" [Works and results of the antimalarial mission of the Armée d'Orient]. Special issue, *Bulletin de la Société de Pathologie Exotique* 11, no. 6 (1918).

Triantaphyllakos, D., and G. Oeconomou. *Le paludisme et les moustiques à Helos de Lacédémone. Contribution aux recherches microscopiques sur les parasites de la malaria intense* [Malaria and mosquitoes in Elos of Lakedaimon. Contribution to microscopic research on the parasites of intense malaria]. Athens: Hestia, 1901.

Tsiamis, Costas, Evangelia-Theophano Piperaki, and Athanassios Tsakris. "The History of the Greek Anti-Malaria League and the Influence of the Italian School of Malariology." *Le Infezioni in Medicina* 1 (2013): 60–75.

Typaldos, Ioannis. "Statistikai pliroforiai peri tis en to Elliniko strato epikratiseos tis elonosias mekhri tou etous 1905" [Statistical information on malaria prevalence in the Greek Army until 1905]. In *I elonosia en Elladi kai ta pepragmena tou Syllogou*, ed. Konstantinos G. Savvas and Ioannis P. Kardamatis, 383-411. Athens: Typografeion Paraskeva Leoni, 1907.

Valaoras, Vasileios G. "A Reconstruction of the Demographic History of Modern Greece." *The Milbank Memorial Fund Quarterly* 38 (1960): 115–39.

———. *Stoikheia viometrias kai statistikis. Dimografiki meleti tou plithysmou tis Ellados* [Elements of biometrics and statistics: Demographic study of the population of Greece]. Athens: Vafeiadakis, 1943.

———. *To dimografikon provlima tis Ellados kai i epidrasis ton prosfygon* [The demographic problem of Greece and the impact of the refugees]. Athens, 1939.

Valassopoulos, I. "Nosologiki geografia tis Lakedaimonos" [Disease geography of Lakedaimon]. In *Praktika tis en Athinais Synodou ton Ellinon Iatron (1882)*, ed. N. Makkas and Kh. G. Rallis, 71–84. Athens: Typografeion Adelfon Perri, 1883.

Vamvas, I. "Peri dimosias ygeias" [On public health]. In *Praktika tis en Athinais Synodou ton Ellinon Iatron (1882) ekdidomena en onomati tou grafeiou*, ed. N. Makkas and Kh. G. Rallis, 311–17. Athens: Typografeion Adelfon Perri, 1883.

Van der Hoogte, Arjo Roersch, and Toine Pieters. "Quinine, Malaria, and the Cinchona Bureau: Marketing Practices and Knowledge Circulation in a Dutch Transoceanic Cinchona-Quinine Enterprise (1920s–30s)." *Journal of the History of Medicine and Allied Sciences* (2015): 1–29.

Vassiliou, Maria. "Politics, Public Health, and Development: Malaria in 20th Century Greece." DPhil, Oxford University, 2005.

Velissarios, G. "Genikos iatrostatistikos pinax ton dimon tis dioikiseos Euboias" [General medico-statistical table of the administration of Euboea]. *Ellinikos Takhydromos* Supplement, no. 81 (1839).

Velonakis, M. N. *Syllogi apanton ton nomon, diatagmaton, diataxeon, kanonismon kl. ton aforonton tin astykin en genei ygeionomian, tin iatrikin, tin farmakeftikin kai ta syngeni touton epangelmata en Elladi, adeia tou ypourgeiou ton esoterikon syllegenton kai ekdothenton* [A collection of all the laws, decrees, regulations, etc. pertaining to civilian hygiene, medicine, pharmaceutics and related occupations in Greece, collected and published with permission from the Interior Ministry]. Athens: Eirinidis, 1860.

Veremis, Th. "O taktikos stratos stin Ellada tou 19ou aiona" [The regular army of Greece in the nineteenth century]. In *Opseis tis ellinikis koinonias tou 19ou aiona*, ed. G. Tsasousis, 165–76. Athens: Estia, 1984.

Vine, J. M. "Malaria Control with DDT on a National Scale, Greece, 1946." *Proceedings of the Royal Society of Medicine* 40 (1946–47): 841–48.

Vladimiros, L., and Kh. Franghidis. "To 'Panellinion Iatrikon Synedrion' tou 1901. Iatrika dromena, ygeionomika provlimata kai koryfaioi iatroi prin apo enan aiona" [The Panhellenic Medical Congress of 1901: Medical proceedings, sanitary problems and prominent doctors a century ago]. *Arkheia Ellinikis Iatrikis* 19, no. 6 (November–December 2002): 700–709.

Vondra, Hana. "Die Malaria: ihre Problematik und Erforschung in Heer und Luftwaffe" [Malaria: Its problems and research in the army and air force]. In *Sanitätswesen im Zweiten Weltkrieg*, ed. Ekkehart Guth, 108–26. Herford: Verlag E. S. Mittler & Sohn, 1990.

Vouros, Ioannis. "Nosologiki katastasis ton Kykladon kata to 1834 etos" [The disease situation of the Cyclades in 1834]. *Asklipios* 11 (1 June 1837): 369–88.

Vouros, Ioannis, Xavier Landerer, and Joseph Sartori. *Elliniki farmakopoiia kata vasilikin diatagin kai kat'engkrisin tou B. Iatrikou Symvouliou ekdotheisa* [Greek pharmacopoeia, published by royal commission and with the approval of the Royal Medical Council]. Athens: Vasiliki Typografia, 1837.

Walpole, Robert, ed. *Memoirs Relating to European and Asiatic Turkey: Edited from Manuscript Journals*. London: Longman, Hurst, Rees, Orme, and Brown, 1817.

Warrell, David A., William M. Watkins, and Peter A. Winstanley. "Treatment and Prevention of Malaria." In *Essential Malariology*, ed. David A. Warrell and Herbert M. Gilles, 268–312. London: Arnold, 2002.

Watts, Sheldon. *Epidemics and History: Disease, Power and Imperialism*. New Haven, CT: Yale University Press, 1997.

Weatherall, D. J. *Thalassaemia: The Biography*. Oxford: Oxford University Press, 2010.

Weatherall, D. J., and J. B. Clegg. "Genetic Variability in Response to Infection: Malaria and After." *Genes and Immunity* 3, no. 6 (September 2002): 331–37. http://www.nature.com/gene/journal/v3/n6/pdf/6363878a.pdf.

Weatherall, D. J., et al. "Malaria and the Red Cell." *Hematology. Education Program of the American Society of Hematology*, no. 1 (2002): 35–57.

Webb, James L. A., Jr. *Humanity's Burden: A Global History of Malaria*. Cambridge: Cambridge University Press, 2009.

———. "Malaria and the Peopling of Early Tropical Africa." *Journal of World History* 16, no. 3 (September 2005): 269–91.

Weindling, Paul. "From Moral Exhortation to the New Public Health, 1918–45." In *The Politics of the Healthy Life: An International Perspective*, ed. Esteban Rodriguez-Ocaña, 113–30. Sheffield: European Association for the History of Medicine and Health Publications, 2002.

Wellcome Trust Sanger Institute, "Out of Africa: The Evolution of *Plasmodium Vivax*." Wellcome Trust Sanger Institute website, 21 February 2014. http://www.sanger.ac.uk/news/view/2014-02-21-out-of-africa-the-evolution-of-em-plasmodium-vivax-em-.

Wenyon, C. M. "Malaria in Macedonia. Part I." *Journal of the Royal Army Medical Corps* 37, no. 2 (August 1921).

Wenyon, C. M., Anderson, A. G., K. McLay, T. S. Hele, and J. Waterston. *Malaria in Macedonia, 1915–1919, Part I–Part V*. Reprinted from the *Journal of the Royal Army Medical Corps*. London, 1921–22.

Willoughby, William George, and Louis Cassidy. *Anti-Malaria Work in Macedonia among British Troops*. London: H. K. Lewis, 1918.

Wolf, Eric R. *Europe and the People without History*. Berkeley: University of California Press, 1982.

Woodbridge, George. *UNRRA: The History of the United Nations Relief and Rehabilitation Administration*. 3 vols. New York: Columbia University Press, 1950.

Worboys, Michael. "Manson, Ross and Colonial Medical Policy: Tropical Medicine in London and Liverpool, 1899–1914." In *Disease, Medicine and Empire: Perspectives on Western Medicine and the Experience of European Expansion*, ed. Roy McLeod and Milton Lewis, 21–37. London: Routledge, 1988.

World Health Organization. *World Malaria Report 2015*. Geneva: World Health Organization, 2015. http://apps.who.int/iris/bitstream/10665/200018/1/9789241565158_eng.pdf.

World Health Organization and the Interregional Conference on Malaria for the Eastern Mediterranean and European Regions. *Information on the Malaria Control Programme in Greece.* Geneva: World Health Organization, 1956. WHO/Mal/163–8.

Ypourgeion Esoterikon. *Peri promitheias kininou entha epikratousi dialeipontes pyretoi.* Ar. engyk.144 epi tou arith. 22313. Pros tous nomarkhas tou Kratous [On the supply of quinine where intermittent fevers prevail. Circular number144/22313 to Prefects]. Athens, 13 October 1854.

Ypourgeion Oikonomikon, Statistikon Grafeion. *Emporion tis Ellados meta ton xenon epikrateion* [The trade of Greece with foreign countries]. Athens: Imprimérie Nationale, 1891–1920.

Zavitsianos, Spyridon K. "Iiatriki en Eptaniso kata ton pro tis Enoseos khronon" [Medicine in the Ionian Islands before the Unification]. In *Praktika tou en Kerkyra Protou Panioniou Synedriou (20–22 Maïou 1914) kai ai en afto anakoinoseis,* 204–30. Athens, 1915.

Zeiss, Heinz, ed. *Seuchen-Atlas* [Atlas of diseases]. Gotha: Perthes, 1942–45.

Zylberman, Patrick. "Mosquitoes and the Komitadjis: Malaria and Borders in Macedonia (1919–1938)." In *Facing Illness in Troubled Times: Health in Europe in the Interwar Years, 1918–1939,* ed. Iris Borowy and Wolf D. Gruner, 305–43. Frankfurt am Main: Peter Lang, 2005.

—–. "A Transatlantic Dispute. The Etiology of Malaria and the Redesign of the Mediterranean Landscape." In *Shifting Boundaries of Public Health: Europe in the Twentieth Century,* ed. Solomon, Susan Gross, Lion Murard, and Patrick Zylberman, 269–97. Rochester, NY: University of Rochester Press, 2008.

NAME INDEX

SUBJECT INDEX